Japanese
for Healthcare
Professionals

An Introduction to Medical Japanese

Shigeru Osuka

TUTTLE Publishing

Tokyo | Rutland, Vermont | Singapore

Published by Tuttle Publishing, an imprint of Periplus Editions (HK) Ltd.

www.tuttlepublishing.com

Library of Congress Cataloging-in-Publication Data

Osuka, Shigeru.
 Japanese for healthcare professionals : an introduction to medical Japanese / by Shigeru Osuka. —1st ed.
    p. cm.
 Includes index.
 ISBN 978-4-8053-1109-7
 1. Japanese language—Conversation and phrase books (for medical personnel) 2. Japanese language—Textbooks for foreign speakers—English. I. Title.
 PL538.M3O88 2011
 495.6'8242102461—dc22
                           2010053841

ISBN 978-4-8053-1109-7

Distributed by

North America, Latin America & Europe
Tuttle Publishing
364 Innovation Drive
North Clarendon, VT 05759-9436 U.S.A.
Tel: 1 (802) 773-8930
Fax: 1 (802) 773-6993
info@tuttlepublishing.com
www.tuttlepublishing.com

Asia Pacific
Berkeley Books Pte. Ltd.
61 Tai Seng Avenue #02-12
Singapore 534167
Tel: (65) 6280-1330
Fax: (65) 6280-6290
inquiries@periplus.com.sg
www.periplus.com

Japan
Tuttle Publishing
Yaekari Building, 3rd Floor
5-4-12 Osaki Shinagawa-ku
Tokyo 141 0032
Tel: (81) 3 5437-0171
Fax: (81) 3 5437-0755
sales@tuttle.co.jp
www.tuttle.co.jp

First edition
15 14 13 12 11   1103TP
10 9 8 7 6 5 4 3 2 1

Printed in Singapore

CONTENTS

INTRODUCTION

In a world shrinking due to advancements in transportation and communication technology, it is crucial that healthcare professionals be prepared for a multicultural society. *Japanese for Healthcare Professionals: An Introduction to Medical Japanese* is designed to facilitate effective communication between Japanese patients and English-speaking healthcare professionals who have not previously studied the Japanese language. Over the past few decades, Japanese interest in overseas travel has grown. Nearly twenty million Japanese people a year travel abroad, and some of them have experienced emergency situations requiring medical care. In addition, there are large Japanese expatriate communities in many English-speaking countries. Yet very few places are qualified to help Japanese patients because of the language barrier. This book will serve as a valuable tool in breaking down such barriers in an ever more globalizing society.

Japanese for Healthcare Professionals is a proficiency-based conversation textbook, created specifically for healthcare professionals who want to communicate with Japanese-speaking clients to provide quality service. It focuses on the language needed to communicate symptoms, illnesses, medications, and medical-related instructions in everyday interactions with Japanese patients, and it's contents are centered around typical provider-patient conversations one would find in clinics and hospitals. Because of this, the vocabulary used in this book is very different from that found in ordinary Japanese-language textbooks. However, basic grammar is covered thoroughly here, as are more sophisticated grammatical elements that are used in everyday speech. Often in the past, parts of speech that have no exact counterpart in English have been ignored by Japanese-language textbooks, but this book aims to teach normal, everyday, idiomatic communication in the healthcare context by including passive forms, onomatopoeias, adverbs, and compound verbs.

Japanese for Healthcare Professionals is also distinctive in that it reflects the national Standards for Foreign Language Learning in the 21st Century, established by the American Council on the Teaching of Foreign Languages (ACTFL). Known as the Five Cs, these standards are summarized as Communication, Culture, Connections, Comparisons, and Communities. First, by providing real situational dialogues, this book emphasizes what healthcare professionals can *do* with the Japanese language rather than what they must know about it in some abstract way. Second, because cultural understanding is a vital part of language learning, each lesson has culture notes that facilitate a better understanding of Japanese ways of thinking and values. Third, this book connects not only with ordinary daily life but with healthcare settings. Fourth, through the cultural and language notes, it offers comparisons between the Japanese and English-speaking Western healthcare fields that allow the learner to discover both similarities and differences. These comparisons may prepare the provider to understand better a Japanese patient's responses and behavior patterns, while illuminating certain uniquely Japanese concepts. Finally, after studying this book, healthcare professionals will find that their ability to reach out to the community of Japanese patients is vastly improved.

This book is in five parts: Parts One (Lessons 1–10) and Two (Lessons 11–20) focus on general aspects of healthcare and the medical process that can be utilized by all providers. Part Three (Lessons 21–30) emphasizes areas of medical specialization, from internal medicine to pediatrics, as well as dentistry. Part Four comprises an English-Japanese dictionary of approximately 1,500 medical terms for when the healthcare professional needs to find the right words for conversation. It also includes the Japanese script for the term, which may be shown to a patient if the occasion requires. The appendices in Part Five include a sample bilingual medical questionnaire, a glossary of onomatopoetic Japanese expressions for common complaints   and other helpful lists, together with answers to quizzes on comprehension and the exercises in each chapter.

In the first three parts, each lesson introduces a list of thirty new vocabulary words, which can be practiced with the help of the CD that comes with this book. A short dialogue provides situational conversation models between healthcare professionals and the patients that anticipate the content and objective of each lesson. The dialogue is followed by grammatical explanations that will help the learner to understand and acquire the basic structures and patterns of the Japanese language. For each lesson, useful expressions and high-frequency words from ordinary conversational Japanese supplement the healthcare-oriented vocabulary. Language and culture notes offer insights about Japanese society, lifestyles, and values.

Learning to speak Japanese requires not translating from English to Japanese but doing the exercises and practicing the grammatical structures in Japanese, and the accompanying CD is included for that purpose. In addition to the repetition exercises for the vocabulary, dialogue, and useful expressions, this book provides oral practice for sentence structures and exercises testing the learner's knowledge and ability to respond in a conversation. Each lesson also has a section on comprehension in the form of a short quiz.

Lessons 1 to 30 teach more than 1,200 Japanese words, which is sufficient for practical medical Japanese conversation of the type providers might encounter every day. Each lesson, when reviewed with the CD, is designed for approximately ninety minutes of study, for a total of forty-five hours from Lesson 1 to Lesson 30. However, studying a language is like consuming daily nourishment.

When you've eaten a meal, you will eventually become hungry again and need to eat another. For language study as well, it is not enough to study only once. You must continue to exercise the knowledge you've acquired through this book and practice speaking with Japanese patients. Five to ten minutes of study every day will make you into a different person in the future. As the maxim says, endurance is the power of life (keizoku wa chikara-nari).

Finally, I would like to take this opportunity to thank the many people who contributed to the publication of this book: Cal Barksdale, Sandra Korinchak, Nancy Goh, and Cheng Har of Tuttle Publishing, Willis Sumargo for the illustrations, Felicia Kazin, Wendy Sue Williams, Hiroko Ogino, Fumiko Bacon, Sevan Simon and Jesse Rosso of Seton Hall University, and the following, whom I met at the University of Hawai'i at Manoa where I taught the course "Japanese for Healthcare Practitioners": Paulette C. Feeney, Dean S. Obayashi, Richard Ridao, Molly H. Hara, Sherly Ikeda, Alisa H. Au, Jill M. Beadles, Maria Chen, Lucille N. Holzgans, Susan J. Hunt, Marilyn E. Ige, Betty Iwai, David Kaku, Joni Kawano, Wendy T. Miyamoto, Nora S. Nagai, Amy Moriguchi, Doris Morishige, Harry Yoshino, Albert I. Yamakawa, Francis Terada, and Carol K. Hirano. Those wonderful healthcare professionals have remained vivid in my memory for nearly fifteen years. I would also like to express my gratitude to the many good spiritual friends who shared a great moment in my life: Shoshin Ichishima, Enshin Saito, Kokuryo Tachi, Shunwa Yamada, Gensho Okuyama, Victor Kobayashi, George Tanabe, the late David Chappell, Masayoshi Sando, Shigetaka Ishii, Hiroshi Suda, Denji Suzuki, Hiroshi Ogawara, Eriko Osuka, and Sora Skye Osuka. The initial writing of this book was made possible in part by a Seton Hall University Research Council Grant.

HOW TO USE THIS BOOK

The purpose of this book is to enhance communication between healthcare professionals and their patients who speak Japanese. Although the contents of each lesson follow a natural progression, the book can be customized to individual styles of study. Please read and understand the following points before beginning in order to achieve your maximum level of proficiency.

1. **Basic Vocabulary**

   The thirty words chosen as the basic vocabulary are the most useful for the topic of the chapter and the situation presented in the dialogue. Listen to the CD to practice pronouncing each word and repeat it. Familiarize yourself with the words as best you can, but do not feel that you need to learn all the words by heart immediately. As you continue on to subsequent chapters, the words will appear again and, through repetition and familiarity, you will learn them naturally. It is suggested that you make vocabulary flash cards or notes in order to study at times when it would be inconvenient to carry your book.

2. **Dialogue**

   The dialogues provide an example of how to communicate with your Japanese patients in a typical conversation. For each dialogue, listen to the CD and repeat. As necessary, make sure you understand the meaning of sentences by checking against the English translation. However, it is important that you not linger in the dialogue section. After you've completed the subsequent parts of the chapter, return here one more time to practice.

3. **Grammar**

   This section gives an overview of the grammatical concepts extracted from the dialogue. The main grammar points in each chapter's dialogue have been boldfaced for your convenience. It is important to read the grammatical explanations and the examples carefully, and then, when you have grasped the grammar points, return to the dialogue. At your leisure, you can create new sentences by substituting different vocabulary words.

4. **Useful Expressions**

   These ten frequently used expressions have been chosen to help expand your vocabulary of ordinary Japanese idioms. In order to practice recognizing and pronouncing them, listen to the CD and repeat in the space allowed. The expressions in this section may not be directly related to the grammatical explanations, but they are commonly used and may prove handy in the medical office.

5. **Key Sentences**

The five key sentences have been selected to demonstrate the grammar. You can enhance your understanding of the grammatical structures by familiarizing yourself with these sentences. If you have difficulty understanding them, review the grammar section one more time, then listen to the CD to practice hearing and pronouncing them.

6. **Additional Words**

The thirty basic vocabulary words consist of nouns, but to speak normally you also need to use verbs, adjectives, adverbs, particles, and so forth. This section supplements the vocabulary words with other parts of speech taken mainly from the sentences in the Dialogue, Grammar, Useful Expressions, and Key Sentences, and Language Notes.

7. **Language Notes**

The Language Notes consider different aspects of Japanese words and expressions to help you understand the language better and use it more effectively. All the information in this section has a direct healthcare application. Be patient and enjoy it.

8. **Language Roots**

The Japanese language has many homonyms—words that sound the same but have different meanings—which can be confusing, but when these words are written in Japanese script the meaning is clear. Since, rather than Japanese characters, this book uses Romanization, which reflects the sound of spoken Japanese, it might sometimes be difficult to distinguish between homonyms. In the Language Roots section, more than sixty key words have been selected to help the learner make this kind of distinction. This section attempts to overcome the limitation of using romaji (Romanized Japanese). It also relates different words or expressions having the same root and thus points out word families, which can help in memorization.

9. **Culture Notes**

With language study alone, it would not be possible to communicate with patients. It is essential to understand their cultural background and perspectives. This section touches on social, cultural, and linguistic themes covered in the chapter and is meant to expand the healthcare professional's awareness of the Japanese way of thinking.

10. Comprehension

This section of short quizzes will help you to identify and test your understanding of the information in the lesson. An answer key is provided in the Appendix. After you have successfully completed the comprehension quizzes, you should begin to feel confident in your ability to communicate with Japanese patients.

11. Practice

This section emphasizes the important basic words, dialogue content, and expressions in the lesson and includes dialogue comprehension and free response questions.

12. Exercises

The Exercises section is likewise designed to assist you in reviewing the content of the chapter, especially the handy, frequently used expressions. An answer key is provided in the Appendix. It is strongly suggested that you complete all the exercises. This will help you acquire Japanese in a natural way and ensure your ability to speak the language in a variety of situations.

13. MP3 Disc

The accompanying MP3 disc ties in to the Writing and Pronunciation Guide that follows this section and to the lessons. For each lesson, it covers the Basic Vocabulary, Dialogue, Useful Expressions, and Key Sentences. The disc provides an opportunity to listen to and speak along with native Japanese speakers. Each lesson on the disc is preceded by music and a reading of the lesson title.

JAPANESE WRITING AND PRONUNCIATION GUIDE

Japanese for Healthcare Professionals: An Introduction to Medical Japanese is intended for English-speaking healthcare professionals who have not previously studied the Japanese language. For this reason, the book is uses romaji, the Romanization of Japanese speech, rather than Japanese characters—hiragana, katakana, and kanji—which require a lot of time to master. For advanced Japanese learners and native speakers, however, the basic vocabulary in each chapter does provide hiragana, katakana, and kanji for the instant recognition of words. Historically, it is interesting that Japanese was a spoken language first and later adopted a written language from Chinese, which led to a difference between pronunciation and the written language. For example, Tokyo is pronounced as "Too-kyoo" (と お き ょ お) but written as **Toukyou** (と う き ょ う) in hiragana. In order to provide the most authentic native Japanese pronunciation, this book adopts the revised Hepburn system of pronunciation ("Tookyoo") and uses the diacritical mark called the macron ˉ to indicate the doubled, or long, vowel. Thus, the long vowel "oo" is represented as **ō**, as in **Tōkyō**, and similarly for the long vowels **ā**, **ī**, **ū**, and **ē**. When the vowel sequence is **ei**, Japanese pronunciations becomes like "ee." To help in word recognition, however, this book utilizes the **ei** spelling for this pronunciation, to match the **ei** sequence in **sensei** (doctor/teacher), **gakusei** (student), **seito** (student), **keitai-denwa** (cell phone), et cetera.

English has twenty-six characters, whereas Japanese has forty-six characters/syllables plus modified syllables and consonants. To begin practicing Japanese pronunciation, listen first to track 0 on the CD and familiarize yourself with the sounds you hear. There are five vowels in Japanese: **a**, **i**, **u**, **e**, and **o**.

> **a** (あ) is similar to the sound of *a* in "about."
> **i** (い) is similar to the sound of *i* in "innocent."
> **u** (う) is similar to the sound of *oo* in "cookie."
> **e** (え) is similar to the sound of *e* on "engine."
> **o** (お) is similar to the sound of *o* in "orange."

The following five charts show all the possible Japanese sounds and Romanized characters.

(CD 0: 1-5) Listen to the CD and repeat the Japanese syllables or sounds in 1-5.

1. Forty-six basic syllables: vowel, consonant plus vowel, and **n.**

	a （あ）	i （い）	u （う）	e （え）	o （お）
k	ka （か）	ki （き）	ku （く）	ke （け）	ko （こ）
s	sa （さ）	shi （し）	su （す）	se （せ）	so （そ）
t	ta （た）	chi （ち）	tsu （つ）	te （て）	to （と）
n	na （な）	ni （に）	nu （ぬ）	ne （ね）	no （の）
h	ha （は）	hi （ひ）	fu （ふ）	he （へ）	ho （ほ）
m	ma （ま）	mi （み）	mu （む）	me （め）	mo （も）
y	ya （や）	-	yu （ゆ）	-	yo （よ）
r	ra （ら）	ri （り）	ru （る）	re （れ）	ro （ろ）
w	wa （わ）	-	-	-	wo （を）
n	n （ん）				

Notes:

1) Over the last one thousand years of Japanese tradition, the following pronunciations have changed: "si" to "**shi**," "ti" to "**chi**," "tu" to "**tsu**," and "hu" to "**fu**." The characters/syllables yi, ye, wi, wu, and we have disappeared.

2) The first sound, "**a**," is said with an open mouth, and the last sound, "**n**," is said with a closed mouth. In Japanese culture, *a* and *n* symbolize the beginning and end or birth and death in natural phenomena. Most Japanese religious sites have a pair of human or animal guardians in front of their gates, one of whom has an open mouth and the other a closed mouth, to symbolizes the boundary between secular and holy spaces.

3) *N* is an independent consonant and does not have to combine with a vowel. In the Hepburn system of Romanization, if *n* is followed by syllables beginning with *m*, *p*, or *b*, it is pronounced as an *m*. However, for consistency and in order to help understanding, this book uses *n* in all Romanizations. For example, not **komban**, but **konban** (ko-n-ba-n) "this evening."

4) The Romanization of **i**-adjectives ends with an **-i**. For example: **itai** (i-ta-i) "pain." However, in sentences with the verb **desu**, Japanese speakers pronounce as follows: **itai(n) desu** (i-ta-i-n-de-su), including the "n" sound immediately after "i." For this reason, the Romanization in this book is represented as

itai(n) desu. In conversation, adding the "n" sound makes for an expression with more feeling and emotion. Both pronunciations **itai/itai(n)** are acceptable in Japanese conversation.

2. Twenty-five modified syllables: consonant plus basic vowel.

g	ga (が)	gi (ぎ)	gu (ぐ)	ge (げ)	go (ご)
z	za (ざ)	ji (じ)	zu (ず)	ze (ぜ)	zo (ぞ)
d	da (だ)	ji (ぢ)	zu (づ)	de (で)	do (ど)
b	ba (ば)	bi (び)	bu (ぶ)	be (べ)	bo (ぼ)
p	pa (ぱ)	pi (ぴ)	pu (ぷ)	pe (ぺ)	po (ぽ)

Note that the two instances respectively of **ji** and **zu** each have the same pronunciation, and in romaji it is difficult to identify which character is being used. There are rules for their representation in hiragana characters, but for the Romanization used in this book these rules do not apply.

3. Thirty-three modified syllables: consonant plus **ya**, **yu**, and **yo**.

kya (きゃ)	kyu (きゅ)	kyo (きょ)
sha (しゃ)	shu (しゅ)	sho (しょ)
cha (ちゃ)	chu (ちゅ)	cho (ちょ)
nya (にゃ)	nyu (にゅ)	nyo (にょ)
hya (ひゃ)	hyu (ひゅ)	hyo (ひょ)
mya (みゃ)	myu (みゅ)	myo (みょ)
rya (りゃ)	ryu (りゅ)	ryo (りょ)
gya (ぎゃ)	gyu (ぎゅ)	gyo (ぎょ)
jya (じゃ)	jyu (じゅ)	jyo (じょ)
bya (びゃ)	byu (びゅ)	byo (びょ)
pya (ぴゃ)	pyu (ぴゅ)	pyo (ぴょ)

4. Four double consonants: small **tsu**.

kk (っ)	pp (っ)	ss (っ)	tt (っ)

Note: The sound represented by the small **tsu** (っ) between two syllables is described as a double consonant. The first of the two consonants is given one syllable in length of pronunciation. The small **tsu** is realized as a little pause after the first consonant and before the second one is pronounced. For example: **kekka** けっか (result); **tatte** たって (stand up).

5. Five double vowels

ā（ああ）	ī（いい）	ū（うう）	ē（ええ）	ō（おお）

Note: Ā is similar in sound to "ah"; ī is similar sound to "ee" in *sweet*; ū is similar in sound to "oo" in *goods*; ē is similar in sound to "a" in *paper*; ō is similar in sound to *oh*.

For Romanization purposes, this book applies three particles in the following way: を is written as **o**; へ is written as **e**; and は is written as **wa**. In the Japanese language, each character has one syllable in length except the modified syllables; consonants plus **ya**, **yu**, and **yo** each have two syllables but are described as having one length.

In order to enhance readability, this book also uses the hyphen symbol "-" between syllables if a word is long and has a specific meaning. The words connected by hyphens are considered one word. For example, **shoku-yoku-fushin** (loss of appetite/anorexia): **shoku** is "eat"; **yoku** is "desire"; and **fushin** is "slump." Or **eiyō-busoku** (malnutrition): **eiyō** is "nutrition"; and **busoku/fusoku** is "shortage." Or **hana-ji** (nose bleeds): **hana** is "nose"; and **ji/chi** is "blood."

It is hoped that these protocols may make it easier for healthcare professionals to practice pronunciation and writing. If you take the time to listen to the CD and practice pronouncing the words as well as the sentences, you will be able to speak Japanese like a near native speaker.

THE JAPANESE LANGUAGE: AN OVERVIEW

Learning Japanese, like any foreign language, requires a grasp of the customs and ways of thinking of its native speakers as well as an understanding of their country's history, society, and culture. The language learner must open his or her mind to the linguistic and cultural differences, while setting aside the rules that govern English. The following discussion introduces eleven characteristics of the Japanese language that are distinct from English. Understanding these basic differences may help you in your study of *Japanese for Healthcare Professionals*.

1. The Japanese language was originally only a phonetic and spoken language until written characters were introduced from China in the sixth century. Consequently, there are certain differences between the spoken and written languages. The learner of Japanese will encounter many homonyms, words with the same pronunciation but different meanings, which complicates the study of the language. Also, for some sounds, pronunciation and dictionary spellings diverge. As indicated earlier, this book acknowledges such difference between actual pronunciation and the written language by using the macron. When looking up words in a Japanese dictionary, however, you must remember that the romaji will follow a different convention, and the learner will see such spellings as **Toukyou** (Tokyo), **byou-in** (hospital), **koumon** (anus), and **nou-geka** (brain surgery). Please keep in mind that native Japanese speakers do not pronounce "**Toukyou**," "**byou-in**," et cetera but rather "**Tōkyō**," "**byō-in**," "**kōmon**," and "**nō-geka**" as rendered in this book.

2. Japanese word order is different from English word order. Languages are commonly classified as being either of two types: SVO (Subject + Verb + Object) type and SOV (Subject + Object + Verb) type. English is SVO; Japanese is SOV. In the map of world languages, SOV languages like Japanese are more numerous than the SVO type. For example:

    English: The patient has an operation.
              S   V   O
    Japanese: **Kanjya wa shujyutsu o shimasu.**
              S   O   V
    (**kanjya**=patient, **shujyutsu**=operation, **shimasu**=do)

3. The subject/subject pronoun can be omitted in Japanese if it is understood from the context or redundant. For example, "I will place a stethoscope on your chest" can be expressed without **Watakushi** (I) or **anata no** (your):

   Watakushi wa anata no mune ni chōshinki o atete-mimasu.
   Watakushi wa mune ni chōshinki o atete-mimasu. ("anata no" omitted)
   Anata no mune ni chōshinki o atete-mimasu. ("Watakushi wa" omitted)
   Mune ni chōshinki o atete-mimasu. ("Watakushi wa anata no" omitted)

   (**mune** = chest, **chōshin-ki** = stethoscope, **atemasu** = place)

   In most cases, Japanese speakers will prefer the last example when conveying this message.

4. The verb must be located at the end of the sentence in Japanese. Japanese word order is relatively free except for this requirement. For example, "Sometimes I feel dizzy in the morning at home" can be expressed in the following sentences, all of which are acceptable:

   Tokidoki, watakushi wa asa uchi de memai ga shimasu.
   Watakushi wa tokidoki asa uchi de memai ga shimasu.
   Asa tokidoki uchi de watakushi wa memai ga shimasu.
   Watakushi wa memai ga tokidoki asa uchide shimasu.

   (**tokidoki** = sometimes, **watakushi** = I, **asa** = morning, **uchi** = home, **memai** = dizziness)

5. Verbs have only two tenses, the present (non-past) and past. There is no future tense. The verb endings for these two tenses are -**masu** (present/non-past) and -**mashita** (past), except there are separate endings for "let's" (-**mashō**) and "shall we" (-**mashō ka**). The present tense is used to express the future, and time indicators or context will suggest which is meant.

6. Nouns contain no concept of person/gender or number. Japanese nouns do not determine the verb, and there is no conjugation for person (I am; you are). Plurals are expressed with counters, which comprise a number plus a suffix that is a counter expression. For example, in English we say, "The doctor is treating many patients today." In Japanese, this idea is expressed as "**Kyō, ishi wa takusan no kanjya o chiryō shimasu**," where **ishi** = medical doctor, **takusan** = many, **kanjya** = patient, and **chiryō** = treatment. The Japanese verb and noun have no plural markers. Notice also that **ishi** has no article correspond-

ing to *the*. Nouns in Japanese do not take articles. There are neither definite nor indefinite articles in Japanese.

7. Japanese is able to be so flexible in sentence word order because it uses particles to mark key parts of speech. The particles, which generally follow the word they mark, allow interlocutors to understand the function of individual words in the syntax of the sentence, no matter what their position relative to the verb. Among the particles, first are the so-called topic/subject-markers **wa** and **ga**, which identify the topic or subject of a sentence. **Wa** and **ga** have no meaning in themselves, except that **ga** places more emphasis on the topic and subject while **wa** just identifies it, and **wa** is also reserved for negative sentences. Generally speaking, though, Japanese tends to use both **wa** and **ga** interchangeably. Second is the direct object marker **o**, which also has no intrinsic meaning but calls out the direct object of a transitive verb. Third, the substitute marker **mo** can replace **ga**, **wa**, and **o**. The particle **mo** translates as "also," "too," or, in negative sentences, "either" in English, but it doesn't change the word order or need an additional word to convey this meaning. Fourth, the particle **no** relates one noun to another and expresses affiliation or possession. Fifth, the particle **ni** is used with time expressions. **Ni** has the same meaning as *at* or *on* in English and immediately follows the word indicating time. The particle **ni** marks specific time, but general time expressions are stated without **ni**. Sixth, when used with the verbs **ikimasu** (go), **kimasu** (come), or **kaerimasu**, (return), the particles **e** or **ni** indicate directional movement or action toward the noun that precedes them. They translate as "to" or "toward" in English. Japanese use **e** and **ni** almost interchangeably, but **ni** is used for emphasis on place. Japanese has other markers that you'll encounter, including sentence-final particles for expressing the speaker's emotions or substituting for verbs when the meaning is clear from the context.

8. Japanese adjectives, unlike English adjectives, have tenses, similar to verbs. They can also end sentences (informal) like Japanese verbs and express observations. For example, **itai** (pain/sore/hurt/ache) and **akai** (red) are adjectives, but they can act as verbs or express the speaker's feelings.

9. Japanese society places great value on politeness both as a reflection of one's human quality and as essential for social order. For example, Japanese may say **O-mizu** rather than **mizu** for "water." Putting the prefix **O-** before a noun makes the noun polite. Moreover, when introducing oneself, saying "NAME **to mōshi-masu**" is more polite than "NAME **desu**." As another example, the question "Do you have any complaints today?" can be said in several different ways in Japanese:

Kyō wa dō shita no. (informal)
Kyō wa dō shimashita ka. (ordinary)
Kyō wa dō nasare-mashita ka. (polite)

(**kyō** = today, **ka** = question marker)

10. The Japanese passive voice is unlike the English passive in three essential aspects. First, the passive in Japanese doesn't alter the S-V-O sentence order and instead is expressed by adding the suffix **-rareru** (present)/**-rareta** (past) to the verb. For example, **tasukeru** means "save," while **tasuke-rareru** means "was saved."

> **Kanjya wa ishi ni tasuke-rareta.**   The patient was saved by the doctor.

Second, the passive is used to express an action or event that happens to a person (the object of the action) without being the result of that person's will, expectation, or intention. For example, **Sensei ni mirareta.** (*lit.*, Doctor examined (me).); **Kanjya o miserareta.** (*lit.*, Am required to take patient.) Neither of these sentences would be considered passive in the English sense. Third, the passive is used to express politeness in Japanese. Adding the suffix **-rareru** or **-rareta** to the verb makes it polite. For example, **Sensei wa kanjya o mirareta.** (Doctor examined patient.); **Kango-shi wa myaku o torareta.** (Nurse took pulse.); **Go-ryōshin ga korareta.** (Parents came.) Furthermore, there are two other words for expressing the passive: **koto ni naru** (present)/ **koto ni natta** (past) and **morau** (present)/**moratta** (past).

11. Japanese frequently use onomatopoetic expressions (sound symbolism) to reduce tension or encourage smooth communication. English too has onomatopoetic expressions, like *glug glug* (drinking or pouring sound), *bark* (dog), *meow* (cat), and so on. However, except when their onomatopoetic origin has simply been forgotten or normalized, they are felt to be childish, comical, or informal and in such cases are avoided in ordinary conversation. In contrast, Japanese use onomatopoeia frequently in their daily lives. Most Japanese language textbooks exclude onomatopoetic expressions that don't correspond to concepts in English. However, since onomatopoeia are common in spoken Japanese, this book includes them as much as possible.

Keep these characteristics in mind as you use this book, and you may find it helps you in your study of Japanese.

PART ONE

Self-Introduction
(Jiko-shōkai)

Basic Vocabulary (CD 1-1)

Listen to the CD and repeat the vocabulary.

1.	name	**(o)namae**	（お）名前
2.	I	**watakushi**	私
3.	you	**anata**	貴方
4.	he	**kare(shi)**	彼（氏）
5.	she	**kano-jyo**	彼女
6.	Mr./Miss/Mrs./Ms.	**-san**	－さん
7.	sir/madam	**-sama**	様
8.	head (chief) doctor	**i-in-chō**	医院長
9.	doctor/teacher	**sensei**	先生
10.	specialized doctor/specialist	**senmon-i**	専門医
11.	medical doctor	**i-shi/(o)i-sha(san)**	医師／（お）医者（さん）
12.	dentist	**shika-i-shi(san)**	歯科医師（さん）
13.	nurse	**kango-shi(san)**	看護師（さん）
14.	healthcare worker	**kaigo-shi(san)**	介護士（さん）
15.	office worker	**jimu-in(san)**	事務員（さん）
16.	counselor	**kaunserā(san)**	カウンセラー
17.	receptionist	**uketsuke(gakari)**	受付（係り）
18.	information	**an-nai**	案内
19.	patient/client	**kanjya(san)**	患者（さん）
20.	attendant	**tsukisoi-nin**	付添人
21.	private nurse	**tsukisoi-kango-shi**	付添看護師
22.	emergency	**kinkyū**	緊急
23.	translator	**tsūyaku**	通訳
24.	illness/disease	**byōki**	病気
25.	name of illness	**byōmei**	病名
26.	hospital	**byōin**	病院
27.	clinic	**kurinikku**	クリニック
28.	job/work	**(o)shigoto**	（お）仕事
29.	initial medical examination	**shoshin**	初診
30.	family	**(go)kazoku**	（御）家族

Dialogue (CD 1-2)

Listen to the CD and repeat the dialogue.

In the Waiting Room

Mr. Suzuki (patient):	**Kon-nichi wa.** Hello.
Sandra (receptionist):	**Kon-nichi wa. Onamae wa nan desu ka.** Hello. What's your name, please?
Mr. Suzuki:	**Suzuki Kenji desu. Hajime-mashite.** I'm Suzuki Kenji. How do you do?
Sandra:	**Sandra desu. Hajime-mashite.** I'm Sandra. How do you do?
Mr. Suzuki:	**Sandra-san wa kango-shi-san desu ka.** Are you a nurse, Sandra?
Sandra:	**Iie, kango-shi dewa arimasen.** No, I'm not a nurse.
	Uketsuke no Sandora desu. I'm the receptionist, Sandra.
	Suzuki-san wa shoshin desu ka. Is this your initial medical examination, Mr. Suzuki?
Mr. Suzuki:	**Hai, shoshin desu.** Yes, this is my initial examination.

Grammar

1.   NOUN **+ desu means "this is, it is."**

The word **desu** is used at the end of a sentence. **Desu** is the equivalent of *be* (*am*, *are*, *is*, and *it is*) in English but is a unique feature of the Japanese language. Adding a noun to **desu** (NOUN + **desu**) is sufficient to make a Japanese sentence.

Suzuki desu.	I am Suzuki.
Sandora desu.	I am Sandra.
I-shi desu.	I am a doctor.
Kango-shi desu.	I am a nurse.
Uketsuke desu.	I am a receptionist.
Kanjya desu.	I am a patient.

Tsukisoi-nin desu.	I am an attendant.
Byōin desu.	It's a hospital, *or* This is a hospital.
Kinkyū desu.	It's an emergency.
Shoshin desu.	This is my initial medical exam.
Pen desu.	This is a pen.
Sofā desu.	This is a sofa.

2. NOUN + **dewa arimasen**

Dewa arimasen is the negative form of **desu** and means "this is not; it's not; I am not." To make a statement negative, first drop **desu** and add **dewa arimasen**. The informal negative is **jyā arimasen**.

Suzuki dewa arimasen.	I am not Suzuki.
Sandora dewa arimasen.	I am not Sandra.
I-shi dewa arimasen.	I am not a doctor.
Kango-shi dewa arimasen.	I am not a nurse.
Uketsuke dewa arimasen.	I am not a receptionist.
Byōin dewa arimasen.	It is not a hospital, *or* This is not a hospital.
Shoshin jyā arimasen.	This isn't my first medical exam.
Pen jyā arimasen.	This is not a pen.
Sofā jyā arimasen.	This is not a sofa.

3. The particle **wa**

The particle **wa** is used to indicate the subject or topic of a sentence: X **wa** Y **desu** means "X is Y." However, if the subject is clear from the context, it will often be omitted in speech. Sentences without subjects are common in Japanese, and speakers will often drop such pronouns as **watakushi** (I), **anata** (you), **kare** (he), and **kano-jyo** (she) when the speaker and listener are likely to understand the subject.

(Watakushi wa) Sandora desu.	I am Sandra.
(Kare wa) Oisha-san desu.	He is a doctor.
(Kanojyo wa) Kango-shi-san desu.	She is a nurse.

Of course, sometimes specifying the subject is the purpose of using the construction X **wa** Y **desu**.

Suzuki-san wa kanjya desu.	Mr. Suzuki is a patient.
Kanjya wa Suzuki-san desu.	The patient is Mr. Suzuki.
Sandora-san wa uketsuke desu.	Sandra is a receptionist.
Uketsuke wa Sandora-san desu.	The receptionist is Miss Sandra.
(Watakushi no) Namae wa Suzuki desu.	My name is Suzuki.

4. The particle **no**

The particle **no** is used to indicate the affiliation of a person with a country, state, city, organization, position, or role in the construction AFFILIATION **no** Y **desu** (I am Y of AFFILIATION). Note that the word order in Japanese is the opposite of what it is in English, but the Japanese **no** is often equivalent to the English *of* or the possessive suffix *'s*.

Kango-shi no Maria desu.	I am Nurse Maria.
I-shi no Harisu desu.	I am Doctor Harris.
Amerika no X Byōin no i-shi no Harisu desu.	I am Dr. Harris at X Hospital in America.

5. The question marker **ka**

The particle **ka** is placed at the end of sentence to form a question. In Japanese, the word order doesn't change as it does in English, nor is a question mark used to punctuate written questions. In speech, the intonation usually rises on **ka**.

(Anata wa) Kanjya-san desu ka.	Are you a patient?
Sandora-san wa uketsuke desu ka.	Is Sandra a receptionist?
Kinkyū desu ka.	Is this an emergency?

6. The tag question-marker **ne**

The particle **ne** is placed at the end of a sentence to form a tag question. **Ne** in Japanese sentences is friendlier and more expressive than **ka**. Intonation usually rises on **ne**.

Sensei desu ne.	You're a doctor, aren't you?
Kanjya-san desu ne.	You're a client/patient, aren't you?
Sandora-san wa uketsuke desu ne.	Sandra is a receptionist, isn't she?

7. **Nan desu ka** means "What is it?"

The Japanese question word for "what" has two variants, **nan** and **nani**. **Nan** is used with **desu**, and **nani** is used as a subject or noun.

Namae wa nan desu ka.	What is your name?
Shigoto wa nan desu ka.	What is your job/work?
Byōki wa nan desu ka.	What is your illness?
Nani ka.	What?
(Hokani) nani ka.	Any questions?/Anything else?

Useful Expressions (CD 1-3)

Listen to the CD and repeat the following greetings.

1. **Ohayō gozaimasu.** Good morning.
2. **Kon-nichi wa.** Good afternoon/Good day/Hello.
3. **Kon-ban wa.** Good evening.
4. **Oyasumi nasai.** Good night.
5. **Sayōnara.** Good-by.
6. **Dō(ka) shimashita ka.** Do you have any complaints? (*lit.*, What happened?)
7. **Odaiji-ni.** Take care of yourself.
8. **Arigatō-gozaimasu.** Thank you very much.
9. **Hajime-mashite.** How do you do? (*lit.*, This is a first time.)
10. **Dōzo yoroshiku.** Nice to meet you.

Key Sentences (CD 1-4)

Listen to the CD and repeat the sentences.

1. **Kango-shi desu.** I am a nurse *or* This is a nurse.
2. **I-shi no Harisu desu.** I am Dr. Harris *or* This is Dr. Harris.
3. **Uketsuke no Sandora desu.** This is/I am the receptionist, Sandra.
4. **Kanjya no Suzuki-san desu ka.** Are you the patient Suzuki?
5. **(O)namae wa nan desu ka.** What is your name?

Additional Words

hai yes
nani/nan what
Nihon Japan
Nihon-go Japanese language
ocha tea
gohan meals/steamed rice
sofā sofa

iie no
odaiji-ni take care
Nihon-jin Japanese people
goshujin your husband
omizu water
pen pen
hokani another/other/anything else

Language Notes

1. **Watakushi** is equivalent to *I* and is used to refer to oneself in formal situations, while **watashi** is used in informal situations. **Watashi** expresses a gentler feeling than **watakushi**. **Watashi** has been used by women only in the modern period. Men may also use **ore** in informal situations; young men use **boku**, and girls use **watashi**.

2. The suffix -**san** is a respectful title attached to names. It should never be used when referring to yourself or your own name. When referring to someone else, use the structure NAME + -**san**. -**sensei** is also a respectful title, attached to doctors/teachers/or similar professionals deserving of respect. -**sama** is a respectful title used to express politeness in business situations and in the service industry. Children (male and female) are referred to as -**chan** from an early age until about elementary school. Then boys use -**kun** until high school, and girls use -**san**, the same suffix as for adults.

Kato-san	Mr./Mrs./Miss/Ms. Kato
Kangoshi-san	Mr./Mrs./Miss (used to address or refer to a nurse)
Harisu-sensei	Doctor Harris
Kato-san desu ka.	Are you Mr./Mrs./Ms./Miss Kato?
Kanjya-san desu ka.	Are you a client/patient?
Suzuki-sama desu ka.	Are you Mr./Mrs./Ms./Miss Suzuki? (very polite)

3. The polite prefixes **o-** and **go-** are used with nouns to express the speaker's respect, modesty, and politeness. These markers are called honorific because they convey respect for others.

(for other people)	
onamae	your name
Odaiji-ni.	Please take care of yourself.
go-shujin	your husband
(for things)	
ocha	tea
omizu	water
go-han	meals/steamed rice

4. **Hai** means "yes" or agreement in response to a yes-no question. **Hai** is formal, while **Ee** is informal. **Iie** means "no" or disagreement in response to a yes-no question.

Suzuki-san desu ka.	Are you Mr./Mrs./Miss Suzuki?
Hai, Susuki-desu.	Yes, I am Suzuki.
Iie, Suzuki dewa arimaen.	No, I'm not Suzuki.
Kango-shi-san desu ka.	Are you a nurse?
Hai, kango-shi desu.	Yes, I am a nurse.
Iie, kango-shi dewa arimasen.	No, I'm not a nurse.

5. Japanese has four polite expressions conveying different levels of gratitude.

Dōmo.	Thanks.
Arigatō.	Thank you.
Arigatō gozaimasu.	Thank you very much.
Dōmo arigatō gozaimasu.	Thank you very much indeed.

6. The expression **Dō ka shimashita ka** (Is anything the matter?/Do you have any complaints?) comes from the term **dō ka**, which means "unusual condition." Literally, **Dō ka shimashita ka** means "Do you have an unusual condition?" **Dō ka shimashita ka** is sometimes expressed as **Dō shimashita ka**, with the first question marker **ka** is elided or dropped.

    Dō ka shimashita ka. (formal)
    Dō (ka) shimashita ka. (informal)

7. In greetings, Japanese often abbreviates sentiments more fully expressed by the phrases **Ikaga desu ka** (How about?); **Genki desu ka** (Are you fine/How are you?); and **Shite kudasai** (Please do), as in the following:

Kon-nichi wa.	Hello/Good day/Good afternoon.
Kon-nichi wa ikaga desu ka.	How are things today?
Kon-nichi wa genki desu ka.	Are you fine today?/How are you today?
Konban wa.	Good evening
Konban wa ikaga desu ka.	How are things this evening?
Konban wa genki desu ka.	Are you fine tonight?/How are you tonight?
Odaiji-ni.	Take care of yourself.
Odaiji-ni shite kudasai.	Please respect yourself/your body/your health.

8. There are many other professionals involved in healthcare facilities besides those listed in the basic vocabulary. Some others are:

kaigo-fukushi-shi	healthcare worker
soshiaru wākā	social worker
shika-eisei-shi	dental hygienist
shika-gikō-shi	dental technician
hōsha-sen-gishi	radiology technician
kensa-gishi	laboratory technician
rigaku-ryōhō-shi	physical therapist
sagyō-ryōhō-shi	occupational therapist
shinō-kunren-shi	orthoptist

gengo-chōkaku-shi	speech therapist
kango-jyoshi	nurse assistant
jo-san-shi	licensed midwife
eiyō-shi	nutritionist
chōri-shi	licensed chef/cook
hoiku-shi	pediatrics instructor
iryō-hisho	medical clerk
shinryō-jyōhō-kanri-shi	health information management professional
keibi-in	security guard

9. Japanese natives pronounce the name of their country "**Nippon**" or "**Nihon**" (日本 "sun origin"). The name derives from the fact that Japan is located to the east of China, where, from China's perspective, the sun rises. When the Portuguese arrived in Japan in the sixteenth century, they pronounced **Nippon** as "**Japão**," substituting the "j" sound for the Japanese "n." Because of this, English refers to the country as Japan. Placing the suffix -**jin** after the name of a country forms the word for its people, and doing the same with the suffix -**go** forms the word for its language.

Countries, Peoples, and Languages

ENGLISH NAME	COUNTRY	PEOPLE (-JIN)	LANGUAGE (-GO)
Japan	Nihon	Nihon-jin	Nihon-go
USA	Amerika	Amerika-jin	Ei-go
Korea	Kankoku	Kankoku-jin	Kankoku-go
China	Chūgoku	Chūgoku-jin	Chūgoku-go
Canada	Kanada	Kanada-jin	Ei-go/Fransu-go
Philippines	Firipin	Firipin-jin	Tagaaru-go
Australia	Ōsutoraria	Ōsutoraria-jin	Ei-go
England	Igirisu	Igirisu-jin	Ei-go
France	Furansu	Furansu-jin	Fransu-go
Germany	Doitsu	Doitsu-jin	Doitsu-go
Italy	Itaria	Itaria-jin	Itaria-go
Spain	Supein	Supein-jin	Supein-go
India	Indo	Indo-jin	Hindē-go
Russia	Roshia	Roshia-jin	Roshia-go
Indonesia	Indoneshia	Indoneshia-jin	Indoneshia-go

Watakushi wa Amerika-jin no i-shi desu.
I am an American doctor.

(Watakushi wa) Kanada-jin no kango-shi desu.
I am a Canadian nurse.

(Anata wa) nihon-jin no kanjya-san desu ka.
Are you a Japanese patient?

10. Kinship relations: Japanese culture makes a clear distinction among family members between *my* relatives and *your/other's* relatives, as can be seen on the following chart. Some of the terms incorporate expressions for respect. Note that, in nouns, Japanese makes no distinction for number and has no single or plural forms. To express whether something is singular or plural, Japanese employs counters, which will be studied later.

ENGLISH MEANING	MY (WATAKUSHI NO ~)	YOUR (ANATA NO ~)	SIR/MADAM (POLITE *YOUR*~)
family	kazoku	go-kazoku	go-kazoku-sama
parents	ryōshin	go-ryōshin-sama	go-ryōshin-sama
father	chichi	otō-san	otō-sama
father-in-law	giri no chichi	giri no otō-san	giri no otō-sama
mother	haha	okā-san	okā-sama
mother-in-law	giri no haha	giri no okā-sama	giri no okā-sama
grandparents	so-fubo	go-sofubo	go-sofubo-sama
grandfather	sofu	ojii-san	ojii-sama
grandmother	sobo	obā-san	obā-sama
great grand-parents*	sō-sofubo	sō-sofubo-san	sō-sofubo-sama
uncle*	oji	oji-san	oji-sama
aunt*	oba	oba-san	oba-sama
child/children	ko/kodomo	oko-san/ kodomo-san	oko-sama/ kodomo-sama
son*	musuko	musuko-san	musuko-sama
daughter*	musume	musume-san	musume-sama
grandchild	mago	o-mago-san	o-mago-sama
husband	otto	go-shujin	go-shujin-sama
wife	kanai	oku-san	oku-sama
older brother	ani	onii-san	onii-sama
older sister	ane	onē-san	onē-sama
younger brother*	otōto	otōto-san	otōto-sama
younger sister*	imōto	imōto-san	imōto-sama
sibling	kyōdai	go-kyōdai	go-kyōdai-sama
nephew	oi	oigo-san	oigo-sama
niece	mei	meigo-san	meigo-sama
cousin	itoko	o-itoko-san	o-itoko-sama
infant/baby	aka-chan	aka-chan	aka-chan
friend	tomodachi	o-tomodachi	go-yū-jin
guardian	hogo-sha	hogo-sha-san	hogo-sha-sama

Note: ▸ *The same expression is used with the addition of the suffixes **-san/-sama**.

The prefix **giri no** expresses the meaning of "in-law." For example, **giri no haha** means "mother-in-law," and **giri no chichi** means "father-in-law."

(Watakushi no) Kanai desu.	This is my wife.
Suzuki-san no oku-san desu.	This is Mr. Suzuki's wife.
Suzuki-san no oku-sama desu ka.	Are you Mr. Suzuki's wife? (polite form)
Suzuki-san no go-shujin-sama desu ka.	Are you Mrs. Suzuki's husband? (polite form)
Suzuki-san no giri no otō-sama desu ka.	Are you Mr. Suzuki's father-in-law?

Language Roots

The word **byō** (病) indicates illness and disease and is used both as a prefix and a suffix.

byō-ki	illness = disease + feeling
byō-in	hospital = illness + institution
byō-mei	name of a disease = disease + name
shinzō-byō	heart disease = heart + disease
hai-byō	lung disease = lung + disease
densen-byō	infectious disease = infection + disease

The suffix **-shi** (師) indicates a person who has extensive knowledge and learning or one of superior social standing.

i-shi	medical doctor
kango-shi	nurse
eiyō-shi	nutritionist
hoken-shi	public health nurse
bengo-shi	lawyer

Culture Notes

The world and Japanese populations

The estimated world population is approximately 6 billion 788 million, and the population of Japan is approximately 127 million (male: 62 million; female: 65 million). Japan is third among industrial nations in gross domestic product and the tenth most populous country following China (1 billion 333 million), India (1 billion 169 million), the United States (307 million), Indonesia (229 million), Brazil (191 million), Pakistan (167 million), Bangladesh (162 million), Nigeria (154 million), and Russia (141 million). (SOURCE: United Nations 2009)

The Japanese bow is called the **ojigi.**

The Japanese usually bow to each other in greeting when they meet and to say good-bye. A Japanese bow is called an **ojigi.** The lower the bow, the more formal it is.

Statistics for Japanese nationals overseas

According to the *Annual Report of Statistics on Japanese Nationals Overseas* by the Ministry of Foreign Affairs, the estimated population of Japanese residing overseas is more than one million and of Japanese overseas for stays less than three months (including travel for tourism) is more than 16 million annually in recent years.

The most popular Japanese family names

When Japanese give their full names, they say their family name first and given name last. Japanese typically introduce themselves using their family name alone. When meeting a Japanese patient for the first time, use the last name to summon them; it is not customary to use a Japanese adult's first name. You may correctly address the person using his or her last name followed by -**san**, for example Yamada-**san**, Suzuki-**san**, or Sato-**san**. The most common Japanese family names are: Sato, Suzuki, Takahashi, Tanaka, Watanabe, Ito, Yamamoto, Nakamura, Kobayashi, Saito, Kato, Yoshida, Yamada, Sasaki, and Yamaguchi.

The origin of the expression **arigatō** (thank you)

Literally, **arigatō** means "uncommon in opportunity" or "rare in existence." In ancient times, Japanese had no expression for "thank you." There is no historic or linguistic evidence for this, but it is thought that when Francis Xavier (1506–1552) arrived with Portuguese merchants on Tanega-shima Island in 1549, he introduced Christianity, Western medicines, and European culture to Japan. Among the novelties was the Portuguese word *obligado* (thank you), which eventually evolved into **arigatō** as an expression of thanks. The Japanese assimilated the new concept by "concept matching," as they would do later, during the Meiji Period (1868–1912).

Comprehension

Answer the following questions.

1. Which of the following could NOT be used as a translation for **kon-nichi wa?**
   a. Hello   b. Good afternoon
   c. Good morning   d. Good day

2. Which of the following best completes the sentence below?
   Watakushi (   ) Kango-shi desu.
   a. **o**   b. **wa**
   c. **de**   d. **ni**

3. Which of the following could be used as a translation for **Dō shimashita ka?**
   a. Thank you very much.   b. How do you do?
   c. Please take care.   d. Do you have any complaints?

4. Which of the following self-introductions is correct?
   a. **Watakushi wa Sandra-san desu.**
   b. **Watakushi wa o-isha-san no Harisu desu.**
   c. **Watakushi wa o-isha-san desu.**
   d. **Watakushi wa i-sha no Harisu desu.**

5. You are a healthcare professional. What do you say when a patient is leaving the hospital?
   a. **Konnichi wa.**   b. **Hajime-mashite.**
   c. **Odaiji-ni.**   d. **Arigatō.**

6. Which of the following best completes the sentence below?
   Watakushi wa kango-shi (   ) Maria desu.
   a. **no**   b. **de**
   c. **wa**   d. **ni**

7. How do you say *hospital* in Japanese?
   a. **Biyōin**   b. **Byōin**
   c. **Byōki**   d. **Byōmei**

Practice

Respond to the following using the cues that have been provided.

1. Greetings: How do you respond?
   (Patient)   (Healthcare professional)
   1. **Ohayō gozaimasu.**   _____
   2. **Kon-nichi wa.**   _____
   3. **Konban wa.**   _____
   4. **Oyasumi nasai**   _____
   5. **Sayōnara**   _____

2. Self-introduction: How do you respond?
   (Patient)   (Healthcare professional)
   1. **Hajime-mashite.**   _____ (reply with a greeting)
   2. **Suzuki desu.**   _____ (name only)
   3. **Kanjya no Suzuki desu.** _____ (reply with affiliation)

3. Giving your name/affiliation: How do you respond?
   (Patient)   (Healthcare professional)
   1. **Onamae wa nan desu ka.** _____ (name only)
   2. **Onamae wa nan desu ka.** _____ (affiliation)

4. Asking name/affiliation.
   (Healthcare professional)   (Patient/colleague)
   1. _____   **Sandora desu.**
   2. _____   **Tsūyaku desu.**
   3. _____   **Kango-shi no Maria desu.**

5. Dialogue comprehension. Based on the dialogue, answer the following.
   1. **Kanjya-san no namae wa nan desu ka.** _____
   2. **Uketsuke no namae wa nan desu ka.** _____
   3. **Suzuki-san wa shoshin desu ka.** _____
   4. **Suzuki-san wa oisha-san desu ka.** _____
   5. **Sandora-san wa kango-shi desu ka.** _____

6. Free response questions.
   (Question)   (Answer)
   1. **Onamae wa nan desu ka.**   _____
   2. **Oshigoto wa nan desu ka.** _____
   3. **Nihon-jin desu ka.**   _____
   4. **Uketsuke desu ka.**   _____
   5. **Byōki dusu ka.**   _____

Exercises

1. Say the following expressions in Japanese.
   A. Good morning.   _____
   B. Good afternoon.   _____
   C. Good evening.   _____
   D. Good night.   _____
   E. Good-by.   _____
   F. Is anything the matter? _____

      G. Take care of yourself.   _____

      H. What is your name?   _____

2. Introduce yourself by using **desu**.
   Q: **(O)namae wa nan desu ka.**
   A: _____

3. Introduce yourself by using **no**, as in: (Position) **no** (Your name) **desu**.
   Q: **(O)namae wa nan desu ka.**
   A: _____

4. Respond to each question by using **Hai** or **Iie**.
   A. **Oisha-san desu ka.**   _____
   B. **Kango-shi-san desu ka.**   _____
   C. **Uketsuke desu ka.**   _____
   D. **Tsukisoi-nin desu ka.**   _____
   E. **Kanjya-san desu ka.**   _____
   F. **Nihon-jin desu ka.**   _____

5. What is the meaning of the following words?
   A. **Namae**   _____
   B. **I-sha**   _____
   C. **Kinkyū**   _____
   D. **Okā-san**   _____
   E. **Tsūyaku**   _____

6. Say the following in Japanese.
   A. I am not a doctor.   _____
   B. You are not a nurse.   _____
   C. Are you a patient?   _____
   D. Is this your initial medical exam?   _____

Appointment I
(Yoyaku)

Basic Vocabulary (CD 2-1)

Listen to the CD and repeat the vocabulary.

1.	appointment/reservation	**yoyaku**	予約
2.	window/counter	**mado-guchi**	窓口
3.	address	**(go)jyūsho**	ご住所
4.	age	**(o)toshi/nenrei**	お年／年齢
5.	birth date	**(o)tanjyō-bi**	誕生日
6.	sex	**sei-betsu**	性別
7.	man	**otoko/danshi**	男／男子
8.	woman	**on-na/jyoshi**	女／女子
9.	adult	**sei-jin**	成人
10.	elderly person/people	**(o)toshiyori**	お年寄り
11.	outpatient	**gairai/gairai-kanjya**	外来／外来患者
12.	occupation	**shoku-gyō**	職業
13.	nationality	**kokuseki**	国籍
14.	insurance	**hoken**	保険
15.	insurance company	**hoken gaisha**	保険会社
16.	health insurance	**kenkō hoken**	健康保険
17.	car insurance	**jidōsha hoken**	自動車保険
18.	travelers insurance	**ryokō-sha hoken**	旅行者保険
19.	overseas travelers insurance	**kaigai ryokō-sha hoken**	海外旅行者保険
20.	number	**bangō**	番号
21.	telephone number	**denwa-bangō**	電話番号
22.	cell phone	**keitai-denwa**	携帯電話
23.	insurance number	**hoken-bangō**	保険番号
24.	room number	**heya-bangō**	部屋番号
25.	doctor's office/clinic	**i-in**	医院
26.	general hospital	**sogō-byōin**	総合病院
27.	specialized hospital	**senmon-byōin**	専門病院
28.	emergency hospital	**kinkyū-byōin**	緊急病院
29.	health center	**hoken-jyo**	保健所
30.	ambulance	**kyūkyū-sha**	救急車

Byōin no Uketsuke (Hospital Registration)

i-shi/(o)i-sha(san) (doctor)

kango-shi(san) (nurse)

kanjya(san) (patient)

uketsuke (receptionist)

mado-guchi (window)

denwa (telephone)

Dialogue (CD 2-2)

Listen to the CD and repeat the dialogue.

At the reception desk: Getting a patient's information.

Sandra: **Dō shimashita ka.**
Do you have any complaints?

Mr. Suzuki: **Netsu ga arimasu.**
I have a fever.

Yoyaku o onegai shimasu.
I would like to make an appointment.

Sandra: **Netsu wa nan-do gurai desu ka.**
About how high is the fever?

Mr. Suzuki: **Hyaku ichi (101) do gurai desu.**
It's about 101°F.

Sandra: **Onamae wa nan desu ka.**
What's your name?

Mr. Suzuki: **Suzuki Kenji desu.**
I am Suzuki Kenji.

Sandra: **Odenwa-bangō wa nan-ban desu ka.**
What's your telephone number?

Mr. Suzuki:	**Hachi-zero-ni no nana-nana-san no kyū-hachi-zero-ichi desu (802 no 773 no 9801 desu).**
	It's 802-773-9801.
Sandra:	**Hoken ga arimasu ka.**
	Do you have insurance?
Mr. Suzuki:	**Iie, hoken wa arimasen.**
	No, I don't have insurance.

Grammar

1. **The particle ga: the construction** NOUN/SUBJECT **ga arimasu means "to have (something), there is (something)."**

The particle **ga** is a subject marker and indicates the existence of an object. The **wa** and **ga** particles are interchangeable in Japanese. However, if someone asks, "**Nani ga arimasu ka.**" (What do you have?), the response must use the particle **ga**.

Netsu ga arimasu.	I have a fever.
Kenkō-hoken ga arimasu.	I have health insurance.
Yoyaku ga arimasu.	I have an appointment.
Keitai-denwa ga arimasu.	There is/I have a telephone.

2. **The particle wa is used for all negative statements.**

The particle **wa**, which we studied in Lesson 1, is always used to mark the topic in a negative statement, even if the question to which it is a response uses the particle **ga**.

Netsu wa arimasen.	I don't have a fever.
Ryokō-sha hoken wa arimasen.	I don't have insurance.
Senmon-byōin wa arimasen.	There is no specialized hospital.
Byōki wa airmasen.	I don't have an illness.

3. **The particle wa in what-questions**

The particle **wa** is used to identify the subject in a what-question in the construction SUBJECT **wa nan desu ka**.

(O)namae wa nan desu ka.	What's your name?
Shigoto wa nan desu ka.	What is your job?
(O)denwa-bangō wa nan-ban desu ka.	What's your telephone number?
Kokuseki wa nan desu ka.	What's your nationality?
Hoken wa nan desu ka.	What insurance do you have?

4. The verb **arimasu** means "to have, there is."

The verb of existence **arimasu** is often associated with the meaning "to have" in the sense of "to own (something)," with the particle **ga** marking the object or thing possessed.

Denwa ga arimasu.	I have a telephone.
Yoyaku ga arimasu.	I have an appointment.
Ryokō-sha hoken ga arimasu.	I have traveler's insurance.
Jidō-sha hoken ga arimasu ka.	Do you have car insurance?

In addition to the meaning "to have" or "to own (something)," **arimasu** can describe things that exist or events that take place.

Uketsuke-madoguchi ga arimasu.	There is a reception desk/window.
Sōgō-byōin ga arimasu.	There is a general hospital.
I-in ga arimasu.	There is a clinic.
Kyūkyū-sha ga airmasu.	There is an ambulance.
Kensa ga arimasu.	There is an examination.

5. The negative form of **arimasu** is **arimasen.**

The negative form of the verb of existence is **arimasen**. In Japanese, changing the suffix -**masu** to -**masen** makes the verb negative. This is a regular rule.

Hoken ga arimasu.	**Hoken wa arimasen.**
I have insurance.	I don't have insurance.
Netsu ga arimasu.	**Netsu wa arimasen.**
I have a fever/You have a fever.	I don't have a fever/You don't have fever.
Byōin ga arimasu.	**Byōin wa arimasen.**
There is a hospital.	There is no hospital.

6. The particle **o**

The particle **o** is an object marker and is used to indicate the direct object in a sentence. A direct object occurs with a transitive verb and is the person, thing, or matter that receives the action of the verb. In other words, it is the object of the verb's action. Note that the particle follows the direct object, which precedes the verb in Japanese but usually follows it in English.

(Watakushi wa) Yoyaku o onegai shimasu.
I would like to make an appointment.

(Watakushi wa) (o)mizu o nomimasu.   I will drink water.
(Watakushi wa) gohan o tabemasu.   I will eat a meal.

7. The expression **onegai shimasu**

The expression **onegai shimasu** literally means "Do me a favor" or "Please give me" and is a common way to say "please" or "do me a favor" or "I would like to" in Japanese. The usual construction is NOUN/OBJECT **o onegai shimasu**. **Onegai** is formed from the verb **negau/negaimasu** (wish).

Denwa-bangō o onegai-shimasu.	Please give me your phone number.
Onamae o onegai-shimasu.	Please give me your name.
Hoken-gaisha o onegai-shimasu.	Please tell me your insurance company.
Kyūkyū-sha o onegai-shimasu.	Please send me an ambulance.
Yoyaku o onegai-shimasu.	I would like to make an appointment.

8. WH words + **desu ka**

The adverbs *where* (**doko**), *what* (**nani/nan**), *who* (**dare**), *why* (**naze**), *when* (**itsu**), *which* (**dore**), *how old/many* (**ikutsu**), *how much* (**ikura**), and *how come* (**dōshite**) are used with **desu ka** to form a question. In conversation, **desu ka** is sometimes dropped and just saying the WH word suffices. The intonation usually rises on the last syllable.

Doko desu ka.	Where?	**Nan desu ka.**	What?
Dare desu ka.	Who?	**Naze desu ka.**	Why?
Itsu desu ka.	When?	**Ikutsu desu ka.**	How old/many?
Ikura desu ka.	How much?	**Dōshite desu ka.**	How come?

9. **Gurai** and the construction NOUN or NUMBER + **gurai**

Gurai means "about" or "approximately." Note that, in the construction NOUN or NUMBER + **gurai**, **gurai** follows the noun or number, whereas English *about* precedes them, as in the phrase "about 100 degrees." **Gurai** is also pronounced **kurai** (not to be confused with the adjective **kurai**, meaning "dark")

Nan-do gurai desu ka.
About how high is your temperature?

Nan-do gurai arimasu ka.
Approximately what (how much) temperature do you have?

Hyaku (100) do gurai desu.
It's about 100 degrees.

Hyaku (100) do kurai arimasu.
I have a temperature of about 100 degrees.

Nenrei wa nan-sai gurai desu ka.
About how old you?

San-jyū-san (33) sai gurai desu.
About 33 years old.

Yoyaku wa nan-ji gurai ga ii desu ka.
What time would you like to make an appointment?

Gozen jyū ichi (11) ji gurai ga ii desu.
I prefer about 11 a.m.

Useful Expressions (CD 2-3)

Listen to the CD and repeat the sentences.

1. **Yoyaku ga arimasu ka.** Do you have an appointment?
2. **Kaigai ryokō-sha hoken ga arimasu ka.**
   Do you have overseas travel insurance?
3. **Kenkō-hoken wa arimasen.** I don't have health insurance.
4. **Onamae wa nan desu ka.** What is your name?
5. **Odenwa-bangō wa nan desu ka.** What's your telephone number?
6. **(Go) jyūsho wa doko desu ka.** Where is your address?
7. **Netsu wa nan-do desu ka.** What is your temperature?
8. **Netsu wa nan-do gurai desu ka.** Approximately how high is your fever?
9. **Gairai-kanjya wa dare desu ka.** Who is the outpatient?
10. **Dō itashi-mashite.** You're welcome. Don't mention it.

Key Sentences (CD 2-4)

Listen to the CD and repeat the sentences.

1. **Onamae wa nan desu ka.** What is your name?
2. **Keitai-denwa-bangō wa nan desu ka.** What is your cell phone number?
3. **Netsu ga arimasu ka.** Do you have a fever?
4. **Hyaku do gurai desu.** It's about 100 degrees.
5. **Denwa-bangō wa XXX desu.** The telephone number is XXX.

Additional Words

netsu fever
gurai about
kashi Fahrenheit
dansei male
kensa examination/exam/test
tabe-masu eat
negai-masu wish

do degree
sesshi centigrade
doko where
josei female
shigoto job/work
nomi-masu drink

Language Notes

1. List of numbers (**kazu** 1–99):

0 **zero, rei**	10 **jyū**	20 **ni jyū**
1 **ichi**	11 **jyū ichi**	30 **san jyū**
2 **ni**	12 **jyū ni**	40 **yon jyū**
3 **san**	13 **jyū san**	50 **go jyū**
4 **yon, shi**	14 **jyū yon, jyū shi**	60 **roku jyū**
5 **go**	15 **jyū go**	70 **shichi jyū, nana jyū**
6 **roku**	16 **jyū roku**	80 **hachi jyū**
7 **shichi, nana**	17 **jyū shichi, jyū nana**	90 **kyū jyū**
8 **hachi**	18 **jyū hachi**	95 **kyū jyū go**
9 **kyū**	19 **jyū kyū**	99 **kyū jyū kyū**

2. List of numbers (**kazu** 100–90,000):

100	**hyaku**	1,000	**sen**	10,000	**ichi man**
200	**ni hyaku**	2,000	**ni sen**	20,000	**ni man**
300	**san byaku**	3,000	**san zen**	30,000	**san man**
400	**yon hyaku**	4,000	**yon sen**	40,000	**yon man**
500	**go hyaku**	5,000	**go sen**	50,000	**go man**
600	**ro ppyaku**	6,000	**roku sen**	60,000	**roku man**
700	**nana hyaku**	7,000	**nana sen**	70,000	**nana man**
800	**ha ppyaku**	8,000	**ha ssen**	80,000	**hachi man**
900	**kyū hyaku**	9,000	**kyū sen**	90,000	**kyū man**

   When saying numbers in Japanese, there are several irregularities:

   300 (**san byaku**); 600 (**ro ppyaku**); 800 (**ha ppyaku**)
   3,000 (**san zen**); 8,000 (**ha ssen**)

   Also, 10 (**jyū**), 100 (**hyaku**), and 1,000 (**sen**) are not said as *ichi-jyū, *ichi-hyaku, and *ichi-sen, but ichi is used starting with 10,000 (**ichi-man**).

3. List of numbers (**kazu** 100,000–100,000,000):

100,000 **jyū man**	1,000,000 **hyaku man**	10,000,000 **i ssen man**
200,000 **ni jyū man**	2,000,000 **ni hyaku man**	20,000,000 **ni sen man**
300,000 **san jyū man**	3,000,000 **san byaku man**	30,000,000 **san zen man**
400,000 **yon jyū man**	4,000,000 **yon hyaku man**	40,000,000 **yon sen man**
500,000 **go jyū man**	5,000,000 **go hyaku man**	50,000,000 **go sen man**
600,000 **roku jyū man**	6,000,000 **ro ppyaku man**	60,000,000 **roku sen man**
700,000 **nana jyū man**	7,000,000 **nana hyaku man**	70,000,000 **nana sen man**
800,000 **hachi jyū man**	8,000,000 **ha ppyaku man**	80,000,000 **ha ssen man**
900,000 **kyū jyū man**	9,000,000 **kyū hyaku man**	90,000,000 **kyū sen man**

The following are also irregular forms:

> 3,000,000 (**san byaku man**); 6,000,000 (**ro ppyaku man**); 8,000,000 (**ha ppyaku man**); 10,000,000 (**i ssen man**); 30,000,000 (**san zen man**); 80,000,000 (**ha ssen man**)

In addition to the above, 100,000,000 is **ichi-oku**.

4. How to count and pronounce Japanese numbers:

11 = 10 + 1 **jyū + ichi**	126 = 100 + 20 + 6 **hyaku + ni jyū + roku**
12 = 10 + 2 **jyū + ni**	203 = (2 x100) + 3 **ni x hyaku + san**
13 = 10 + 3 **jyū + san**	350 = (3 x100) + (5x10) **san byaku + go jyū**
14 = 10 + 4 **jyū + yon**	809 = 8 x 100 + 9 **ha ppyaku + kyū**
15 = 10 + 5 **jyū + go**	1,957 = 1,000 + (9 x100) + (5 x 10) + 7
19 = 10 + 9 **jyū + kyū**	**sen + kyū hyaku + go jyū + nana**
20 = 2 x 10 **ni x jyū**	3,333 = (3 x1,000) + (3 x100) + (3 x10) + 3
21 = 2 x 10 + 1 **ni x jyū + ichi**	**san zen + san byaku + san jyū + san**
30 = 3 x 10 **san x jyū**	8,247 = (8 x1,000) + (2 x100) + (4 x10) + 7
90 = 9 x10 **kyū x jyū**	**ha ssen + ni hyaku + yon jyū + nana**
99 = 9 x 10 + 9 **kyū x jyū + kyū**	

The several irregular forms are pronounced as follows:

> 347 = **san-byaku yon-jyū-nana**
> 689 = **ro-ppyaku hachi-jyū-kyū**
> 826 = **ha-ppyaku ni-jyū-roku**
>
> 3,000 (**san zen**); 8,000 (**ha ssen**)
> 3,794 = **san-zen nana-yaku-kyū-jyū-yon**
> 8,380 = **ha-ssen san-byaku-hachi-jyū**

Note: Japanese terms for calculations are **keisan** and **tasu** (addition), **hiku** (subtraction), **kakeru** (multiplication), **waru** (division), and **wa** (equals).

$$1 + 1 = 2$$ **(Ichi tasu ichi wa ni desu.)**
$$5 - 1 = 4$$ **(Go niku ichi wa yon desu.)**
$$6 \times 7 = 42$$ **(Roku kakeru nana wa yon-jyū-ni desu.)**
$$8 \div 2 = 4$$ **(Hachi waru ni wa yon desu.)**

5. A Comparative Chart for Fahrenheit and Centigrade

°F	96	97	98	99	100	101	102	103	104	105	106	107	108
°C	35.5	36.1	36.6	37.2	37.7	38.3	38.8	39.4	40.0	40.5	41.1	41.6	42.2

In Japan, only the Celsius (centigrade) system is used to measure temperature. To specify which system you are using, you can say **sesshi** (centigrade) or **kashi** (Fahrenheit). For example, 37.2°C (**sesshi san jyū nana ten ni do**) is equal to 96°F (**kashi kyū jyū roku do**). [Fahrenheit = (°C x 1.8) + 32. Centigrade = (°F - 32)/1.8] To indicate the decimal point when giving the temperature, the Japanese word **ten** is equivalent to the English *point*.

> **kashi** 98.2 (**kyū jyū hachi ten ni-do**)
> **kashi** 100.5 (**hyaku ten go-do**)
> **sesshi** 39.3 (**san jyū kyū ten san-do**)
> **sesshi** 40.2 (**yon jyū ten ni-do**)

Japanese has another way of expressing the temperature: another term for degree is **do**, and the decimal point is **bu**.

> 37.2 °C = (**sesshi san jyū nana ten ni do**)
> 37.2 °C = (**sesshi san jyū nana do ni bu**)

6. The question **Onamae wa** does not always end in **ka**. In formal Japanese, questions do end in **ka**, but an informal style of spoken question often omits **nan desu ka/arimasu ka**. **Onamae wa nan desu ka** becomes **Onamae wa**. The intonation is on **wa**.

> **Onamae wa (nan desu ka).**   What's your name?
> **Go-jyūsho wa (nan desu ka).**   What's your address?
> **Keitai-denwa-bangō wa (nan desu ka).** What's your cell phone number?
> **Hoken wa (arimasu ka).**   Do you have insurance?

7. The honorific prefix **o-** or **go-** is used to refer to someone else's name, address, age, and so on. Remember to drop these prefixes when speaking about your own name, address, age, and so on, or about family members or colleagues.

(Anata no) Onamae wa nan desu ka.	What is your name?
(Watakushi no) Namae wa Suzuki desu.	My name is Suzuki.
(Anata no) Gojyūsho wa doko desu ka.	Where is your address?
(Watakushi no) Jyūsho wa Honorure desu.	My address is Honolulu.

8. When saying telephone numbers in Japanese, the hyphenated part of the number is read as **no**.

201-592-1316	**ni zero ichi no go kyū ni no ichi san ichi roku desu.**
808-594-2557	**hachi zero hachi no go kyū yon no ni go go nana desu.**

9. Car insurance is called **jidōsha hoken**. There are two expressions for "car": **kuruma** (car) and **jidōsha** (automobile). When you use the word **kuruma** in speaking about car insurance, you must use the particle **no** (of) as in **kuruma no hoken**.

jidōsha hoken	automobile insurance
kuruma no hoken	car insurance

10. A company is called a **kaisha**. However, an insurance company is pronounced **hoken gaisha**. **Kaisha** changes to **gaisha** when describing a profession.

hoken gaisha	insurance company
ryokō gaisha	travel company (travel agency)
honyaku gaisha	translation company
denwa gaisha	telephone company

Language Roots

The suffix -**sha**/-**jya** (者) indicates a person.

ryokō-sha	traveler
kan-jya	patient
gairi-kan-jya	outpatient

There are many homonyms in Japanese. For example, -**sha** (車) indicates a car, and -**sha** (社) indicates a company. The following are examples of some words using the above homonyms.

kyūkyū-sha	ambulance
jidō-sha	automobile
kai-sha	company
hoken-gai-sha	insurance company

The word **ban** (番) means "number" in a series and is used as either a prefix or a suffix.

yoyaku-ban-gō   reservation number
denwa ban-gō   telephone number
jun-ban   sequential order/number

Culture Notes

Countries with the Highest Life Expectancy at Birth for 2005–2010 and 2045–2050

2005–2010	2045–2050
1. Japan 82.7	1. Japan 87.2
2. China, Hong Kong SAR 82.2	2. China, Hong Kong SAR 86.8
3. Switzerland 81.8	3. Switzerland 86.6
4. Iceland 81.8	4. Australia 86.2
5. Australia 81.5	5. France 86.0
6. France 81.2	6. Iceland 86.0
7. Italy 81.2	7. China, Macao SAR 85.7
8. Sweden 80.9	8. Spain 85.5
9. Spain 80.9	9. Italy 85.4
10. Israel 80.7	10. Israel 85.4

SOURCE: Population Division of the Department of Economic and Social Affairs of the United Nations Secretariat (2009)

According to the World Health Organization (WHO), life expectancy at birth for Japanese males was 76 years in 1990, 78 in 2000, and 79 in 2007, and for females was 82 years in 1990, 85 in 2000, and 86 in 2007.

Lucky and unlucky numbers in Japanese culture

The number eight is considered lucky because of its kanji shape:

8 (**hachi** 八 has an open base, which make for a stable standing figure.)

Two numbers are considered unlucky because of their Japanese pronunciations:

4 (**shi** 死 means death)
9 (**ku** 苦 means suffering)

Comprehension

Answer the following questions.

1. Which of the following does NOT belong with the others?
    a. **byōin**   b. **i-in**
    c. **bangō**   d. **hoken-jyo**

2. Which of the following could be used as a translation for "**Yoyaku ga arimasu ka**"?
    a. How are you?   b. Do you have an appointment?
    c. What's your name?   d. How do you do?

3. Which of the following best completes the sentence below?
    Keitai-bangō wa (   ) desu ka.
    a. **itsu**   b. **doko**
    c. **nan**   d. **dare**

4. Which statement is TRUE?
    a. Japanese frequently use their family name only.
    b. Japanese culture prizes the number 4.
    c. In Japanese, **hoken-jyo** means "insurance."
    d. In Japanese, **byōki** means "hospital."

5. With which sentence are you asking for a telephone number?
    a. **(O)tanjyōbi wa itsu desu ka.**
    b. **(O)denwa bangō wa nan desu ka.**
    c. **(Go)jyusho wa doko desu ka.**
    d. **(O)toshi wa ikutsu desu ka.**

Select the appropriate Japanese pronunciation.

6. Number 4
    a. **yon**   b. **hachi**
    c. **go**   d. **ni**

7. Number 9
    a. **roku**   b. **kyū**
    c. **shi**   d. **san**

8. Number 2
   a. **go**   b. **ni**
   c. **ichi**   d. **nana**

9. Number 65
   a. **ni jyū go**   b. **roku jyū go**
   c. **san jyū go**   d. **go jyū go**

10. Number 91
    a. **san-jyū**   b. **nana jyū ichi**
    c. **kyū jyū ichi**   d. **hachi jyū ichi**

Select the correct meaning in Japanese.

---

11. Car insurance
    a. **shōgai hoken**   b. **jidōsha koken**   c. **seimei hoken**

12. General hospital
    a. **kodomo byōin**   b. **sōgō byōin**   c. **hoken-jyo**

13. Telephone number
    a. **hoken bangō**   b. **uketsuke bangō**   c. **denwa bangō**

Practice

Respond to the following in Japanese using the cues that have been provided.

---

1. Asking for a patient's information.
    (Healthcare professional)   (Patient)
    1. _____ (name)   **Suzuki Kenji desu.**
    2. _____ (temperature)   **99 do desu.**
    3. _____ (telephone number)   **XXX**
    4. _____ (address)   **New York desu.**
    5. _____ (insurance company)   **XXX hoken desu.**
    6. _____ (type of insurance)   **Ryokō-sha hoken desu.**
    7. _____ (sex)   **Otoko desu.**
    8. _____ (nationality)   **Nihon desu.**

2. Reading telephone numbers. Say the telephone number in Japanese.
    (Patient's number)
    1. **Denwa-bangō wa** 802-763-4930 **desu.** _____
    2. **Denwa-bangō wa** 808-592-0451 **desu.** _____
    3. **Denwa-bangō wa** 201-469-3700 **desu.** _____

3. Understanding numbers and temperatures. Say the temperature in Japanese.
    (Healthcare professionals)   (Patient's temperature)
    1. **Netsu wa nan-do desu ka.** (98°F)   _____
    2. **Netsu wa nan-do gurai desu ka.** (About 99°F)   _____
    3. **Netsu wa nan-do desu ka.** (39.3°C)   _____
    4. **Ikutsu desu ka.** (62)   _____
    5. **Ikutsu desu ka.** (85)   _____

4. Dialogue comprehension. Based on the dialogue at the beginning of the chapter, answer the following.
    1. **Kanjya wa dare desu ka.** _____
    2. **Denwa-bangō wa nan-ban desu ka.** _____
    3. **Kyō wa dō shimashita ka.** _____
    4. **Netsu wa nan-do gurai desu ka.** _____
    5. **Suzuki-san wa hoken ga arimasu ka.** _____

5. Free response questions.
    (Questions)   (Answers)
    1. **Onamae wa nan desu ka.** _____
    2. **Denwa-bangō wa nan ban desu ka.** _____
    3. **Go-jyū-sho wa doko desu ka.** _____
    4. **Kokuseki wa nan desu ka.** _____
    5. **Arigatō gozai-mashita.** _____

Exercises

1. What are the meanings of the following words?
    A. **Kenkō hoken** _____
    B. **Hoken-jyo** _____
    C. **Denwa-bangō** _____
    D. **Sogō-byōin** _____
    E. **Kyūkyū-sha** _____

2. Say the following expressions in Japanese.
   A. Do you have an appointment? _____
   B. Do you have a fever? _____
   C. Do you have insurance? _____
   D. What is your name? _____
   E. What's your telephone number? _____
   F. What is your address? _____
   G. What is your temperature? _____
   H. You're welcome. _____

3. What do the following expressions mean?
   A. **Hoken ga arimasu ka.** _____
   B. **Onamae wa nan desu ka.** _____
   C. **Denwa-bangō wa nan desu ka.** _____
   D. **(Go) jyūsho wa doko desu ka.** _____
   E. **Netsu wa nan-do gurai desu ka.** _____

4. Read the following telephone numbers.
   A. 807-594-3650 _____
   B. 201-857-2089 _____
   C. 1-800-201-986-9713 _____

5. Read the following temperatures.
   A. **Kashi 97 do desu.** (97°F) _____
   B. **Sesshi 37.2 do desu.** (37.2°C) _____
   C. **Kashi 100 do desu.** (100°F) _____
   D. **Sesshi 38.7 do desu.** (38.7°C) _____
   E. **Kashi 102 do desu.** (102°F) _____

Appointment II
(Yoyaku)

Basic Vocabulary (CD 3-1)

Listen to the CD and repeat the vocabulary.

1.	date of birth	**seinen gappi**	生年月日
2.	medical examination	**shinsatsu**	診察
3.	consultation	**sōdan**	相談
4.	re-examination	**sai-kensa/sai-shin**	再検査/再診
5.	physical (examination)	**kenkō-shindan**	健康診断
6.	doctor's note	**shindan-sho**	診断書
7.	referral	**shōkai-jyō**	紹介状
8.	referrer/recommender	**shōkai-sha**	紹介者
9.	injured/wounded person	**fushō-sha**	負傷者
10.	visitor	**menkai-nin**	面会人
11.	years old (suffix)	**-sai**	ー才
12.	cancel	**torikeshi**	取り消し
13.	year	**nen**	年
14.	month (suffix)	**-gatsu**	月
15.	day (suffix)	**-nichi**	日
16.	time	**ji(kan)**	時(間)
17.	hour (suffix)	**-ji**	時
18.	minute (suffix)	**-fun/pun**	分
19.	second (suffix)	**-byō**	秒
20.	a.m.	**gozen(chū)**	午前(中)
21.	p.m.	**gogo**	午後
22.	now	**ima**	今
23.	today	**kyō**	今日
24.	tomorrow	**ashita**	明日
25.	the day after tomorrow	**asatte**	明後日
26.	the third day after today	**shi-asatte**	明明後日
27.	yesterday	**kinō**	昨日
28.	the day before yesterday	**ototoi**	一昨日
29.	convenience/condition/situation	**tsugō**	都合
30.	condition	**chōshi**	調子

Dialogue (CD 3-2)

Listen to the CD and repeat the dialogue.

At the Reception Desk: Confirming an appointment

Sandra (receptionist): **Shoshin desu ka. Onamae wa nan desu ka.**
Is this your first visit? What is your name?

Mr. Suzuki (patient): **(Namae wa) Suzuki Kenji desu.**
My name is Suzuki Kenji.

Sandra: **Shōkai-sha wa imasu ka.**
Did someone refer you?

Mr. Suzuki: **Hai, hoken-jyo no Kim-sensei desu.**
Yes, Dr. Kim at the health center recommended me.

Sandra: **Yoyaku wa itsu ga ii desu ka.**
When do you want to make an appointment?

Mr. Suzuki: **Ashita ga ii desu.**
Tomorrow is good for me.

Gozen-chū wa aite imasu ka.
Do you have an opening in the morning?

Sandra: **Iie, gozen wa yoyaku de ippai desu.**
No, we are fully booked with appointments in the morning.

Gogo 3-ji-han wa dō desu ka.
How about 3:30 p.m.?

Mr. Suzuki: **Hai, kekko desu. 3 ji-han ni onegai shimasu.**
Yes, that's fine. Please make it at 3:30.

Sandra: **Ashita no gogo 3 ji han ni kite kudasai.**
Then please come tomorrow at 3:30 p.m.

Omachi-shite-imasu.
We will be waiting for you.

Grammar

1. The expression **ii desu ka**

The expression **ii desu ka** asks for a preference or choice. The literal meanings of **ii** are "good, excellence, convenience." The formal form of **ii** is **yoi**. Japanese use **ii** in ordinary conversation, but **yoi desu ka** is used for formal situations.

Nan-ji ga ii desu ka.	What time do you like?
Nan-nichi ga ii desu ka.	What day do you prefer?
Itsu ga ii desu ka.	When would you like (to be seen)?
Ashita ga yoi desu ka.	Would you like tomorrow?
Gozen ga ii desu ka, gogo ga ii desu ka.	Do you prefer a.m. or p.m.?

2. The particle ni

The particle **ni** (at) is used to indicate a specific point in time. Only time words that are specific, for example a date or number (October 15, seven o'clock) take the particle **ni**. Words indicating relative time (today, tomorrow, everyday, morning, afternoon, etc.) do not take **ni** and are indicated with X in the following examples.

Gozen ku-ji ni onegai shimasu.	I would like (to be seen at) nine a.m.
Gogo roku-ji ni onegai shimasu.	I prefer (to be seen at) six p.m.
Kyō [X] onegai shimasu.	I prefer today.
Gogo [X] aite imasu.	It's open in the afternoon.
Ashita [X] yoyaku o onegai shimasu.	Please make the appointment tomorrow.

3. The construction PLACE + ni

The construction PLACE/LOCATION plus the PARTICLE **ni** conveys the meaning of "to the place, toward the place."

Byōin ni ikimasu.	I'm going to the hospital.
Kanjya-san ga uketsuke ni kimashita.	The patient came to the reception desk.
Ashita shinsatsu ni ikimasu.	I will go to the medical examination tomorrow.
Ima uchi ni kaerimasu.	Now I am going home.

4. The particle de

The particle **de** is used to indicate a causal reason and translates as "because of, due to."

Kinkyū-byōin wa fushō-sha de ippai desu.
The emergency hospital is fully occupied with (*lit.*, due to) injured people.

Netsu de chōshi ga warui desu ka.
Are you feeling bad because of a fever?

Shigoto no tsugō de yoyaku no torikeshi o onegai shimasu.
I would like to cancel my appointment because of my work (condition).

The particle **de** also indicates a means, method, or instrument and translates as "by, with, in."

> **Kyūkyū-sha de byōin ni ikimasu ka.**
> Are you going to the hospital by ambulance?

> **Denwa de yoyaku o shimasu.**
> I am making an appointment by telephone.

> **Nihon-go de hanashimasu.**
> I will speak in Japanese.

5. The interrogative **nan de**

The interrogative **nan de** is used to ask the reason or means for something and translates as "why" or "how."

Nan de byōin ni kimashita ka.	Why did you come to the hospital? (asking the reason)
Nan de kensa o shimasu ka.	Why am I having this test?
Nan de byōin ni kimashita ka.	How did you come to the hospital? (asking the means)

6. The verb **arimasu/imasu**

The verb **arimasu** or **imasu** is used at the end of a sentence to convey the meaning "there is/are." **Arimasu** (from the stem verb **aru**) is used for in-animate subjects or abstract nouns such as body parts, plants, time, foods, books, telephones, problems, causes, etc. In English, body parts and plants are considered living, but for the Japanese language they are non-animate. The polite form of **arimasu** is **gozaimasu**. **Imasu** (from the stem verb **iru**) is used for living or animate beings such as people, dogs, fish, birds, and so on. The polite form of **imasu** is **irasshai-masu**. We will study what a stem verb (or dictionary form) is in Lesson 13.

Netsu ga arimasu.	I/You have a fever.
Shōkai-jyō ga arimasu.	I have a referral.
Jikan ga arimasu.	I have time.
Okane ga airmasu.	I have money.
Kurejito-kādo ga gozaimasu ka.	Do you have credit card?
Suzuki-san ga imasu.	There is Mr. Suzuki
Shōkai-sha ga imasu ka.	Who referred you? (*lit.*, Do you have a referrer?)
Menkai-nin ga imasu.	There is a visitor.
Go-kazoku ga irasshai-masu ka.	Do you have family? (polite expression)

7. The expressions **dō-desu ka** and **ikaga-desu ka**

The expression **dō-desu ka** means "how about" and is commonly used to ask someone how things are going. **Ikaga-desu ka** (Would you like . . . ?), which sounds more polite, is also used.

4 ji wa dō-desu ka.	How about 4 o'clock?
4 ji wa ikaga-desu ka.	Would you like it at 4 o'clock?
Netsu wa dō-desu ka.	How is your fever?
Omizu wa ikaga-desu ka.	Would you like to have water?
Chōshi wa ikaga-desu ka.	What is your condition? (polite form)
Sōdan wa ikaga-desu ka.	Would you like to have consultation?
Muryō-sōdan wa dō-desu ka.	How about free consultation?

8. The present/future tense verb ending **-masu** and past tense verb ending **-mashita**

Japanese verbs in the present/future tense end with **-masu**. Verbs in the past tense end with **-mashita**. No distinction is made between the present and future tenses in verb endings, and the Japanese will judge which sense is meant from the context of a statement. This reflects a Japanese cultural perception that the present is equal to the future. Living fully in the present moment is considered to equal to living in the future.

Netsu ga ari-masu.	I/you have a fever.
Netsu ga ari-mashita.	I/you had a fever.
Jikan ga ari-masu ka.	Do you have the time?
Jikan ga ari-mashita ka.	Did you have the time?
Kanjya ga i-masu.	There is a patient.
Kanjya ga i-mashita.	There was a patient.
Menkai-nin ga i-masu ka.	Do you have a visitor?
Menkai-nin ga i-mashita ka.	Did you have a visitor?

9. The expression **-te kudasai**

Japanese verbs ending with **-te** are called **te**-form verbs. The construction **te**-FORM VERB + **kudasai** expresses a request. For example, **kite kudasai** means "Please come."

Yoyaku o shite kudasai.	Please make an appointment.
Denwa o kakete kudasai.	Please call on the telephone.
Shinsatsu o shite kudasai.	Please have a medical examination.
Kenkō-shindan ukete kudasai.	Please have a physical examination.
Kite kudasai.	Please come.

To make the **te**-form, the following verbs drop the -**masu** ending and add -**te**.

ENGLISH	-MASU FORM	TE-FROM
to do/play	shi-masu	shi-te
to come, to wear clothes	ki-masu	ki-te
to see/look/watch/examine/check up	mi-masu	mi-te
to show	mise-masu	mise-te
to speak	hanashi-masu	hanashi-te
to eat	tabe-masu	tabe-te
to lend	kashi-masu	kashi-te
to turn on	tsuke-masu	tsuke-te
to turn off/erase	keshi-masu	keshi-te
to wake-up/rise-up	oki-masu	oki-te
to push	oshi-masu	oshi-te
to teach	oshie-masu	oshie-te
to open (mouth, eye, door, window, hole)	ake-masu	ake-te
to call (phone)	kake-masu	kake-te
to close (door, window)	shime-masu	shime-te
to close (mouth, eye, ear, hand, legs, book, hole)	toji-masu	toji-te
to stop/park	tome-masu	tome-te
to sleep/lie down	ne-masu	ne-te
to receive	uke-masu	uke-te

Note: The **te**-form by itself is used to express an informal request, command, and order. For example: **mite** (see me), **misete** (show me), **oshiete** (tell me), **okite** (wake up/rise up), **nete** (sleep/lie down), etc.

10. The construction **(o) shite imasu** conveys the present progressive tense.

The **te**-form used with **imasu** expresses the present progressive tense. For example, the sentence **Omachi-shite imasu** means "(We) are waiting (for you)."

Byōki o kensa shite imasu.	I am conducting an examination. (*lit.*, I am examining an illness.)
Byōin wa aite imasu.	The hospital is open.
Yoyaku wa aite imasu.	There is an opening in the reservations.

Useful Expressions (CD 3-3)

Listen to the CD and repeat the sentences.

1. **Kenkō-shindan desu ka.** Is this about your physical?
2. **Tsugō ga warui(n) desu.** That's not a good time for me.
3. **Shōkai-sha no (o)namae wa.** What's the name of the refered person?
4. **Seibetsu wa nan desu ka.** What is your sex?
5. **Itsu ga ii desu ka.** When is the best time for you?
6. **Gozen 9-ji wa ikaga desu ka.** Would you like it for nine o'clock?
7. **Gogo 2-ji ni omachi-shite imasu.** We will be waiting for you at 2 p.m.
8. **Gozen 10-ji ni kite kudasai.** Please come at 10 a.m.
9. **Nan-sai desu ka.** How old are you?
10. **Seinen-gappi wa itsu desu ka.** What is your date of birth?

Key sentences (CD 3-4)

Listen to the CD and repeat the sentences.

1. **Nan-ji ga ii desu ka.** What time would you like to come?
2. **Nan-sai desu ka.** How old are you?
3. **Seinen-gappi o oshiete kudasai.** Please tell me your date of birth.
4. **Itsu ga ii desu ka.** When is the best time for you?
5. **Gogo 3-ji ni omachi-shite imasu.** We will be waiting for you at 3 p.m.

Additional Words

matsu/machimasu wait
ippai full
warui bad
kekkō fine/sufficient/nice/wonderful
kekka result
saki-ototoi three days ago
muryō-sōdan free consulation
uchi home

kakeru/kakemasu call
ii/yoi good
itsu when
dō how about
kibun feeling
han half/30 minutes
okane money
ie house

Language Notes

1. Understanding age
   -sai is a suffix for indicating age. Since nouns in Japanese have no plural, Japanese uses counters in sentences. "Twenty years old" is **nijyu-ssai** or **hatachi** in Japanese.

i-ssai	1 year old	**roku-sai**	6 years old	**jyu i-ssai**	11 years old
ni-sai	2 years old	**nana-sai**	7 years old	**jyu ni-sai**	12 years old
san-sai	3 years old	**ha-ssai**	8 years old	**hatachi**	20 years old
yon-sai	4 years old	**kyū-sai**	9 years old	**ni jyu ssai**	20 years old
go-sai	5 years old	**jyu-ssai**	10 years old	**ni jyu i-ssai**	21 years old

The following are some examples of counters for: cylindrical objects (bottles, pens, belts, syringes, ropes, etc), floors, and animals.

NUMBER	CYLINDRICAL OBJECTS (PON/BON)	FLOORS (KAI/GAI)	ANIMAL (HIKI/BIKI)
1	i ppon	i kkai	i piki
2	ni hon	ni kai	ni hiki
3	san bon	san gai	san biki
4	yon hon	yon kai	yon hiki
5	go hon	go kai	go hiki
6	ro pon	ro kai	ro piki
7	nana hon	nana kai	nana hiki
8	ha pon	ha kai	ha piki
9	kyū hon	kyū kai	kyū hiki
10	jyū pon	jyū kai	jyū piki

Chūsha-ki ga san-bon arimasu.	There are three syringes.
Kanjya wa san-gai ni imasu.	The patients are staying on the third floor.
Inu ga san-biki imasu.	There are three dogs.

2. Understanding years

The word for "year" in Japanese is **nen**. Place **nen** after the number. There are three ways to ask someone's birthdate.

Tanjyō-bi wa itsu desu ka.	When is your birthday?
Seinen-gappi wa itsu desu ka.	What is your date of birth?

Tanjyō-bi wa nan-nen, nan-gatsu, nan-nichi desu ka.
What is the year, month, and date of your birth?

1952	**Sen kyū-hyaku go-jyū ni nen desu.**
1993	**Sen kyū-hyaku kyū-jyū san nen desu.**
2010	**Ni sen jyū nen desu.**

3. Understanding months
   For the names of the months, the suffix **gatsu** is affixed to numbers from one to twelve except for the irregular numbers four (**shi**) and nine (**ku**).

ichi gatsu	January	**shichi gatsu**	July
ni gatsu	February	**hachi gatsu**	August
san gatsu	March	**ku gatsu**	September
shi gatsu	April	**jyū gatsu**	October
go gatsu	May	**jyū-ichi gatsu**	November
roku gatsu	June	**jyū-ni gatsu**	December

4. Understanding days
   To say the date or count days, **nichi** or **-ka** is placed after the number, except for the first ten days of the month, which use **-tachi** for the first day and **-ka** or **-kka** for the rest.

tsui-tachi	first day	**nano-ka**	seventh day
futsu-ka	second day	**yō-ka**	eighth day
mi-kka	third day	**koko-no-ka**	ninth day
yo-kka	fourth day	**tō-ka**	tenth day
itsu-ka	fifth day	**jyū ichi nichi**	eleventh day
mui-ka	six day	**jyū ni nichi**	twelfth day

   The days after the tenth use the suffix **-nichi** except:

jyū-yo-kka	fourteenth day
hatsu-ka	twentieth day
ni-jyū-yo-kka	twenty-fourth day

   Japanese has two counting systems: the Sino-Japanese number system, as in **ichi**, **ni**, **san**, **yon**, **go**, etc., as we studied in Lesson 2; and, for the numbers 1 to 10, the Japanese number system. After 10, the Japanese system uses the Sino-Japanese number system. The following chart shows the traditional Japanese numbers from 1 to 10. The suffix **-tsu** is the counter for objects of indefinite shape; **-ri/-nin** is used for counting persons; and **-tsuki/-ka-getsu** is used for duration of months.

NUMBER	TRADITIONAL	NUMBER (-TSU)	PERSON (RI/NIN)	MONTH (-TSUKI/-KA-GETSU)
1	**hito**	**hito-tsu**	**hito-ri**	**hito-tsuki**
2	**futa**	**futa-tsu**	**futa-ri**	**futa-tsuki**
3	**mi**	**mi-ttsu**	**san-nin**	**san-ka-getsu**

NUMBER	TRADITIONAL	NUMBER (-TSU)	PERSON (RI/NIN)	MONTH (-TSUKI/-KA-GETSU)
4	yo	yo-ttsu	yo-nin	yon-ka-getsu
5	itsu	itsu-tsu	go-nin	go-ka-getsu
6	mu	mu-ttsu	roku-nin	ro-kka-getsu
7	nana	nana-tsu	nana-nin	nana-ka-getsu
8	ya	ya-ttsu	hachi-nin	hachi-ka-getsu
9	koko	koko no tsu	kyū-nin	kyū-ka-getsu
10	tō	tō	jyū-nin	jyū-kka-getsu

Note: The numbers 9 and 10 are irregular. The counter for person changes from **-ri** to **-nin** beginning with number 3, and at that point uses the regular number system as well.

5. Understanding the time/hour
   The counter **-ji** is used for hour and time, with the numbers for 4 o'clock and 9 o'clock being irregular. **Ima nan-ji desu ka** (What time is it now?) is used to ask the time.

ichi ji	1 o'clock	**shichi ji**	7 o'clock
ni ji	2 o'clock	**hachi ji**	8 o'clock
san ji	3 o'clock	**ku ji**	9 o'clock
yo ji	4 o'clock	**jyū ji**	10 o'clock
go ji	5 o'clock	**jyū-ichi ji**	11 o'clock
roku ji	6 o'clock	**jyū-ni ji**	12 o'clock

6. Understanding time/minutes
   The counters **-fun** and **-pun** is used for minutes; **-han** (half) is used for the half-hour; and **san-jyu-ppun** is used for 30 minutes.

i ppun	1 minute	**jyū i ppun**	11 minutes
ni fun	2 minutes	**jyū ni fun**	12 minutes
san pun	3 minutes	**jyū san pun**	13 minutes
yon pun	4 minutes	**jyū yon pun**	14 minutes
go fun	5 minutes	**jyū go fun**	15 minutes
ro ppun	6 minutes	**san jyu ppun**	30 minutes
nana fun	7 minutes	**han**	30 minutes
ha ppun	8 minutes	**yon jyū go fun**	45 minutes
kyū fun	9 minutes	**go jyū ha ppun**	58 minutes
jyu ppun	10 minutes	**roku jyu ppun**	60 minutes

7. Understanding seconds
The Japanese expression for seconds is **byō**, and it is placed after the number as a suffix. There is no irregular form for seconds.

ichi byō	1 second	**kyū byō**	9 seconds
ni byō	2 seconds	**jyū-byō**	10 seconds
san byō	3 seconds	**jyū-ichi byō**	11 seconds
yon byō	4 seconds	**jyū-ni byō**	12 seconds
go byō	5 seconds	**san-jyū byō**	30 seconds
roku byō	6 seconds	**yon-jyū-go byō**	45 seconds
nana byō	7 seconds	**roku-jyū byō**	60 seconds
hachi byō	8 seconds		

8. Time expressions
The following words indicate relative times. These general expressions for time don't require the particle **ni** (at) in sentences.

saki ototoi	three days ago
ototoi	the day before yesterday
kinō	yesterday
kyō	today
ima	now
ashita	tomorrow
asatte	day after tomorrow
shi-asatte	three days from now
mai-nichi	every day

Ashita (x) **kensa ga arimasu.**	There is an examination tomorrow.
Kinō (x) **kensa o shimashita.**	I conducted an examination yesterday.
Ima (x) **kekka o mimasu.**	I will look at the results now.

However, in specific time expressions the particle **ni** (at) is required.

Gogo 2 ji ni kensa o shimasu.	You have an examination at two p.m.
Ashita no 10 ji ni kite kudasai.	Please come at ten tomorrow.

Language Roots

The suffix -**in** (院) indicates an institution, especially a government office, school, hospital, or institute of higher learning.

byō-in	hospital
i-in	clinic

nyū-in	hospitalized/admitted to a hospital
daigaku-in	graduate school

The word -**ki** (気) indicates feelings, mood, spirit, mind, and heart.

ki-mochi	feeling
ki-bun	feeling/mood (formal)
byō-ki	illness (*lit.*, illness feelings)
gen-ki	healthy (*lit.*, original feelings)
tan-ki	short temper
kachi-ki	unyielding sprit
yowa-ki	faint-hearted

Culture Notes

Yaku-doshi is the bad luck year for the Japanese.

The age of 33 for a woman and 42 for a man are called **yaku-doshi** ("bad luck year"). This may have to do with the physical changes in a woman's or man's life. During that year, most Japanese visit a Shinto shrine or Buddhist temple for **yaku-barai** (a purification rite for the bad luck year).

Appointment system in Japan

Most Japanese hospitals and clinics don't take appointments. Patients are treated on a first-come-first-served basis. For the Japanese, generally speaking, making appointments is not customary.

The first day of the month

The first day of the month is called **tsui-tachi**, which comes from **tsuki-tachi** (literally "moon-stand"), when the new moon appears to be standing up.

Comprehension

Select the appropriate Japanese expression for the following situations.

1. Address a patient who is approaching you:
   a. **Dō shimashita ka.**   b. **Hajime mashite.**   c. **Irasshai mase.**

2. "Do you have an appointment?"
   a. **Yoyaku arimasu ka.**
   b. **Yoyaku ga arimaus ka.**
   c. **Yoyaku o arimasu ka.**

3. Which of the following is an expression for "What time do you like?"
   a. **Nan-ji ga ii desu ka.**
   b. **Nan-ji oshiete kudasai.**
   c. **Nan-ji ni kimasu ka.**

4. Which of the following expressions is WRONG.
   a. **Netsu ga arimasu.**
   b. **Sensei ga arimasu.**
   c. **Uketsuke ga arimasu.**

5. Which of the following is NOT an expression for "How about tomorrow?"
   a. **Ashita wa dō desu ka.**
   b. **Ashita wa ikaga desu ka.**
   c. **Ashita onegai shimasu.**

Select the appropriate Japanese term for the following:

---

6. September:
   a. **Kyū-gatsu**   b. **Ku-gatsu**

7. Nine years old:
   a. **Kyū-sai**   b. **Ku-sai**

8. Nine o'clock:
   a. **Kyū-ji**   b. **Ku-ji**

9. Nine minutes:
   a. **Kyū-fun**   b. **Ku-fun**   c. **Kyū-pun**

10. Ninth day of the month:
    a. **Kyū-nichi**   b. **Ku-nichi**   c. **Kokonoka**

Select the correct meaning in English.

---

11. **Seibetsu**
    a. male   b. female   c. sex

12. **Otona**
    a. adult   b. child   c. mother

13. **Seinen-gappi**
    a. address   b. date of birth   c. certificate

14. **Shinsatsu**
    a. certificate   b. recommendation   c. examination

15. **Kenkō-shindan**
    a. emergency   b. physical examination   c. recommendation

Practice

Respond to the following in Japanese using the cues that have been provided.

1. Making an appointment.
   (Patient)   (Healthcare professional)
   1. **Itsu ga aite imasu ka.**   _____ Which day would you like?
   2. **Raishū wa aite imasu ka.**   _____ No, we are full.
   3. **Asatte wa aite imasu ka.**   _____ Yes, what time would you like?
   4. **Gozen 10-ji wa aite imasu ka.** _____ No, we have only 4 p.m.
   5. **Gogo 4 ji wa aite imasu ka.** _____ Yes, we have an opening.

2. Checking available space.
   (Patient)   (Healthcare professional)
   1. **Ashita wa aite imasu ka.**   _____ Yes, there's an opening.
   2. **Asatte wa aite imasu ka.**   _____ No, it's full.
   3. **Gozen 10-ji wa aite imasu ka.** _____ Yes, there's an opening.
   4. **Gogo 4 ji wa aite imasu ka.** _____ No, it's full.

3. Suggesting available date/time.
   (Healthcare professional)   (Patient)
   1. _____ How about the 9th [day]?   **Hai, kekkō desu.**
   2. _____ How about the day after tomorrow?   **Iie, dame desu.**
   3. _____ How about 11 a.m.?   **Hai, onegai shimasu.**

4. Read the year, month, day and time.
   (Questions)   (Healthcare professional)
   1. 1993   _____
   2. October   _____
   3. 12 o'clock   _____
   4. 35 minutes   _____

5. Dialogue comprehension. Based on the dialogue, answer the following.
   1. **Kanjya-san no namae wa nan desu ka.**

   _____

   2. **Shōkai-sha wa dare desu ka.**

   _____

   3. **Yoyaku wa itsu desu ka.**

   _____

   4. **Yoyaku wa nan-ji desu ka.**

   _____

   5. **Gozen-chū wa aite imashita ka.**

   _____

6. Free response questions.
   (Questions)   (Answers)
   1. **Kyō wa nan-gatsu, nan-nichi desu ka.**   _____
   2. **Tanjyō-bi wa itsu desu ka.**   _____
   3. **Ima nan-sai desu ka.**   _____
   4. **Ashita wa nan-nichi desu ka.**   _____
   5. **Ima nan-ji desu ka.**   _____

Exercises

1. Express the following in Japanese.
   A. Is this your first visit?   _____
   B. How old are you?   _____
   C. Please tell me your birth date.   _____
   D. We will wait for you at 3 p.m.   _____
   E. When is the best time?   _____

2. Read the following days and times in Japanese.
   A. August 2, 1970   _____
   B. April 10, 1968   _____
   C. January 15, 2001   _____
   D. 9:45 p.m.   _____
   E. 4:30 a.m.   _____

3. How do you say the following words in Japanese?
   A. Today   _____
   B. Yesterday   _____
   C. Tomorrow   _____
   D. The day after tomorrow   _____
   E. Every day   _____

4. How do you read the following ages in Japanese?
   A. One year old _____
   B. Three years old _____
   C. Four years old _____
   D. Nine years old _____
   E. Ten years old _____

5. Say the following in Japanese.
   A. Please tell me your sex. _____
   B. Please tell me your address. _____
   C. Please tell me your telephone number. _____
   D. Please come at April 5 at 3 p.m. _____
   E. Please come tomorrow at 9 a.m. _____

LESSON 4

Admissions
(Nyū-in tetsuzuki)

Basic Vocabulary (CD 4-1)

Listen to the CD and repeat the vocabulary.

	English	Romaji	Japanese
1.	admission	**nyū-in**	入院
2.	procedure	**tetsuzuki**	手続き
3.	name (full name)	**shimei**	氏名
4.	birthplace, place of birth	**shussei-chi**	出生地
5.	town or city of origin	**shusshin-chi**	出身地
6.	insurance subscriber's name	**hoken kanyū-sha**	保険加入者
7.	occupation	**shoku-gyō**	職業
8.	religion	**shū-kyō**	宗教
9.	spouse	**haigū-sha**	配偶者
10.	closest relative	**kinshin-sha**	近親者
11.	relation to patient	**kanjya tono kankei**	患者との関係
12.	patient information	**kanjya jyōhō**	患者情報
13.	marital status	**kekkon-reki**	結婚暦
14.	married	**kikon**	既婚
15.	divorced	**rikon**	離婚
16.	single	**dokushin**	独身
17.	medical questionnaire	**monshin-hyō**	問診表
18.	informed consent	**dōi-sho**	同意書
19.	insured person	**hi-hoken-sha**	被保険者
20.	employer	**yatoi-nushi**	雇い主
21.	registration window	**uketsuke mado-guchi**	受付窓口
22.	cashier	**kaikei**	会計
23.	visiting hours	**menkai jikan**	面会時間
24.	company employee	**kaisha-in**	会社員
25.	student	**seito/gakusei**	生徒/学生
26.	baggage	**nimotsu**	荷物
27.	explain	**setsumei**	説明
28.	fill in, complete (a form)	**kinyū**	記入
29.	contact information	**renraku-saki**	連絡先
30.	doctor's fee	**chiryō-dai/hi**	治療代/費

Dialogue (CD 4-2)

Listen to the CD and repeat the dialogue.

At the Registration Desk

| Sandra (receptionist): | **Yoyaku wa shite armasu ka.** |
| | Do you have an appointment? |

Mr. Suzuki (patient): **Hai, gogo 3-ji han ni kochira no byōin ni yoyaku ga shite arimasu.**
Yes, I have a reservation for 3:30 p.m. at this hospital.

Sandra: **Hoken ga arimasu ka.**
Do you have insurance?

Mr. Suzuki: **Hai, arimasu. X hoken-gaisha desu.**
Yes, I do. It's with X insurance company.

Sandra: **Hoken-kanyū-sha wa dare desu ka.**
Who is the insurance subscriber?

Mr. Suzuki: **Watakushi no kanai desu.**
My wife is.

Sandra: **Uketsuke-hyō ni kinyū shita koto ga arimsu ka.**
Have you ever filled out the patient information form?

Mr. Suzuki: **Iie, arimasen.**
No, I have not.

Sandra: **Dewa, kanjya jyōhō o kinyū shite kudasai.**
Then, please fill in your patient information.

Mr. Suzuki: **Hai, kinyū shite okimasu.**
Yes, I will fill in the form.

Grammar

1. The location words **ko**, **so**, **a**, and **do**

The location words **koko** (here/this place), **soko** (there/that place), **asoko** (over there/that place over there), and **doko** (where) are used to refer to locations. **Koko** refers to locations nearest the speaker, **soko** to locations next closest to the speaker, and **asoko** to locations farthest from the speaker. When the speaker is not sure of the relative location, **doko** is used.

Monshin-hyō wa koko desu.	The medical questionnaire is here.
Seito wa soko desu.	The student is there.
Uketsuke madoguchi wa asoko desu.	The registration window is over there.
Shussei-chi wa doko desu ka.	What is your place of birth?

In polite expressions, **ko-chira** (here), **so-chira** (there), **a-chira** (over there), and **do-chira** (where) are used.

Monshin-hyō wa kochira desu.	The medical questionnaire is here.
Seito wa sochira desu.	The student is there.
Uketsuke madoguchi wa achira desu.	The registration window is over there.
Shussei-chi wa dochira desu ka.	What is your place of birth?

2. The particle de

In Lesson 3, we studied the particle **de** used to indicate causality. The particle **de** also indicates a specific location and translates as "at, in, on."

Uketsuke-madoguchi de kanjya-jōhō o kinyū shite kudasai.
Please fill in your patient information at the registration window.

Kaikei de chiryō-hi o haratte kudasai.
Please pay the doctor's fee at the cashier.

Uketsuke de nyūin tetsuzuki no setsumei o shimasu.
I will explain the admissions procedure at registration.

3. The te-form + aru/arimasu

The **te**-form used with **aru/arimasu** expresses a condition that has resulted from an intentional action. It is translated as "has been (done)," or "had been (done)" and is usually used in conjunction with the subject marker **wa** or **ga**. Sometimes, the object maker **o** is used or the subject marker **wa/ga** is omitted because the subject is unknown, obvious, or unimportant.

Yoyaku ga shite arimasu.
I have an appointment. (*lit.*, Appointment has been made.)

Namae ga kinyū shite arimasu.
The name has been filled in.

Nyūin tetsuzuki wa setsumei shite arimasu.
The admissions procedure has been explained.

Kanjya wa shinsatsu shite arimasu.
The patient has been examined.

Kensa wa shite arimasu.
The examination has been conducted.

Gohan wa tabete arimasu.
I had already eaten the meal.

Byōin o shōkai shite arimasu.
The hospital has been (was) referred.

4. The **masu** form and stem verb (dictionary) form of Japanese verbs

The Japanese verb has a number of different forms, including the **masu** form and the stem verb (dictionary) form, which in the present ends in **-ru**. The **masu** form ends with **-masu** and is the polite form of the verb used in everyday Japanese. The stem verb is informal and is used when conjugating sentences. In the present tense it is also used for the dictionary listing, which is why it's also called the dictionary form. To make the past tense of the stem verb, drop the suffix **-ru** and replace it with **-ta**. The stem verb by itself can express a question without the question marker **ka**. The intonation usually rises on **-ru** or **-ta**.

| **Denwa o suru.** | Do you want to call? |
| **Denwa o shita.** | Did you call? |

The following are examples of the two verb forms.

ENGLISH	MASU FORM	STEM VERB	STEM VERB (PAST)
there is/I have (non-animate subject)	ari-masu	aru	a-tta
there is/I have (animate-subject)	i-masu	iru	i-ta
do/play	shi-masu	suru	shi-ta (irregular)
see/look/watch/ examine/check up	mi-masu	miru	mi-ta
teach	oshie-masu	oshieru	oshie-ta
eat	tabe-masu	taberu	tabe-ta

5. The construction STEM VERB PAST TENSE + **koto ga aru/arimasu**

The expression **koto ga aru/arimasu** (have been, have ever/never been) may be placed after the stem verb in the past tense to express an experience, fact, or event in the past.

Nyūin o shita koto ga arimasu.
I have been admitted before.

Kenkō-shindan o shita koto ga arimasen.
I have never had a physical examination before.

Hoken-gaisha ni renraku shita koto ga arimasu ka.
Have you ever contacted the insurance company ?

Kochira ni rai-in shita koto ga arimasu ka.
Have you ever visited this hospital before?

6. The construction STEM VERB PRESENT TENSE + **koto ga arimasu**

However, the stem verb in the present tense plus **koto ga aru/arimasu** expresses the idea that something happens sometimes or occasionally and translates literally as "there are times when."

Kenkō-shindan suru koto ga aru.
I have had physicals before. (*lit.*, There are times when I have had physical examinations.)

Monshin-hyō ni kinyū shita koto ga arimasu.
I have sometimes completed medical questionnaires before.

Byōin de seito o miru koto ga arimasu.
I see students occasionally.

7. The construction **te**-FORM + **oku/okimasu**

The **te**-form plus **oku/okimasu** is used to express an action done in preparation for future events or for convenience or generally something done in advance. The literal meaning of **oku** is "put, place, leave." However, the meaning changes in the **te**-form. When used with a causative verb, the **te**-form plus **oku** can express the idea "Let's do something." For past actions, use the past tense **oki-mashita**.

Yoyaku o shite okimasu.
I will make an appointment ahead of time.

Yoyaku o shite okimashita.
I made an appointment ahead of time (for the sake of convenience).

Kanjya o mite okimasu.
I will observe the patient beforehand.

Kanjya o mite okimashita.
I watched the patient in advance.

Kenkō-shindan o shite okimasu.
I will have a physical examination beforehand.

Kenkō-shindan o shite okimashita ka.
Have you had a physical examination before?

Kensa o shite okimashō.
Let's do a test in advance.

8. The interrogatives **dare** (who); **dore** (which); **doko** (where); **naze** (why); **itsu** (when); **nan** (what)

In Lesson 2, WH-question words were introduced briefly. The interrogative **dare** (who) is used for asking about people; **dore** (which/which one) for asking about things, concepts, and events; **doko** (where) for asking about places; **naze** (why) for asking about reasons; **itsu** (when) for asking about time; and **nan** (what) for asking about general topics.

Haigū-sha wa dare desu ka.	Who is your spouse?
Yatoi-nushi wa dare desu ka.	Who is your employer?
Fuku wa dore desu ka.	Which ones are your clothes?
Uketsuke-madoguchi wa doko desu ka.	Where is the registration counter?
Nyūin wa naze desu ka.	Why have you been hospitalized?
Menkai-jikan wa itsu desu ka.	When are visiting hours?
Shokugyō wa nan desu ka.	What is your occupation?

9. The interjection **dewa**

The interjection **dewa** (then, well, so, well then) is commonly used to change topics or introduce a subject in conversation. Sometimes it is used simply to make for smooth conversation

Dewa, mimashō.	Well then, let's see/take a look.
Dewa, shinsatsu shimashō.	Well then, let's do a checkup/have an examination.
Dewa, hakarimashō.	Let's measure.
Dewa, tabemashō.	So, let's eat.
Dewa, machimashō.	Well then, let's wait.

Useful Expressions (CD 4-3)

Listen to the CD and repeat the expressions.

1. **Shussei-chi wa doko desu ka.** What is your place of birth?
2. **Nyūin-bi wa itsu desu ka.** What is your date of admission?
3. **Hoken-gaisha wa nan desu ka.** What is your insurance company?

4. **Haigū-sha wa dare desu ka.** Who is your spouse?
5. **Monshin-hyō wa setsumei shite arimasu.** I already explained the medical questionnaire.
6. **Nyūin shita koto ga arimasu ka.** Have you ever been hospitalized?
7. **Nyūin tetsuzuki o shite okimasu.** I will arrange for your admission in advance.
8. **Shūkyō wa nan desu ka.** What is your religion?
9. **Fuku o kite kudasai.** Please put on your clothes.
10. **Dewa, omachi kudasai.** Then, please wait.

Key Sentences (CD 4-4)

Listen to the CD and repeat the sentences.

1. **Yoyaku ga shite arimasu ka.** Do you have a reservation ? (*lit.*, Has your reservation been made?)
2. **Haigū-sha wa dare desu ka.** Who is your spouse?
3. **Fuku o nuide kudasai.** Please take off your clothes.
4. **Kenkō shindan shite okimasu.** I will have a physical examination in advance.
5. **Nyūin shita koto ga arimsu ka.** Have you ever been hospitalized?

Additional Words

setsumei explanation
kiru/kimasu wear/put on (for clothing that is worn above the belt line)
nugu/nugimasu take off (clothes)
harau/haraimasu pay
tsukeru/tsukemasu attach/put on (accessories)
toru/torimasu take off
wakaru/wakarimasu understand
kakaru/kakarimasu spend/cost/charge
rai-in hospital visit
shomei signature
makura pillow
yubi-wa ring
fuku clothes
shita-gi underwear
kutsu-shita socks

haku/hakimasu wear/put on (for clothing that is worn below the belt line)
kigaeru/kigaemasu change clothes
hazusu/hazushimasu take off (accessories)
hakaru/hakarimasu measure
kakeru/kakemasu hang up/put on
miru/mimasu see/look/watch/examine
miseru/misemasu show
nyū-in hospitalization
megane eyeglasses
tokie watch
bōshi cap/hat
zubon trousers/pants
kutsu shoes
shufu housewife

Language Notes

1. The expression **nuide kudasai** means "please take off, remove" and applies to all clothing such as dresses, pants, jackets, shirts, underwear, etc.

Fuku o nuide kudasai.	Please take off your clothes.
Shatsu o nuide kudasai.	Please take off your shirt.
Zubon o nuide kudasai.	Please take off your trousers.
Kutsu o nuide kudasai.	Please take off your shoes.
Shita-gi o nuide kudasai.	Please take off your underwear.
Kutsu-shita o nuide kudasai.	Please take off your socks.

2. The expression **kite kudasai** (please put on/wear) is used only for upper body clothing.

Fuku o kite kudasai.	Please put on your clothes.
Shatsu o kite kudasai.	Please put on your shirt.
Jaketto o kite kudasai.	Please put on your jacket.

3. The expression **kigaete kudasai** (please change your clothes) is used for any clothing but not for shoes and accessories. Literally, **ki-gaeru** is a composite of **kiru** (wear) and **kaeru** (change).

Fuku o kigaete kudasai.	Please change your clothes .
Shatsu o kigaete kudasai.	Please change your shirt.
Shita-gi o kigaete kudasai.	Please change your underwear.

When changing into different clothes, Japanese uses the particle **ni** (to).

Kensa-gi ni kigaete kudasia.	Please change into examination clothes.
Gaun ni kigaete kudasai.	Please put on/change into this gown.
Pajyama ni kigaete kudasai.	Please put on/change into pajamas.

4. For changing shoes and accessories, Japanese uses the construction OBJECT **o kaete kudasai** (Please change/replace OBJECT.)

Kutsu o kaete kudasai.	Please change your shoes.
Megane o kaete kudasai.	Please change your eyeglasses.
Makura o kaete kudasai.	Please change your head rest/pillow/cushion.

5. The expression **haite kudasai** (please put on /wear) is used only for articles of clothing worn below the belt, including shoes.

Kutsu o haite kudasai.	Please put on your shoes.
Kutsu-shita o haite kudasai.	Please put on your socks.
Zubon o haite kudasai.	Please wear your trousers.
Sukāto o haite kudasai.	Please put on your skirt.

6. The expression **hazushite kudasai** (please take off, remove) is used only for accessories or articles, such as jewelry, attached to the body.

Tokei o hazushite kudasai.	Please take off your watch.
Yubi-wa o hazushite kudasai.	Please take off your ring.
Iya-ringu o hazushite kudasai.	Please take off your earring.
Bura-jyā o hazushite kudasai.	Please take off your bra.
Megane o hazushite kudasai.	Please take off eyeglasses.
Beruto o hazushite kudasai.	Pleas take off the belt.

7. For eyeglasses or items on or near the head, Japanese uses **kakete kudasai** to express politely the idea of "put on."

Megane o kakete kudasai.	Please put on your eyeglasses.
San-gurasu o kakete kudasai.	Please put on your sunglasses.
Heddo-hōn o kakete kudasai.	Please put on your headphones.
Kubi ni sukāfu o kakete kudasai.	Please put the scarf on your neck.
Beddo ni shītsu o kakete kudasai.	Please cover the sheets on the bed.

8. The expression **tsukete kudasai** (please put on/wear/attach) is used for accessories.

Tokei o tsukete kudasai.	Please put on your watch.
Yubi-wa o tsukete kudasai.	Please put on your ring.
Iya-ringu o tsukete kudasai.	Please put on your earring.
Bura-jyā o tsukete kudasai.	Please put on your bra.

9. For a cap or hat (**bōshi**) or any kind of headgear, Japanese uses the expressions **totte kudasai** (take off), and **kabutte kudasai** (put on).

Bōshi o totte kudasai.	Please take off your cap/hat.
Sukāfu o totte kudasai.	Please take off your scarf.
Bōshi o kabutte kudasai.	Please put on your cap/hat.
Herumetto o kabutte kudasai.	Please put on your helmet.

10. Major occupations (**shigoto/shokugyō**) in Japanese:

student	**seito/gakusei**	farmer	**nō-ka**
housewife	**shufu**	fisher	**ryō-shi**
company employee	**kaisha-in**	teacher	**kyō-in/sensei**
government employee	**kōmu-in**	artist	**geijyutsu-ka**
self-employed person	**jiyū-gyō**	architect	**kenchiku-ka**
lawyer	**bengo-shi**	photographer	**shashin-ka**
accountant	**kaikei-shi**	merchant	**shō-nin**
banker	**ginkō-in**	policeman	**keisatsu-kan**
owner	**keiei-sha**	fireman	**shōbō-shi**
chef	**chōri-shi**	calligrapher	**shodō-ka**
gardener	**zōen-shi**	painter	**ga-ka**

11. Admissions-related expressions:

Wakarimasu ka.	Do you understand?
Eigo ga wakarimasu ka.	Do you understand English?
Eigo de kakemasu ka.	Can you write in English?
Kore o yonde kudasai.	Please read this.
Yukkuri hanashite kudasai.	Please speak slowly.
Katsuji de kaite kudasai.	Please print.
Koko ni namae o kaite kudasai.	Please write your name here.
Koko ni shomei shite kudasai.	Please sign here.
Ikura kakrimasu ka.	What is the cost?
Kādo o misete kudasai.	Please show me your card.

Language Roots

The word **kan** (患) indicates illness, disease, and ailment.

kan-jya	patient
shi-kkan	aliment
kyu-kan	emergency illness

The word **shin** (診) indicates a diagnosis, checkup, examination, and seeing.

shin-satsu	medical examination
shin-satsu-bi	checkup day
mon-shin-hyō	medical questionnaire
shin-ryō	diagnosis

Culture Notes

Traditional Chinese herbal medicine in Japan

The Japanese used to see a pharmacist first in order to get over-the-counter medicines for everyday ailments such as colds and stomachaches. They would consult a physician only if the pharmacist suggested it or the pharmacist's treatment didn't work. Many people also liked to use **kanpō yaku**, traditional Chinese herbal medicine, for minor medical problems. In the modern period, however, Japanese tend to visit clinics or hospitals even for minor ailments.

Three terms for students

Japanese culture emphasizes the importance of education, and this emphasis is reflected in the different terms for students, depending on the grade level. Students in nursery school and kindergarten are called **enji**. In elementary school and high school, they are called **seito**; and in post-secondary schools, they are called **gakusei**.

Comprehension

Answer the following questions.

1. Which of the following could be used as a translation for "Do you have a reservation?"
   a. **Shusshin wa doko desu ka.**   b. **Namae wa nan desu ka.**
   c. **Yoyaku ga arimasu ka.**   d. **Itsu ga iidesu ka.**

2. Which of the following best completes the sentence below?
   Shita-gi ( ) nuide kudasai.
   a. **wa**   b. **ga**
   c. **o**   d. **de**

3. Which of the following is NOT a correct expression in Japanese?
   a. **Kensa-gi o kita koto ga arimasu ka.**
   b. **Osake o nonda koto ga arimasu ka.**
   c. **Yoyaku o shita koto ga arimasu ka.**
   d. **Shussei-chi o matsu koto ga arimasu ka.**

4. In which sentence are you asking about the insurance company's name?
   a. **Hoken-gaisha ga doko desu ka.**
   b. **Hoken-gaisha ga arimasu ka.**
   c. **Hoken-gaisha wa nan desu ka.**
   d. **Hoken-gaisha wa itsu desu ka.**

Select the correct meaning in Japanese.

5. When
   a. **itsu**   b. **dare**   c. **nani**

6. Where
   a. **dare**   b. **doko**   c. **naze**

7. What
   a. **itsu**   b. **doko**   c. **nani**

8. Who
   a. **dare**   b. **naze**   c. **itsu**

9. Why
   a. **nani**   b. **dare**   c. **naze**

Which verb is used for the following items?

10. Underwear
    a. **torimasu**   b. **nugimasu**   c. **hazushimasu**

11. Shoes
    a. **hakimasu**   b. **kimasu**   c. **tsukemasu**

12. Bra
    a. **kakemasu**   b. **kimasu**   c. **tsukemasu**

13. Eyeglasses
    a. **kimasu**   b. **kakemasu**   c. **tsukemasu**

14. Shirt
    a. **nugimasu**   b. **hazushimasu**   c. **torimasu**

Practice

Respond to the following in Japanese using the cues that have been provided.

1. Confirming appointment.

   (Healthcare professional)   (Patient)

   1. _____ (Appointment)   **Hai, shite arimasu.**
   2. _____ (Appointment)   **Iie, shite arimasen.**
   3. _____ (Fill out the form)   **Hai, shimashita.**
   4. _____ (Fill out the form)   **Iie, shite arimasen.**

2. Asking some questions.

   (Healthcare professional)

   1. _____   **Hai, kenkō hoken ga arimasu.**
   2. _____   **X hoken gaisha desu.**
   3. _____   **Shujin desu.**
   4. _____   **1960 nen 4 gatsu 8 ka desu.**
   5. _____   **On-na desu.**

3. Before the examination. What shall I do? (**Dō shimasu ka.**)

   (Patient)   (Healthcare professional)

   1. **Fuku wa dō shimasu ka.**   _____ (Please take off.)
   2. **Kutsu wa dō shimasu ka.**   _____ (Please take off.)
   3. **Yubi-wa wa dō shimasu ka.**   _____ (Please take off.)
   4. **Megane wa dō shimasu ka.**   _____ (Please take off.)
   5. **Kensa-gi wa dō shimasu ka.**   _____ (Please take off.)

4. After the examination. What shall I do? (**Dō shimasu ka.**)

   (Patient)   (Healthcare professional)

   1. **Fuku wa dō shimasu ka.**   _____ (Please put on.)
   2. **Kutsu wa dō shimasu ka.**   _____ (Please put on.)
   3. **Yubi-wa wa dō shimasu ka.**   _____ (Please put on.)
   4. **Megane wa dō shimasu ka.**   _____ (Please put on.)

5. Dialogue comprehension. Based on the dialogue, answer the following.

   1. **Hoken-gaisha no namae wa nan desu ka.**   _____
   2. **Yoyaku wa shite arimasu ka.**   _____
   3. **Nan-ji no yoyaku desu ka.**   _____
   4. **Hoken-kanyū-sha wa dare desu ka.**   _____
   5. **Uketsuke-hyō ni kinyū shita koto ga arimashita ka.** _____

6. Free response questions.
    (Questions)   (Answers)
    1. **Kenkō shindan wa shite arimasu ka.** _____
    2. **Nyū-in shita koto ga arimasu ka.** _____
    3. **Shusshin-chi wa doko desu ka.** _____
    4. **Yatoi-nushi wa dare desu ka.** _____

Exercises

1. Say the following words in Japanese.
    A. Birthplace _____
    B. Insurance company _____
    C. Occupation _____
    D. Cashier _____
    E. Clothes _____

2. What does it means in English?
    A. **Nugimasu** _____
    B. **Hakimasu** _____
    C. **Machimasu** _____
    D. **Hi-hoken-sha** _____
    E. **Kinyū shimasu** _____

3. Say the following expressions in Japanese.
    A. Where is your birthplace? _____
    B. What is your insurance company? _____
    C. Who is your spouse? _____
    D. Please take off your shirt. _____
    E. Please wait. _____

4. Reply to the following questions.

    Q: **Yoyaku wa shite arimasu ka.**
    A: _____

    Q: **Go-jyūsho wa doko desuka.**
    B: _____

    Q: **Hoken ga arimasu ka.**
    C: _____

    Q: **Nyūin shita koto ga arimasu ka.**
    D: _____

LESSON 5 Upper Body Parts
(Jō-han-shin)

Basic Vocabulary (CD 5-1)

Listen to the CD and repeat the vocabulary.

1.	body	**karada**	体
2.	upper body	**jyō-han-shin**	上半身
3.	lower body	**ka-han-shin**	下半身
4.	head	**atama**	頭
5.	hair (on the head)	**kami**	髪
6.	forehead	**hitai**	額
7.	temple	**komekami**	顳
8.	glabella	**miken**	眉間
9.	face	**kao**	顔
10.	cheek	**hoppe(ta)/hoho**	ほっぺ (た)/頬
11.	eye	**me**	目
12.	pupil	**hitomi**	瞳
13.	eyelashes	**matsuge**	睫毛
14.	eyebrows	**mayuge**	眉毛
15.	ear	**mimi**	耳
16.	ear lobe	**mimi-tabu**	耳たぶ
17.	nape of the neck	**kubi-suji**	首筋
18.	nose	**hana**	鼻
19.	mouth	**kuchi**	口
20.	lip	**kuchi-biru**	唇
21.	tongue	**shita/bero**	舌/べろ
22.	tip of tongue	**shita-saki**	舌先
23.	tooth	**ha**	歯
24.	chin	**ago-saki**	顎先
25.	jaw	**ago**	顎
26.	neck	**kubi**	首
27.	throat	**nodo**	喉
28.	shoulder	**kata**	肩
29.	upper back	**senaka**	背中
30.	chest/breast	**mune/kyōbu/chibusa**	胸/胸部/乳房

Kao (Face)

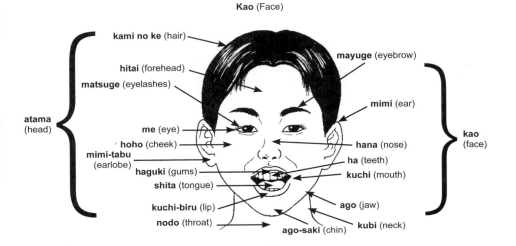

Dialogue (CD 5-2)

Listen to the CD and repeat the dialogue.

At the Initial Screening Room

Kris (nurse):   **Kyō wa dō shimashita ka?**
                  How are you feeling today?

Mr. Suzuki (patient): **Nodo ga itai(n) desu.**
                  I have a sore throat.

Kris: **Itsu kara nodo ga itai(n) desu ka.**
                  How long have you had a sore throat?

Mr. Suzuki: **(Itai nodo wa) sakuya kara desu.**
                  (My sore throat is) Since last night.

Kris: **Mune mo itai(n) desu ka.**
                  Do you have chest pain, too?

Mr. Suzuki: **Iie, mune wa ita-kunai(n) desu.**
                  No, I don't have chest pain.

                  Sukoshi netsu ga arimasu.
                  I have a little fever.

Kris: **Nan-do gurai arimashita ka.**
                  What was your temperature?

Mr. Suzuki: **Kesa wa hyaku-ten-go-do gurai deshita.**
                  It was about 100.5°F this morning.

Grammar

1. ### The i-adjectives modifying nouns

    The words **itai** (pain, sore, hurt), **kayui** (itchy), and **darui** (tired/fatigued) are i-adjectives, meaning they end in **i**. **Itai** is a comprehensive terms for pains anywhere on the body, and it covers all manner of pains conveyed by the English words *sore*, *painful*, and *hurt*.

Atama ga itai desu.	My head is sore. My head hurts. My head is painful. I have headache.
Kao ga kayui desu.	My face is itchy.
Kubi ga darui desu.	My neck is tired.

2. ### Adding n after an i-adjective to convey the feelings and emotion of speaker: -i(n) desu

    In speaking, an (**n**) is placed directly after the **-i** of an i-adjective in the expression **itai(n) desu**. This sounds more natural in Japanese and also invests the adjective with the speaker's emotion or feelings.

Mune ga itai(n) desu.	I have chest pain. (*lit.*, My chest has pain.)
Mimi ga kayui(n) desu.	My ear is itchy.
Ashi ga darui(n) desu.	My leg is tired.

3. ### The construction i-ADJECTIVE + SUFFIX -kunai(n) desu to express the negative

    To make the i-adjectives **itai**, **kayui**, and **darui** negative, first drop the **-i** and add **-kunai(n) desu**. When the sentence is negative, the subject marker changes from **ga** to **wa** generally. However, **ga** may be retained to emphasize the subject. The negative past is **-ku nakkata desu.**

Ha ga itai(n) desu.	I have a toothache.
Ha wa ita-kunai(n) desu.	I don't have a toothache.
Me ga kayui(n) desu.	My eye is itchy.
Me wa kayu-kunai(n) desu.	My eye is not itchy.
Kata ga darui(n) desu.	My shoulder is tired.
Kata wa daru-kunai(n) desu.	My shoulder is not tired.
Karada no chōshi ga ii(n) desu.	My body is in good condition.
Karada no chōshi ga yoku-nakkata desu.	My body was not in good condition.

Jōhan-shin, Mae (Upper Body, Front)

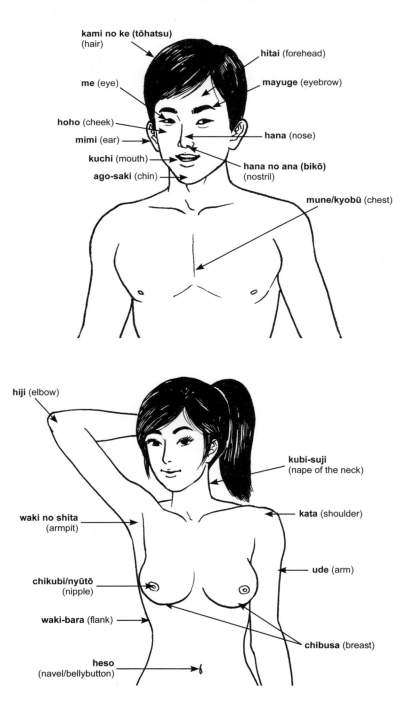

kami no ke (tōhatsu) (hair)

hitai (forehead)

me (eye)

mayuge (eyebrow)

hoho (cheek)

mimi (ear)

hana (nose)

kuchi (mouth)

ago-saki (chin)

hana no ana (bikō) (nostril)

mune/kyobū (chest)

hiji (elbow)

kubi-suji (nape of the neck)

waki no shita (armpit)

kata (shoulder)

ude (arm)

chikubi/nyūtō (nipple)

waki-bara (flank)

chibusa (breast)

heso (navel/bellybutton)

Ii is the informal adjective for "good." The formal adjective is **yoi**. The negative form of **yoi** is **yoku-nai**.

4. The particle **kara**

The particle **kara** indicates a starting point. Placed after a time or place in the construction NOUN OF TIME/PLACE plus **kara**, it means "from" or "since."

> **Hachi-ji kara uketsuke ga hajimarimasu.**
> Registration has been open since 8 o'clock.

> **(O)hiru kara kurinikku wa yasumi desu.**
> Since noon, the clinic has been closed.

> **Getsuyō-bi kara nyūin shimashita.**
> I have been hospitalized since Monday.

> **Senshū kara karada no chōshi ga yokunai(n) desu.**
> Since last week, my condition has not been good.

> **Byōin kara uchi ni kaerimashita.**
> I am back home from the hospital.

> **Go-sai kara byōki desu.**
> Since five years old, she/he has been ill.

5. The particle **mo**

The particle **mo** is similar to English *too* or *also*. In a sentence, it occupies the same position as **wa/ga** and can replace them, adding the sense of "too" or "also."

Netsu mo arimasu ka.	Do you have fever too?
Atama mo itai(n) desu ka.	Do you have headache too?
Nodo mo itai(n) desu.	My throat is also sore.
Kata mo darui(n) desu ka.	Is your shoulder tired too?
Tsugi no yoyaku mo shimasu ka.	Do you want to make your next reservation too?

6. The adverbs **sukoshi, chotto, hontō-ni, tottemo,** and **bimyō-ni**

Sukoshi (a little, somewhat), **chotto** (few), **hontō-ni** (really), **tottemo** (very), and **bimyō-ni** (slightly) are adverbs and are placed before an adjective or verb. Japanese use **chotto** and **sukoshi** interchangeably, and there is very little difference in meaning between them. **Bimyō-ni** expresses a vague or subtle feeling. Using adverbs in Japanese sentences makes for lively and more precise expression.

Kata ga sukoshi kayui(n) desu.	I have a little itch on my shoulder.
Chotto itai(n) desu.	I have a little/small pain.
Kubi ga hontō-ni itai(n) desu.	My neck feels really sore.
Tottemo darui(n) desu.	I feel very tired.
Bimyō-ni itai(n) desu.	I have a slight pain.
Karada ga sukoshi kayui(n) desu.	My body is a little itchy.
Netsu ga sukoshi arimasu.	You have a slight fever.
Jikan ga chotto arimasu.	I have a little time.

Jōhan-shin, Ushiro (Upper Body, Back)

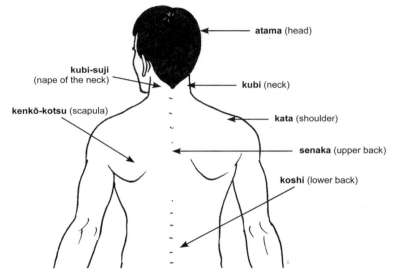

atama (head)

kubi-suji
(nape of the neck)

kenkō-kotsu (scapula)

kubi (neck)

kata (shoulder)

senaka (upper back)

koshi (lower back)

Useful Expressions (CD 5-3)

Listen to the CD and repeat the sentences.

1. **Atama ga itai(n) desu.** I have a headache.
2. **Onaka ga itai(n) desu ka.** Do you have a stomachache?
3. **Mimi ga kayui(n) desu.** My ear is itchy/itches.
4. **Senaka wa itakunai(n) desu.** My back doesn't hurt.
5. **Karada ga darui(n) desu ka.** Is your body tired?
6. **Ashi wa darukunai(n) desu.** My leg/foot isn't tired.
7. **Asa kara ha mo itai(n) desu.** Since this morning, I've had a toothache too.
8. **Nichiyō-bi kara kata ga itai(n) desu.** Since Sunday, I've had a pain in my shoulder.
9. **Kinō no yoru kara kubi ga itai(n) desu.** Since last night, my neck has been sore.
10. **Itsu kara mune ga itai(n) desu ka.** Since when have you had chest pain?

Key Sentences (CD 5-4)

Listen to the CD and repeat the sentences.

1. **Mune ga itai(n) desu ka.** Do you have chest pain?
2. **Itsu-kara nodo ga itai(n) desu ka.** Since when have you had a sore throat?
3. **Karada ga darui(n) desu ka.** Does your body feel tired?
4. **Ashi wa itakunai(n) desu.** My leg/foot doesn't hurt.
5. **Itsu-kara kayui(n) desu ka.** When did you start to itch?

Additional Words

iku/ikimasu go	**naoru/naorimasu** cure/heal
shūmatsu weekend	**sakuya** last night
chikubi/nyū tō nipple	**fuku-tsū** stomachache
tsugi next	**yotei** schedule/plan
kayui itchy	**darui** tiredness/fatigue
taikei fitness, shape	**yasumi** recess/close/rest/absence

Language Notes

1. The days of the week in Japanese relate to natural phenomena: Sunday = sun, Monday = moon, Tuesday = fire, Wednesday = water, Thursday = wood, Friday = metal/gold, and Saturday = earth. To name the days of the week, the suffix **yō-bi** is added to the words for these things. **Nan yōbi desu ka** means "What day of the week is it?"

Nichi-yōbi	Sunday
Getsu-yōbi	Monday
Ka-yōbi	Tuesday
Sui-yōbi	Wednesday
Moku-yōbi	Thursday
Kin-yōbi	Friday
Do-yōbi	Saturday

Getsu-yōbi ni kensa o suru yotei desu.
We have scheduled your examination for Monday.

Ka-yōbi ni yoyaku o onegai shimasu.
I would like to make a reservation for Tuesday.

Nichi-yōbi ni kurinikku wa yasumi masu.
The clinic is closed on Sunday.

2. In Lesson 3, we studied basic time expressions. The following time expressions generally do not require particle **ni** (at).

ima	just now/now	**sakuban**	last evening
sakuya	last night	**sōchō**	early morning
asa	morning	**kesa**	this morning
gozen(-chū)	a.m.	**(o)hiru**	noon
gogo	p.m.	**yūgata**	early evening
ban	evening	**kon-ban**	this evening
yoru	night	**mayonaka**	midnight

Sōchō kara mune ga itai(n) desu.
Since early in the morning, I have had chest pain.

Sakuya kara nodo ga tottemo itai(n) desu ka.
Have you really had a sore throat since the last night?

Kinō komekami wa itaku-nakkata(n) desu.
My temple did not hurt yesterday.

3. The prefixes **sen-** (last), **kon-** (this), **rai-** (next), **sa-** (after next), and **mai-** (every) are used to form expressions with respect to the day, week (**shū**), month (**getsu**), and year (**nen**). For example, "last week" is **sen shū**; and "last month" is **sen getsu**. Kinō, kyō, ashita, asatte, kyonen, and kotoshi are exceptions.

	LAST (**SEN**)	THIS (**KON**)	NEXT (**RAI**)	AFTER NEXT (**SA**)	EVERY (**MAI**)
DAY	kinō	kyō	ashita	asatte	mai-nichi
WEEK (**SHŪ**)	sen shū	kon shū	rai shū	sa rai shū	mai shū
MONTH (**GETSU**)	sen getsu	kon getsu	rai getsu	sa rai getsu	mai tsuki
YEAR (**NEN**)	kyo nen	ko toshi	rai nen	sa rai nen	mai nen

4. The suffix -**matsu** means "end." Accordingly, "weekend" is **shū-matsu**, "end of the month" is **getsu-matsu**, and "end of the year" is **nen-matsu**. Since these words of time are specific, they use the particle **ni** (at) in sentences.

Shū-matsu ni yoyaku o shimasu ka.
Do you need an appointment during the weekend?

Getsu-matsu ni kensa o shimasu.
I will have an examination at the end of the month.

Nen-matsu kara atama ga itai(n) desu.
I've had a headache since the end of the year.

5. The suffix **-ka-kan** is used to express a duration of days.

futsuka-kan	for two days	**mikka-kan**	for three days
yokka-kan	for four days	**itsuka-kan**	for five days

6. The suffix **-shū-kan** is used to express a duration of weeks.

i-shū-kan	for one week	**ni-shū-kan**	for two weeks
san-shū-kan	for three weeks	**yon-shū-kan**	for four weeks
go-shū-kan	for five weeks	**roku-shū-kan**	for six weeks

ni (2) shūkan netsu ga arimasu.	I've had a fever for two weeks.
san (3) shūkan kubi ga itai(n) desu.	I've had neck pain for three weeks.

7. The suffix **-ka-getsu-kan** is used to express a duration of months.

i-kka-getsu-kan	for a month	**ni-kagetsu-kan**	for two months
san-kagetsu-kan	for three months	**yon-kagetsu-kan**	for four months
go-kagetsu-kan	for five months	**ro-kka-getsu-kan**	for six months

8. The suffix **-nen-kan** is used to express a duration of years.

ichi-nen-kan	for one year	**ni-nen-kan**	for two years
san-nen-kan	for three years	**yo-nen-kan**	for four years
go-nen-kan	for five years	**roku-nen-kan**	for six years

Language Roots

The word **ke/ge** (毛) means "hair." The same character is also pronounced **mō**.

kami no ke	head hair
waki-ge	underarm hair
ubu-ge	downy hair
muna-ge	chest hair
sune-ge	leg hair
mayu-ge	eyebrows
matsu-ge	eyelashes
mō-fu	blanket (literally, hair sheet)
datsu-mō	hair removal

The suffix **tsū** (痛) indicates pain, soreness, and hurt. This character is also pronounced **itai**.

zu-tsū headache
kyō-tsū chest pain
me ga itai(n) desu. I have eye pain.

Culture Notes

Japanese geography and a map of Japan with major cities

(This information may help you understand the patient's country of birth.)

Japan has four major islands: Hokkaidō, Honshū, Shikoku, and Kyūshū. The largest, Honshū, is divided into five regions: Tōhoku; Kantō; Chūbu; Kansai; and Chūgoku. There are also about 3,000 smaller islands including Okinawa. Japanese territory is about 146,000 square miles, with more than 70 percent covered by mountains. Japan is approximately 1/26th the size of the United States (3,794,000 square miles), one-half the size of France (261,000 square miles) and smaller than the state of California (164,000 square miles). Japan is bigger than Germany (138, 000 square miles), Italy (116,000 square miles), the Philippines (116,000 square miles),

Map of Japan

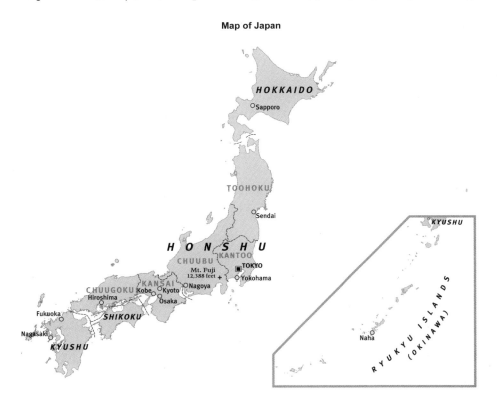

New Zealand (104,000 square miles), and the United Kingdom (94,000 square miles).

The major cities are Sapporo in Hokkaido, Sendai in the Tohoku region in Northern Honshū, Tokyo in the central Kanto region in Honshū, Yokohama (near Tokyo), Nagoya in the Tokai region in Honshū, Kyoto in the Kinki region in Honshū, Osaka (next to Kyoto), Kobe (also in the Kinki region), Hiroshima in the Chūgoku region in West Honshū, Nagasaki in northern Kyūshū, and Naha in Okinawa.

Mount Fuji, the iconic volcano that rises 12,388 feet above sea level, is at the center of the Pacific Ocean side of Honshū.

Comprehension

Select the appropriate Japanese expression for the following situations.

1. Do you have a headache?
   a. **Atama ga itai(n) desu ka.**   b. **Atama ga kayui(n) desu ka.**

2. I am tired.
   a. **Karada ga itai(n) desu.**   b. **Karada ga darui(n) desu.**

3. Which of the following does NOT belong to the expression "My stomach aches"?
   a. **Onaka ga itai(n) desu.**   b. **Onaka ga kayui(n) desu.**

4. Which of the following expressions is WRONG?
   a. **Ashi mo darui(n) desu ka.**   b. **Mimi o itai(n) desu ka.**

5. Which of the following is the Japanese for "Your eyes are not good"?
   a. **Me wa yokunai desu.**   b. **Me ga ii desu.**

Select the appropriate Japanese expression for the following:

6. The duration of six months:
   a. **Roku gatsu-kan**   b. **Rokka-getsu-kan**   c. **Roku shū-kan**

7. The duration of four months:
   a. **Yonka-getsu-kan**   b. **Shigatsu-kan**   c. **Shika-getsu-kan**

8. This morning:
    a. **Sōchō**   b. **Kesa**
    c. **Konban**   d. **Asa**

9. The early evening:
    a. **Ban**   b. **Konban**
    c. **Yūgata**   d. **Yoru**

10. Every day:
    a. **Mai-getsu**   b. **Mai-nen**
    c. **Mai-nichi**   d. **Mai-shū**

Select the correct meaning in English.

---

11. **Kuchi-biru**
    a. lip   b. gums   c. ear

12. **Shita**
    a. mouth   b. tongue   c. tooth

13. **Mune**
    a. nose   b. shoulder   c. chest

14. **Senaka**
    a. upper back   b. lower back   c. chin

15. **Karada**
    a. temple   b. forehead   c. body

Practice

Respond to the following in Japanese using the cues that have been provided.

---

1. Asking about the patient's physical condition.
    (Healthcare professional)   (Patient)
    1. _____(head)   **Sukoshi atama ga itai(n) desu.**
    2. _____(tongue)   **Shita wa itaku nai(n) desu.**
    3. _____(upper back)   **Senaka wa kayuku nai(n) desu.**
    4. _____(neck)   **Kubi ga darui(n) desu.**

2. Asking about the onset of symptoms.
   (Patient)   (Healthcare professional)
   1. **Karada ga itai(n) desu.**   _____ (When did your pain begin?)
   2. **Kubi ga darui(n) desu.**   _____ (When did your tiredness begin?)
   3. **Ago ga itai(n) desu.**   _____ (When did you start feeling sore?)
   4. **Senaka ga kayui(n) desu.** _____ (When did you start feeling these symptoms?)

3. Estimating the time for healing.
   (Patient)   (Healthcare professional)
   1. **Kao wa itsu naorimasu ka.**   _____ (about a month)
   2. **Mimi wa itsu goro naorimasu ka.** _____ (about two weeks)
   3. **Me wa itsu goro naorimasu ka.** _____ (about three months)

4. What would you say for the following days relative to today if today is Monday?
   (Questions)   (Healthcare professional)
   1. **Kinoo wa nan-yōbi deshita ka.** _____ (Sunday)
   2. **Ashita wa nan-yōbi desu ka.** _____ (Tuesday)
   3. **Ototoi wa nan-yōbi deshita ka.** _____ (Saturday)
   4. **Asatte wa nan-yōbi desu ka.** _____ (Wednesday)

5. Dialogue comprehension. Based on the dialogue, answer the following questions.
   1. **Kanjya wa mune ga itai(n) desu ka.** _____
   2. **Itsu kara nodo ga itai(n) desu ka.** _____
   3. **Netsu ga arimasu ka.** _____
   4. **Netsu wa nan-do deshita ka.** _____
   5. **Itsu netsu o hakari mashita ka.** _____

6. Free response questions.
   (Questions)   (Answers)
   1. **Kyō wa nan-nichi deshita ka.** _____
   2. **Kon-getsu wa nan-gatsu desu ka.** _____
   3. **Kon-shū wa nani o shimasu ka.** _____
   4. **Rainen Nihon ni ikimasu ka.** _____
   5. **Senshū wa nani o shimashita ka.** _____

Exercises

1. How do you say the following words in Japanese?
   A. Lower body _____
   B. Temple _____
   C. Face _____
   D. Eyelashes _____
   E. Lip _____
   F. Neck _____
   G. Upper back _____
   H. Jaw _____
   I. Gums _____
   J. Shoulder _____

2. Say following sentences in Japanese.
   A. My eye is itchy.

   _____

   B. Since this morning, I've had a pain in my ear lobe too.

   _____

   C. Since last night, my forehead has been sore.

   _____

   D. My jaw isn't tired.

   _____

   E. I have an earache.

   _____

3. Say the following in Japanese.
   A. Do you have a stomachache?

   _____

   B. Since morning, have you had a toothache too?

   _____

   C. Has your shoulder been in pain since Sunday?

   _____

   D. Since when have you had neck pain?

   _____

   E. Have you had chest pain since last night?

   _____

   F. Do you need an appointment for next week?

   _____

Arms & Lower Body Parts
(Ude to Ka-han-shin)

Basic Vocabulary (CD 6-1)

Listen to the CD and repeat the vocabulary.

#	English	Romaji	Japanese
1.	belly/stomach	hara/onaka	腹/お腹
2.	abdomen	ka-fukubu	下腹部
3.	navel	heso	臍
4.	arm	ude	腕
5.	armpit	waki-no-shita	脇の下
6.	elbow	hiji	肘
7.	hand	te	手
8.	palm	te no hira	掌
9.	wrist	te-kubi	手首
10.	finger	yubi	指
11.	thumb	oya-yubi	親指
12.	forefinger/index finger	hitosashi-yubi	人差し指
13.	middle finger	naka-yubi	中指
14.	ring finger	kusuri-yubi	薬指
15.	little finger	ko-yubi	小指
16.	lower back/hips	koshi	腰
17.	bottom/buttocks	(o)shiri/denbu	(お)尻/臀部
18.	leg/foot	ashi	足
19.	ankle	ashi-kubi	足首
20.	ankle bone	kurubushi	踝
21.	thigh	momo	腿
22.	knee	hiza	膝
23.	shin	sune	脛
24.	calf	fukurahagi	脹脛
25.	heel	kakato	踵
26.	bone	hone	骨
27.	joints	kansetsu	関節
28.	muscle	kin-niku	筋肉
29.	skin	hifu	皮膚
30.	nail	tsume	爪

Ka-han-shin, Mae (Lower Body, Front)

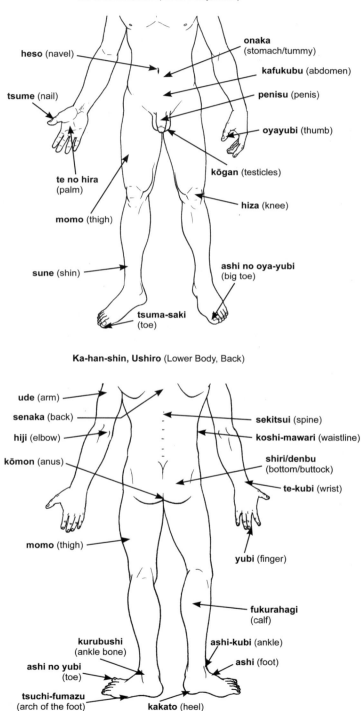

heso (navel)

onaka (stomach/tummy)

kafukubu (abdomen)

tsume (nail)

penisu (penis)

oyayubi (thumb)

te no hira (palm)

kōgan (testicles)

hiza (knee)

momo (thigh)

sune (shin)

ashi no oya-yubi (big toe)

tsuma-saki (toe)

Ka-han-shin, Ushiro (Lower Body, Back)

ude (arm)

senaka (back)

sekitsui (spine)

hiji (elbow)

koshi-mawari (waistline)

kōmon (anus)

shiri/denbu (bottom/buttock)

te-kubi (wrist)

momo (thigh)

yubi (finger)

fukurahagi (calf)

kurubushi (ankle bone)

ashi-kubi (ankle)

ashi no yubi (toe)

ashi (foot)

tsuchi-fumazu (arch of the foot)

kakato (heel)

Dialogue (CD 6-2)

Listen to the CD and repeat the dialogue.

In the Screening Room

Kris (nurse): **Kyō wa dō shimashita ka.**
Do you have any complaints today?

Mr. Suzuki (patient): **Kafukubu ga tottemo itai(n) desu.**
I have a lot of pain in my abdomen.

Kris: **Itsu kara itai(n) desu ka.**
Since when have you had the pain?

Mr. Suzuki: **Kinō no asa kara desu.**
Since yesterday morning (I have had pain).

Kris: **Don-na itami desu ka.**
What kind of pain is it?

Mr. Suzuki: **Sasu itami desu.**
It's a piercing pain.

Kris: **Hokani itai tokoro wa arimasen ka.**
Do you have pain anywhere else?

Mr. Suzuki: **Iie, tokuni arimasen.**
No, nothing in particular.

Grammar

1. **The verb suffix -masen indicates the negative present tense.**

   The negative of the present tense is indicated by placing -**masen** at the end of a verb.

uchi-masu	hit	**uchi-masen**	not hit
kiri-masu	cut	**kiri-masen**	not cut
sashi-masu	pierce	**sashi-masen**	not pierce
shibire-masu	becoming numb	**shibire-masen**	not becoming numb
kanō shimasu	fester	**kanō shi-masen**	not fester
hare-masu	swell	**hare-masen**	not swell

2. **The verb suffix -masen deshita indicates the negative past tense.**

   The negative of the past tense is indicated by placing -**masen deshita** at the end of a verb.

uchi-masu	hit	uchi-masen deshita	did not hit
kiri-masu	cut	kiri-masen deshita	did not cut
sashi-masu	pierce	sashi-masen deshita	did not pierce
shibire-masu	become numb	shibire-masen deshita	did not become numb
kanō-shimasu	fester	kanō shi-masen deshita	did not fester
hare-masu	swell	hare-masen deshita	did not swell

3. The **te**-form + **imasu** for the present progressive tense

The present progressive form **shite** plus **imasu** was introduced in Lesson 3. In order to make the present progressive of the **te**-form, drop -**masu** and add -**te imasu**. This is a very useful form for expressing or asking about ongoing actions or conditions. The following are some examples:

ENGLISH	MASU FORM (PRESENT TENSE)	TE-FORM (TE IMASU)
to numb	shibire-masu	shibire-te-imasu
to swell	hare-masu	hare-te-imasu
to hurt	itame-masu	itame-te-imasu
to broke	ore-masu	ore-te-imasu
to come out/show-up	de-masu	de-te-imasu
to do/play	shi-masu	shi-te imasu

shibire-masu (numb)
Hiji ga shibirete imasu.   My elbow is feeling numb.

kanō shi-masu (fester)
Mimi ga kanō shite imasu.   Your ear is festering.

hare-masu (swell)
Ko-yubi ga harete imasu.   Your baby finger is swelling

4. The **te**-form + **imasen** for the negative of the present progressive tense

The verb ending -**te** plus **imasen** is used to express negative progressive action.

Geri o shite imasen.	I have not had (*lit.*, have not been having) diarrhea.
Kaze o hiite imasen.	I haven't had (*lit.*, have not been having) a cold.
Kusuri o nonde imasen.	I am not taking/drinking medicine.
Nani mo tabete imasen.	I am not eating at all.

5. The present negative -**masen ka** to ask about a condition or invite an action

The negative ending -**masen** and question marker **ka** are used to ask about someone's condition or to invite someone to do something.

shibiremasu (numb)
Te ga shibiremasen ka.   Isn't your hand numb?

kanō shimasu (fester)
Yubi ga kanō shimasen ka.   Aren't your fingers festered?

shokuji o shimasu (have a meal)
Shokuji o shimasen ka.   Won't you have a meal?

6. The **te**-form + **imasen ka** to ask about the present progress of an action

The **te**-form plus **imasen ka** is used to ask about the present progress of an action.

Tekubi ga shibirete imasen ka.   Isn't your wrist becoming numb?
Te-no-hira ga kanō shite imasen ka.   Isn't your palm festering?
Ude ga orete imasen ka.   Isn't your arm broken (*lit.*, breaking)?

For the last example, note that Japanese perceives the broken arm as a continuing action or ongoing condition and therefore requires the present progressive, while English emphasizes the condition of being broken.

7. To make an **i**-adjective into a noun

In order to change an **i**-adjective into a noun, drop the suffix -**i** and replace it with -**mi**.

ita-i   ita-mi   pain
Itami ga arimasu ka.   Do you have pain?

kayu-i   kayu-mi   itchiness
Kayumi ga arimasu ka.   Do you itch? (*lit.*, Do you have itchiness?)

Hiji ni itami ga arimasu.
I have a pain in my elbow.

Hifu ni kayumi ga arimasu.
My skin itches. (*lit.*, I have itchiness on my skin.)

Kansetsu ni itami ga arimasu ka.
Do you have pain in your joints?

Momo ni kayumi ga arimasu ka.
Does your thigh itch? (*lit.*, Do you have itchiness on your thigh?)

Note that Japanese has the noun **tsukare** to express exhaustion and therefore doesn't form a synonym from the adjective **darui** (exhausted, tired).

Ashi ni tsukare ga arimasu.   My legs are exhausted.
Kin-niku ni tsukare ga arimasu ka.   Are your muscles tired?

8. The interrogative pronoun **don-na**

The interrogative **don-na** is usually followed by noun and means "What kind of."

Don-na itami desu ka.   What kind of pain (do you have)?
Don-na yōsu desu ka.   What kind of situation?
Don-na shōjyō desu ka.   What kind of symptom?
Don-na guai desu ka.   What kind of condition?

9. The adverbs **ichiban**, **itsumo**, **tokidoki**, **tamani**, **yoku**, **tsuyoku**, **yowaku**, and **tokuni**

The following adverbs express degree and can be used in both affirmative and negative sentences: **ichiban** (most), **itsumo** (always), **tokidoki** (sometimes), **tamani** (once in a while), **yoku** (often), **tsuyoku** (strongly/hard), **yowaku** (weakly/softly), and **tokuni** (especially/particularly). Notice that these adverbs are not followed by object marker **o**. As adverbs, they modify both adjectives and verbs.

Fukurahagi ga ichiban itai(n) desu.
My calf hurts the most.

Fukurahagi no kin-niku ni itami ga itsumo arimasu.
I always have pain in my calf muscle.

Ude ga tokidoki itai(n) desu.
Sometimes I have pain in my arm.

Onaka ga tamani itai(n) desu.
Once in a while I have a stomachache.

Kakato ga yoku itai(n) desu.
I often have pain in my heel.

Hiji ga tokuni itai(n) desu.
I especially have pain in my elbow.

Waki-no-shita ni tokidoki kayumi ga arimasu.
My armpit sometimes itches. (*lit.*, Armpit sometimes itchiness have = I sometimes have itchiness in my armpit.)

10. The adverbs **zenzen, hotondo,** and **amari**

The adverbs **zenzen** (not at all), **hotondo** (hardly), and **amari** (not much; not very much; not often) convey a negative meaning and are used only in negative sentences.

Yubi ga zenzen itaku arimasen.
I don't have pain in my fingers at all.

Kata ga hotondo itaku arimasen ka.   Don't you have hardly any shoulder pain?
Mune ga amari itaku arimasen.   I don't have much chest pain.

11. The adverb **hokani**

Hokani means "besides; additional; is there anything else?" In ordinary speech, the expression **Hokani nani ka (arimasu ka).** "Do you need anything else?" occurs quite frequently. When used in a complete sentence, **hokani** always takes the verbs phrase **arimasu ka.**

Hokani itai tokoro wa arimasu ka.   Do you have any additional pain?

Hokani, doko ka itai tokoro wa arimasu ka.
Do you have any additional pain in your body?

Useful Expressions (CD 6-3)

Listen to the CD and repeat the sentences.

1. **Te-kubi o itamemashita ka.** Did you hurt your wrist?
2. **Oya-yubi o kirimashita ka.** Did you cut your thumb?
3. **Doko de naka-yubi o hasamimashita ka.** Where did you jam (pinch) your middle finger?
4. **Hiza o tsuyoku uchimashita.** I bumped my knee very hard.
5. **Kusuri-yubi ga harete imasen ka.** Do you have swelling on your ring finger?
6. **Hiji o surimukimashita.** I scraped my elbow.
7. **Inu ni momo o kamaremashita.** I was bitten on the thigh by a dog.
8. **Koko ni suri kizu ga arimasu.** I have an abrasion here.
9. **Kizu ga kanō shite imasu yo.** The wound is becoming infected, isn't it?
10. **Migi-kurubushi o kujiki mashita ka.** Did you sprain your right ankle?

Key Sentences (CD 6-4)

Listen to the CD and repeat the sentences.

1. **Don-na itami desu ka.** What is your pain like?
2. **Hoka ni itai tokoro ga arimasu ka.** Do you have pain anywhere else?
3. **Tokuni itai tokoro wa arimasen.** I don't have any particular pain.
4. **Ude o tsuyoku uchi masen deshita ka.** Didn't you bump your arm very hard?
5. **Migi-ashi ga shibirete imasu ka.** Do you have numbness in your right leg/ foot?

Additional Words

hiku/hikimasu catch/pull
surimuku/ surimukimasu scrap
hikkaku/hikkakimasu scratch
kiru/kirimasu cut
haru/harimasu tighten/enlarge
tokoro place
tsuyoi strong
kaze cold
shokuji meals
guai condition
hidari left
te-no-kō back of one's hand

tsukareru/ tsukaremasu exhaust
hasamu/ hasamimasu pinch
kujiku/kujikimasu sprain
utsu/uchimasu hit
suku/sukimasu be hungry/become less crowded
geri diarrhea
kusuri medicine
yōsu appearance/looks
migi right
te-no-hira palm
kanō fester

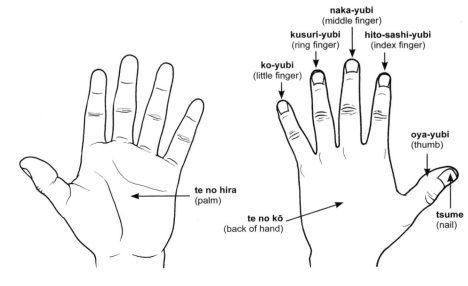

Te, Mae (Hands, Front)

Te, Ushiro (Hands, Back)

naka-yubi
(middle finger)

kusuri-yubi
(ring finger)

hito-sashi-yubi
(index finger)

ko-yubi
(little finger)

oya-yubi
(thumb)

te no hira
(palm)

te no kō
(back of hand)

tsume
(nail)

Language Notes

1. In Lesson 3, we saw how verbs with the present tense ending in -**masu** form the past tense by dropping -**masu** and replacing it with -**mashita**. The following are more examples of verbs that may have relevance in a healthcare setting.

uchi-masu	hit	**uchi-mashita**	hit
kiri-masu	cut	**kiri-mashita**	cut
sashi-masu	pierce	**sashi-mashita**	pierced
shibire-masu	numb	**shibire-mashita**	numbed
kanō shi-masu	fester	**kanō shimashita**	festered
hare-masu	swell	**hare-mashita**	swelled

2. Fingers are called **yubi** in Japanese. Literally, **oya-yubi** (thumb) means "parent finger"; **hito-sashi-yubi** (index finger) mean "pointer finger"; **naka-yubi** (middle finger) means "middle finger"; **kusuri-yubi** (ring finger) means "medicine finger"; and **ko-yubi** (little finger) means "baby finger." Traditionally, the ring finger was used to touch or pick medicines in ancient times. Therefore, the ring finger is called **kusuri-yubi** (medicine finger). A fist or clenched hand is called a **kobushi**.

3. Toes are called **tsumasaki**. The big toe is **ashi no oya-yubi**, the second toe **dai-ni-shi**, the third toe **dai-san-shi**, the fourth toe **dai-yon-shi**, and little toe **ko-yubi**. The word for "arch" is **tsuchi-fumazu** (literally, "not step on soil").

4. For the stomach area, the navel is called the **heso**, and the abdomen is **kafukubu**. The polite word for stomach is **onaka**, which means "inside, center." The informal word is **hara**.

Onaka ga itai(n) desu ka.	Do you have a stomachache?
Onaka ga sukimashita ka.	Are you hungry? (*lit.*, Is your stomach empty?)
Onaka ga peko-peko desu ka.	Are you hungry? (spoken language for children)

Peko-peko is an onomatopoetic expression for indicating hunger that is commonly used in ordinary speech.

5. There are many different kinds of expressions for pain. The following are ones used with the verb **shimasu/arimasu**, as in **Gekitsū ga shimasu ka**. "Do you have severe pain?"

geki-tsū	severe pain/excruciating pain
don-tsū	dull pain
attsū	pressing pain

The following nouns are used with verb **arimasu**, as in **Kafukubu ni tsuyoi itami ga arimasu**. "I have a sharp pain in my abdomen." and **Sasu itami ga arimasu ka**. "Do you have a piercing pain?"

surudoi itami	sharp pain
shitsukoi itami	persistent pain
jyuzoku-shita itami	continuous pain
sakeru-yōna itami	tearing pain
sasu itami	piercing pain
shiku-shiku suru itami	piercing pain
zukin to suru itmi	biting pain
zuki-zuki suru itami	throbbing pain
chiku-chiku suru itami	pricking pain

6. With respect to direction or orientation, the word for "right" is **migi** and "left" is **hidari**, and the word for "both directions" is **ryō**. The "right side" is **migi-gawa**, the "left side" is **hidari-gawa**, and the word for "both sides" is **ryō-gawa**. Directions are always placed in front of the noun. When **gawa** (side) is used to describe the body or parts of the body, use **no** between the direction/orientation and the noun for the body or part.

migi-me	right eye
hidari-me	left eye
migi-gawa no me	right side (of the) eye
migi-te	right hand
hidari-te	left hand
hidari-gawa no te	left side (of the) hand
ryō-me	both eyes
ryō-te	both hands
ryō-gawa no me	both sides of the eyes

7. The Japanese equivalents of the English words for location *here*, *there*, and *over there* require the particle **ni** (at). The relative distance is from the speaker's perspective. The polite forms are **ko-chira** (here), **so-chira** (there), **a-chira** (over there) and **do-chira** (where, who, which).

koko (here)	**soko** (there)	**asoko** (over there)	**doko** (where)
kochira	**sochira**	**achira**	**dochira**

Doko ni itami ga arimasu ka.	Where do you have pain?
Doko ni itami ga aru.	Where do you have pain? (informal)
Koko ni itami ga arimasu.	I have pain here.

Doko ga itai(n) desu ka.	Where do you have pain?
Doko ga itai.	Where do you have pain? (informal)
Dochira ga ita(n) desu ka.	Where do you have pain? (polite)
Koko ga itai(n) desu.	I have pain here.

Language Roots

The prefix **jyō-** (上) means "upper" and "above." It is also pronounced **ue/uwa.**

jyō-hanshin	upper body
jyō-wan-kin	brachial muscle
uwa ago	upper jaw
uwa mabuta	upper eyelid

Naka (中) means "inside, middle, center." The same character is also pronounced **chū,** in which case the meaning becomes "during."

se-naka	middle of back/upper back
naka-yubi	middle finger
gozen-chū	during the morning
shinsatsu-chū	during the medical examination
shujyutsu-chū	during the operation
kensa-chū	during the test

The prefix **ka-** (下) means "lower, below, under." The character is also pronounced **shita** and **ge.**

ka-hanshin	lower body
ka-fukubu	abdomen
waki no shita	armpit
shita ago	lower jaw
ge-ri	diarrhea

Culture Notes

Medical facilities and doctors in Japan

According to the Ministry of Health, Labor and Welfare (2008), the total number of medical facilities in Japan is about 175,000, including about 8,800 hospitals. The approximate number of beds in Japanese hospitals is 20–49 (14%), 50–99 (26%), 100–149 (16%), 150–199 (14%), 200–299 (13%), 300–399 (8.5%), 400–499 (4%),

500–599 (2%), 600–699 (1.4%), and 700–899 (1%). There are about 260,000 physicians in Japan (2.2 doctors per 1,000 in the population); dentists number 98,000; pharmacists 250,000; nurses and assistant nurses 125,000.

Heso-related expressions in Japanese

The Japanese language has many expressions related to **heso** (belly button). Navel fluff is called **heso no goma** (**goma** means "sesame"). The following are some examples in everyday speech.

> **Kanjya ga heso o magemashita.**
> The patient got cranky/became belligerent.

> **Sensei wa heso-kuri ga arimasu.**
> The doctor has secret savings.

> **Ano hito wa heso-guroi desu.**
> That person has an evil mind.

> **Kango-shi-san wa heso de ocha o wakashimasu.**
> That nurse is so funny.

> **Kanjya no heso ga yadogae suru.**
> The patient was convulsing with laughter. (*lit.*, The patient boils tea by the belly button = laughs until the belly hurts.)

> **Sensei wa heso o kanda.**
> The doctor bitterly regretted (it).

Comprehension

Answer the following questions.

1. Which of the following does NOT belong with the others?
   a. **Te**   b. **Te no hira**
   c. **Yubi**   d. **Ashi**

2. Which of the following could be used as a translation for "**Kizu ga kanō shimashita.**"
   a. My finger is swollen.   b. The wound has become infected.
   c. I hit my knee very hard. d. I scraped my hand.

3. Which of the following best completes the sentence below?
   Ashi ga (   ) masu ka.
   a. **Itai**   b. **Tokidoki**
   c. **Shibire**   d. **Itakunai**

4. Which statement is true?
    a. "Big toe" is **naka-yubi**.
    b. "Ring finger" is **kusuri-yubi**.
    c. "Middle finger" is **hitosashi-yubi**.
    d. "Little finger" is **oya-yubi**.

5. How do you pose a question about the symptom?
    a. **Don-na itami desu ka.**   b. **Don-na yōsu desuka.**
    c. **Don-na shōjyō desu ka.**   d. **Don-na onaka desuka.**

Select the correct meaning in Japanese.

---

6. Severe pain
    a. **attsū**   b. **dontsū**   c. **gekitsū**

7. Piercing pain
    a. **shitsukoi itami**   b. **sasu itami**   c. **tsuyoi itami**

8. Sharp pain
    a. **tsuyoi itami**   b. **zukizuki suru itami** c. **shitsukoi itami**

9. Tearing pain
    a. **attsū**   b. **dontsū**   c. **sakeru yoona itami**

10. Pressing pain
    a. **shitsukoi itami**   b. **attsū**   c. **chiku chiku suru itai**

Practice

Respond to the following in Japanese using the cues that have been provided.

1. Asking physical conditions.
    (Healthcare professional)   (Patient)
    1._____ (knee)   **Sukoshi hiza ga shibirete imasu.**
    2._____ (lower back) **Tokidoki koshi ga itai(n) desu.**
    3._____ (hand)   **Te ga harete imasu.**
    4._____ (ankle)   **Ashi-kubi ga harete imasu.**

2. Telling what kind of symptoms.
   (Patient)   (Healthcare professional)
   1. **Kakato ga itai(n) desu.** _____ (swelling)
   2. **Fukurahagi ga itai(n) dusu.** _____ (festering)
   3. **Oya-yubi ga itai(n) desu.** _____ (cutting)
   4. **Koshi ga itain(n) desu.** _____ (broken)

3. Confirming the nature of pains.
   (Patient)   (Healthcare professional)
   1. **Kakato ga itai(n) desu.** _____ (often)
   2. **Momo ga harete imasu.** _____ (always)
   3. **Kansetsu ga shibirete imasu.** _____ (once in a while)

4. How to say the following pains.
   (Questions)   (Healthcare professional)
   1. **Don-na itami desu ka.** _____ (severe pain)
   2. **Don-na shōjyō ga arimasu ka.** _____ (sharp pain)
   3. **Onaka ni don-na itami ga arimasu ka.** _____ (piercing pain)
   4. **Fukurahagi wa don-na guai desu ka.** _____ (dull pain)

5. Dialogue comprehension. Based on the dialogue, answer the following questions.
   1. **Suzuki-san wa doko ga itai(n) desu ka.** _____
   2. **Itsu kara itai(n) desu ka.** _____
   3. **Netsu ga arimasu ka.** _____
   4. **Don-na itami desu ka.** _____
   5. **Hokani itai tokoro ga arimasu ka.** _____

6. Free response questions.
   (Questions)   (Answers)
   1. **Doko-ka itai tokoro wa arimasu ka.** _____
   2. **Ashi wa harete imasu ka.** _____
   3. **Doko ga itai(n) desu ka.** _____
   4. **Kakato wa zenzen itaku nai desu ka.** _____
   5. **Koshi no chōshi wa dō desu ka.** _____

Exercises

1. Say the following body parts in Japanese.
   A. Elbow   _____
   B. Knee   _____

C. Calf _____

D. Arm _____

E. Wrist _____

F. Heel _____

2. Say the following expressions in Japanese.
    A. Did you bump your knee very hard? _____
    B. What kind of pain is it? _____
    C. Is it a piercing pain? _____
    D. Do you have pain anywhere else? _____
    E. Your finger is swollen. _____
    F. Where do you feel numbness? _____

3. Say the appropriate question (Q) for the answer (A).
    A. Q: _____. A: **Migi-ashi ga shibiremasu.**
    B. Q: _____. A: **Kusuri-yubi ga haremashita.**
    C. Q: _____. A: **Tekubi o itame mashitata.**
    D. Q: _____. A: **Hiza o uchimashita.**
    E. Q: _____. A: **Ude o surimukimashita.**

4. Say the following expressions in Japanese.
    A. Sharp pain _____
    B. Persistent pain _____
    C. Dull pain _____
    D. Throbbing pain _____
    E. Pricking pain _____

5. Say the NEGATIVE sentence by using the following words.
    A. I don't have pain in my abdomen at all.
       Zenzen (not at all) _____
    B. I hardly have any joint pain.
       Hotondo (hardly) _____
    C. I don't have much ankle pain.
       Amari (not much) _____
    D. You really do have pain, don't you?
       Hontōni (really) _____

Initial Medical Examination
(Shoshin)

Basic Vocabulary (CD 7-1)

Listen to the CD and repeat the vocabulary.

#	English	Rōmaji	Japanese
1.	weight	**taijyū**	体重
2.	weight scale	**taijyū-kei**	体重計
3.	height	**shinchō**	身長
4.	height scale	**shinchō-kei**	身長計
5.	temperature	**taion**	体温
6.	medical thermometer	**taion-kei**	体温計
7.	blood pressure	**ketsu-atsu**	血圧
8.	sphygmomanometer (blood pressure gauge)	**ketsu-atsu-kei**	血圧計
9.	oxygen	**sanso**	酸素
10.	oxygen mask	**sanso-masuku**	酸素マスク
11.	aspirator	**kyūin-ki**	吸引機
12.	IV drip	**tenteki**	点滴
13.	syringe	**chūsha-ki**	注射器
14.	stethoscope	**chōshin-ki**	聴診器
15.	pulse	**myaku/myaku-haku**	脈／脈拍
16.	feeling	**kibun**	気分
17.	exercise	**undō**	運動
18.	indigestion	**shōka-furyō**	消化不良
19.	nervousness	**shinkei-shitsu**	神経質
20.	tobacco/cigarette	**tabako**	煙草
21.	alcohol	**(o)sake**	お酒
22.	allergy	**arerugī**	アレルギー
23.	physical constitution	**taishitsu**	体質
24.	improvement of constitution	**taishitsu-kaizen**	体質改善
25.	coldness	**hie-shō**	冷え性
26.	period/menstruation	**seiri/gekkei**	生理/月経
27.	pregnant	**ninshin**	妊娠
28.	appetite	**shoku-yoku**	食欲
29.	fatigue	**hirō**	疲労
30.	weakness	**datsu-ryoku-kan**	脱力感

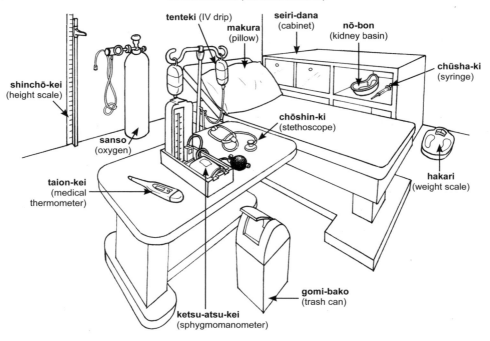

Shinsatsu-shitu (Examination Room)

tenteki (IV drip)

seiri-dana (cabinet)

makura (pillow)

nō-bon (kidney basin)

shinchō-kei (height scale)

chūsha-ki (syringe)

chōshin-ki (stethoscope)

sanso (oxygen)

hakari (weight scale)

taion-kei (medical thermometer)

gomi-bako (trash can)

ketsu-atsu-kei (sphygmomanometer)

Dialogue (CD 7-2)

Listen to the CD and repeat the dialogue.

In the Examination Room

Kris (nurse): **Kyō wa dō shimashita ka.**
Are you concerned about anything today?

Mr. Suzuki (patient): **Kinō kara onaka ga ita(n) desu.**
Since yesterday, I've had a stomachache.

Kris: **Dewa, taion to ketsuatsu o hakarimashō.**
Let me take your temperature and blood pressure.

Kuchi o ōkiku akete (kudasai).
Open your mouth wide.

Mr. Suzuki: **Hai, (onegai shimasu).**
Yes, please.

Kris: **Ketsu-atsu o (ketsuatsu-kei de) hakarimasu kara ude o misete kudasai.**
I will take your blood pressure (with the blood pressure gauge), so please show me your arm.

Geri o shite imasu ka.
Do you have diarrhea?

Mr. Suzuki: **Iie, geri wa shite imasen.**
No, I don't have diarrhea.

Kris: **Ima nani-ka kusuri o nonde imasu ka.**
Are you taking any medication now?

Mr. Suzuki: **Iie, nani mo nonde imasen.**
No, I am not taking any medication.

Grammar

1. The verb ending -mashō

The verb ending -**mashō** is a volitional form that translates as "let's" and expresses the speaker's invitation or suggestion to do something. To make the volitional form, drop the -**masu** ending and replace it with -**mashō**.

Taion o hakarimashō.	Let's take your temperature.
Taijyū o hakarimashō.	Let's measure your weight.
Shinchō o hakarimashō.	Let's measure your height.
Ketsuatsu o hakarimashō.	Let's take your blood pressure.
Myakuhaku o torimashō.	Let's take your pulse.
Chōshin-ki de mimashō.	Let's check you out (with the stethoscope).

2. The te-form + imashita expresses the past progressive tense.

The te-form plus **imashita** expresses a past progressive action. In English this is expressed by *was* + VERB-*ing*, as in "I was sleeping." Note, in the first two examples, that Japanese perceives having had diarrhea or having had a cold as an ongoing progessive action (in the past), whereas in English the simple past tense is more appropriate in these cases.

Geri o shite imashita.	I had diarrhea (*lit.*, I was having diarrhea.)
Kaze o hiite imashita.	I had a cold (*lit.*, I was having a cold.)
Kusuri o nonde imashita.	I was taking medicine.
Ketsuatsu o hakatte imashita.	I was taking (your, his, her) blood pressure.
Taijyū o hakatte imashita.	I was taking (his) weight.
Shinchō o hakatte imashita.	I was taking (her) height.
Taion o hakatte imashita.	I was taking (your) temperature.
Myaku(haku) o totte imashita.	I was taking (your) pulse.

3. The adverb **nani-ka**

The adverb **nani-ka** is used to express the idea of "something else" or "anything (else)?" in a question.

Nani-ka tabemasu ka.	Do you want to eat something?
Nani-ka nomimasu ka.	Do you want to drink anything?

4. **Nani-ka** + VERB **-te imasu ka**

The construction **nani-ka** plus VERB **-te imasu ka** is used to ask a question about the present progress of an action.

Nani-ka tabete imasu ka.	Are you eating something?
Nani-ka nonde imasu ka.	Are you drinking something?
Nani-ka kusuri o nonde imasu ka.	Are you taking any medicine?

5. The particle **to**

The particle **to** (and) is a conjunction for nouns and acts similar to *and* in English. However, it isn't used to join sentences.

Kango-shi to sensei ga imasu.	There are nurses and doctors.
Kaze to geri o shite imasu.	I have a cold and diarrhea.
Atama to kao to te to ashi ga itai(n) desu.	I have pain in my head, face, hands, and legs.

6. Three uses of the conjunction **kara**: NOUN + **kara**; NOUN + **desu/da-kara**; VERB + **kara**

The particle **kara** has three conjunctive forms: NOUN plus **kara**; NOUN plus **desu/da-kara**; VERB plus **kara**. In Lesson 4, we studied the construction NOUN plus **kara**. The following are additional usages that healthcare professionals may encounter.

A) NOUN + **kara** indicates a starting point or source, as expressed by the English *from*, *since*, *after*, *by means of*, and *out of*.

Hokenjyo wa ku-ji kara hajimarimasu.
The health center opens at 9 o'clock.

Hokenjyo kara byōin made ikimashita.
I went from the health center to the hospital.

Shinchō-kei kara shinchō ga wakarimasu.
We can measure your height by means of the height scale. (*lit.*, We understand your height by the height scale.)

B) NOUN + **desu/da-kara** indicates a reason or cause, as in the English *because*, *so*, and *since*. **-desu-kara** is formal; **-da-kara** is informal.

Sensei desu-kara yoku shitteimasu.   He knows well because he's a doctor.

Kyū-jyū hachi (98) -do desu-kara daijōbu desu.
It's 98 degrees, so you're all right.

Tenteki da-kara kowakunai(n) desu.   Since this is an IV drip, it's not scary.

C) VERB + **kara** also indicates a reason or cause, as in the English *so*, *since*, *after*, and *because*.

Fuku o nuide kara kensa o shimasu.
After you take off your clothes, we can examine you.

Kensa o shimashita kara fuku o kite kudasai.
Please put on your clothes, since we've finished examining you.

Taion o hakatta kara kensa o shimasen.
Because we took your temperature, we will not examine you.

Byō-shitsu (Hospital Room)

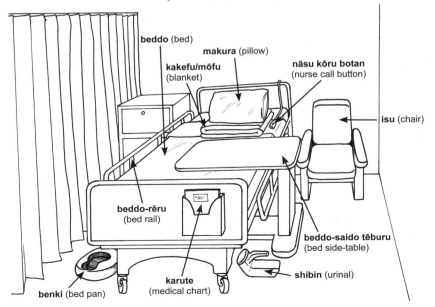

beddo (bed)

makura (pillow)

kakefu/mōfu
(blanket)

nāsu kōru botan
(nurse call button)

isu (chair)

beddo-rēru
(bed rail)

beddo-saido tēburu
(bed side-table)

shibin (urinal)

karute
(medical chart)

benki (bed pan)

Useful Expressions (CD 7-3)

Listen to the CD and repeat the sentences.

1. **Taion o hakarimashō.** Let's take your temperature.
2. **Myaku o torimashō.** Let's take your pulse.
3. **Nani-ka kusuri o nonde imasu ka.** Are you taking any medication?
4. **Tabako o suttte imasu ka.** Do you smoke?
5. **Arerugī ga arimasu ka.** Do you have any allergies?
6. **Seiri wa itsu deshita ka.** When was your last period?
7. **Geri o shite imashita ka.** Had you been having diarrhea?
8. **Kensa o shimashita ka.** Did you have an examination?
9. **Nani mo tabete imasen ka.** Are you sure you're not eating at all?
10. **Nani-ka nomimashita ka.** Did you drink anything?

Key Sentences (CD 7-4)

Listen to the CD and repeat the sentences.

1. **Taion o hakarimashō.** Let me take your temperature.
2. **Myaku to ketsuatsu o hakarimasu.** I will take your pulse and blood pressure.
3. **Tabako o sutte imasu ka.** Do you smoke?
4. **Geri wa itsu kara desu ka.** When did you start having diarrhea?
5. **Nani-ka tabemashita ka.** Did you eat something?

Additional Words

sū/suimasu smoke/inhale
hakari scale
kiro kilogram
guramu gram/g
inchi inch
shita low (location)
osoi slow (motion/speed)
hikui low (position)

haku/hakimasu vomit/exhale
pondo pound/lb.
onsu ounce/oz.
fīto feet
ue high (location)
hayai fast/speedy
takai high (position)
kakari-tsuke no i-sha/shuji-i
  personal/family doctor

Language Notes

1. In Lessons 3 and 5, we studied how to change from the **masu** form to the **te**-form. So far, we've seen only one rule for this. However, there are a total of

five rules for changing from the **masu** to **te**-form, depending on the verb base ending.

a) Drop -**masu** and replace it with -**te**:

ENGLISH	VERB BASE AND MASU FORM (-MASU)	TE-FORM (-TE)
do/play	shi-masu	shi-te
come, to wear clothes	ki-masu	ki-te
see/look/watch/check/examine	mi-masu	mi-te
show	mise masu	mise-te
eat	tabe-masu	tabe-te
lend	kashi-masu	kashi-te
turn on	tsuke-masu	tsuke-te
turn off/erase	keshi-masu	keshi-te
wake up	oki-masu	oki-te
push	oshi-masu	oshi-te
teach	oshie-masu	oshie-te
open (mouth, eye, door, window)	ake-masu	ake-te
close (door, window)	shime-masu	shime-te
close (mouth, eye, ear, hand, legs, book)	toji-masu	toji-te
stop/park	tome-masu	tome-te
turn on/put on	tuke-masu	tsuke-te
unfasten/remove	hazushi-masu	hazush-te
insert	ire-masu	ire-te
take out/get out	dashi-masu	dashi-te
sleep	ne-masu	ne-te
speak	hanashi-masu	hanashi-te
numb	shibire-masu	shibire-te
swell	hare-masu	hare-te
hurt	itame-masu	itame-te
broke	ore-masu	ore-te
come out/show up	de-masu	de-te
loosen	yurume-masu	yurume-te
begin	hajime-masu	hajime-te
hang up/put on	kake-masu	kake-te
tire	tsukare-masu	tsukare-te

b) Drop **-mi masu/-bi masu** and replace it with **-nde**:

ENGLISH	VERB BASE AND MASU FORM (-MASU)	TE-FORM (-TE)
drink	**nomi-masu**	**no-nde**
rest	**yasumi-masu**	**yasu-nde**
bite/chew	**kami-masu**	**ka-nde**
read	**yomi-masu**	**yo-nde**
pinch	**hasami-masu**	**hasa-nde**
call/invite	**yobi-masu**	**yo-nde**
tie	**musubi-masu**	**musu-nde**
tumble/fall down	**korobi-masu**	**koro-nde**

c) Drop **-ri masu**, **-chi masu**, **-i masu** and replace it with **-tte**:

ENGLISH	VERB BASE AND MASU FORM (-MASU)	TE-FORM (-TE)
measure	**hakari-masu**	**haka-tte**
cut	**kiri-masu**	**ki-tte**
cure/recover/heal	**naori-masu**	**nao-tte**
pay	**harai-masu**	**hara-tte**
cost/take	**kakari-masu**	**kaka-tte**
shave/bend backward	**sori-masu**	**so-tte**
scratch	**suri-masu**	**su-tte**
touch	**sawari-masu**	**sawa-tte**
bind	**shibari-masu**	**shiba-tte**
take	**tori-masu**	**to-tte**
shoot/hit	**uchi-masu**	**u-tte**
stand up	**tachi-masu**	**ta-tte**
wait	**machi-masu**	**ma-tte**
wash	**ariai-masu**	**ara-tte**
buy	**kai-masu**	**ka-tte**
smoke	**sui-masu**	**su-tte**
meet	**ai-masu**	**a-tte**
sew/stitch	**nui-masu**	**nu-tte**

d) drop -**ki masu** and replace it with -**ite**:

ENGLISH	VERB BASE AND MASU FORM (-MASU)	TE-FORM (-TE)
write	kaki-masu	ka-ite
listen	kiki-masu	ki-ite
pull	hiki-masu	hi-ite
vomit/to sweep	haki-masu	ha-ite
open space	aki-masu	a-ite
untie/to comb/to solve	toki-masu	to-ite
scratch	hikkaki-masu	hikka-ite
scrap	surimuki-masu	surimu-ite
sprain	kujiki-masu	kuji-ite
wear/put on (under belt)	haki-masu	ha-ite

e) drop -**gi masu** and replace it with -**ide**:

ENGLISH	VERB BASE AND MASU FORM (-MASU)	TE-FORM (-TE)
take off clothes	nugi-masu	nu-ide
swim	oyogi-masu	oyo-ide
smell	kagi-masu	ka-ide
peel off	hagi-masu	ha-ide

2. Japanese use the metric system. They express weight in kilograms and grams and are not familiar with pounds as a measure. Japanese patients will have an easier time understanding if healthcare professionals remember this and refer to the system they are familiar with. The following is a sample comparison chart.

1 lb. = 0.454 kg; 1 kg = 2.2 lb.; 1 oz. = 28.3 g; 1 lb. = 16 oz.

(kg)	(lb)	(kg)	(lb)	(kg)	(lb)	(kg)	(lb)	(kg)	(lb)	(kg)	(lb)	(kg)	(lb)	(kg)	(lb)
1	2	11	24	21	46	31	68	41	91	51	113	61	135	71	156
2	4	12	26	22	49	32	71	42	93	52	115	62	137	72	158
3	7	13	29	23	51	33	73	43	95	53	117	63	139	73	160
4	9	14	31	24	53	34	75	44	97	54	119	64	141	74	162
5	11	15	33	25	55	35	77	45	99	55	121	65	143	75	164

(kg)	(lb)	(kg)	(lb)	(kg)	(lb)	(kg)	(lb)	(kg)	(lb)	(kg)	(lb)	(kg)	(lb)	(kg)	(lb)
6	13	16	35	26	58	36	79	46	102	56	124	66	146	76	166
7	15	17	38	27	60	37	82	47	104	57	126	67	148	77	170
8	18	18	40	28	62	38	84	48	106	58	128	68	150	78	172
9	20	19	42	29	64	39	86	49	108	59	130	69	152	79	174
10	22	20	44	30	66	40	88	50	110	60	132	70	154	80	177

3. Similarly, to measure height, Japanese use meters and centimeters. The following is a sample comparison chart:

1 ft. = 12 in. = 30.48 cm; 1 in =2.54 cm

cm	feet inch	cm	feet inch	cm	feet inch	cm	feet inch	cm	feet inch	cm	feet inch	cm	feet inch	cm	feet inch
101	3'4"	111	3'8"	121	4'0"	131	4'4"	141	4'8"	151	4'11"	161	5'3"	171	5'7"
102	3'4"	112	3'8"	122	4'0"	132	4'4"	142	4'8"	152	5'0"	162	5'4"	172	5'8"
103	3'5"	113	3'9"	123	4'1"	133	4'5"	143	4'9"	153	5'0"	163	5'4"	173	5'8"
104	3'5"	114	3'9"	124	4'1"	134	4'5"	144	4'9"	154	5'1"	164	5'5"	174	5'8"
105	3'6"	115	3'9"	125	4'2"	135	4'6"	145	4'9"	155	5'1"	165	5'5"	175	5'9"
106	3'6"	116	3'10"	126	4'2"	136	4'6"	146	4'9"	156	5'1"	166	5'5"	176	5'9"
107	3'6"	117	3'10"	127	4'2"	137	4'6"	147	4'10"	157	5'2"	167	5'6"	177	5'10"
108	3'7"	118	3'11"	128	4'3"	138	4'7"	148	4'10"	158	5'2"	168	5'6"	178	5'10"
109	3'7"	119	3'11"	129	4'3"	139	4'7"	149	4'11"	159	5'3"	169	5'6"	179	5'10"
110	3'8"	120	3'11"	130	4'4"	140	4'7"	150	4'11"	160	5'3"	170	5'7"	180	5'11"

4. In measuring blood pressure, Japanese express "high" as **ue** and "low" as **shita**, as in **Ketsuatsu no ue wa 110 desu**. "The blood pressure high is 110." When saying or joining two sentences with **desu**, Japanese drop the -**su** of the first **desu** and the second subject, as shown in the examples below:

Ketsuatsu no ue wa 110 desu. Ketsuatsu no shita wa 80 desu.
The blood pressure high is 110, and blood pressure low is 80.

Ketsuatsu no ue wa 110 de (su. Ketsuatsu no) shita wa 80 desu.
Ketsuatsu no ue wa 110 de, shita wa 80 desu.
(Your) blood pressure is 110 over 80.

5. General questions for the initial medical examination:

Osake o nomimasu ka.	Do you drink liquor?
Tabako o suimasu ka.	Do you smoke?
Undō o shimasu ka.	Do you exercise?
Kibun wa dōdesu ka.	How do you feel?
Kibun ga warui desu ka.	Do you feel bad?
Kibun ga ii desu ka.	Do you feel good?
Kuruma no unten o shimasu ka.	Do you drive?
Kakari-tsuke no i-sha wa dare desu ka.	Who is your family/regular doctor?

Language Roots

Kei (計) indicates a measurement, measuring device, or plan.

taion-kei	medical thermometer
taijyū-kei	weight scale
ketsuatsu-kei	sphygmomanometer or blood pressure gauge
kai-kei	account
gō-kei	total
ondo-kei	thermometer

The suffix **-ki** (器) indicates a device, instrument, or container. A different word **-ki** (機) with same pronunciation means "machine."

chūsha-ki	syringe
chōshin-ki	stethoscope
ben-ki	bedpan, chamber pot
kyūin-ki	aspirator
hikō-ki	airplanes
sōji-ki	vacuum cleaner

Culture Notes

Pulmonary tuberculosis in Japan

Pulmonary tuberculosis was the main cause of death in Japan from the1870s to the 1940s. It caused over 100,000 deaths each year, but now more people die from cancer. Currently, tuberculosis infects about 25,000 people each year (50 percent of the infections are over 70 and 25 percent are under 40), and over 2,000 people die from the disease. All Japanese are required to have a BCG (Bacille de Calmette-Guerin) injection within six months of birth. For that reason, if Japanese are administered the tuberculosis skin test in the United States, most show a positive result. However, if they subsequently have an X ray, the result is negative in most cases. (SOURCE: Research Institute of Tuberculosis, Japan Anti-tuberculosis Association).

Health-related Japanese proverbs I

Laughter brings good luck.
Warau kado ni fuku kitaru.
笑う門に福来たる

Doctors not taking care of themselves
(Note the similarity to: Physician, heal thyself.)
Isha no fuyō-jyō.
医者の不養生

Comprehension

Answer the following questions.

1. Which of the following words do NOT use **hakarimasu**?
    a. **Ketsu-atsu**   b. **Myaku-haku**
    c. **Shinchō**   d. **Taijyū**

2. Which of the following could be a translation of "**Geri o shite imasu ka?**"
    a. Are you having your period? b. Do you have an appointment?
    c. Do you have an appetite?   d. Do you have diarrhea?

3. Which of the following best completes the sentence below?
    Taijyū (   ) hakari mashō.
    a. **wa**   b. **ga**
    c. **ni**   d. **o**

4. Which statement is true?
    a. Japanese use pounds.   b. Japanese use kilograms.
    c. Japanese use inches.   d. Japanese use feet.

5. How do you say, "Are you taking any medicine?"
    a. **Nani-ka kusuri o torimasu ka.**
    b. **Nani-ka kusuri o nonde imasu ka.**
    c. **Nani-ka kusuri o nomimasu ka.**
    d. **Nani-ka kusuri o totteimasu ka.**

Select an appropriate **te**-form.

---

6. **Nomi-masu**
   a. **no-mite**   b. **no-nde**
   c. **no-tte**   d. **no-ite**

7. **Mi-masu**
   a. **mi-te**   b. **mi-nde**
   c. **mi-ite**   d. **mi-tte**

8. **Hakari masu**
   a. **haka-ite**   b. **haka-te**
   c. **haka-tte**   d. **haka-nde**

9. **Kiki masu**
   a. **ki-te**   b. **ki-nde**
   c. **ki-tte**   d. **ki-ite**

10. **Nugi masu**
    a. **nu-nde**   b. **nu-tte**
    c. **nugi-te**   d. **nu-ide**

Practice

Respond to the following in Japanese using the cues that have been provided.

---

1. Asking about physical conditions.
   (Healthcare professional)   (Patient)
   1. _____ (diarrhea)   **Sukoshi, geri desu.**
   2. _____ (temperature)   **Netsu wa arimasen.**
   3. _____ (take medicine)   **Hai, nonde imasu.**
   4. _____ (height)   **170 cm desu.**

2. Asking about physical conditions.
   (Patient)   (Healthcare professional)
   1. No appetite   _____
   2. No periods   _____
   3. Coldness   _____
   4. Fatigue   _____

3. Change the verb to the present progressive tense.
   (Present tense)   (Present progressive tense)
   1. **Myaku o torimasu.**   _____
   2. **Ketsu-atsu o hakarimasu.**   _____
   3. **Ninshin o kensa shimasu.**   _____

4. Taking blood pressure and reading the blood pressure values.
   (Questions)   (Healthcare professional)
   1. The high is 120, low is 80   **Ue wa _____ de, shita wa _____ desu.**
   2. The high is 105, low is 70   **Ue wa _____ de, shita wa _____ desu.**
   3. The high is 133, low is 65   **Ue wa _____ de, shita wa _____ desu.**
   4. The high is 154, low is 58   **Ue wa _____ de, shita wa _____ desu.**

5. Dialogue comprehension. Based on the dialogue, answer the following questions.
   1. **Suzuki-san wa doko ga itai(n) desu ka.** _____
   2. **Itsu kara itai(n) desu ka.** _____
   3. **Suzuki-san wa nani o kensa shimasu ka.** _____
   4. **Geri o shite imasu ka.** _____
   5. **Nani-ka kusuri o nonde imasu ka.** _____

6. Free response questions.
   (Questions)   (Answers)
   1. **Taijyū o hakatta koto ga arimasu ka.** _____
   2. **Taijyū wa nan-kiro desu ka.** _____
   3. **Shinchō wa nan-senchi desu ka.** _____
   4. **Ketsuatsu wa ikutsu desu ka.** _____
   5. **Nani-ka kusuri o nonde imasu ka.** _____

Exercises

1. Say the following words in Japanese.
   A. Weight   _____
   B. Height   _____
   C. Temperature   _____
   D. Blood pressure _____
   E. Pulse   _____

2. Ask the following questions in Japanese.
   A. Are you taking any medicine?   _____
   B. Shall we take your temperature? _____

C. Shall we take your pulse? _____

D. Do you smoke? _____

E. Do you have any allergies? _____

3. Take part in the following conversation.

Healthcare practitioner (H): **Dō shimashita ka.**
Patient (P): **Sumimasen, atama ga ita(n) desu. Netsu mo sukoshi arimasu.**

H: A) _____ (When did it start?)
P: **Kinō kara desu.**

H: B) _____ (Open your mouth.)
P: **Hai, onegai shimasu.**

H: **40.5 do desu. Tottemo netsu ga arimasu ne.**
P: **Ee, chotto karada ga furuete imasu.**

4. Read the following numbers in Japanese.
   Ex. The weight is 132 lbs., equals 60 kilograms. (**Taijyū wa 132 pondo de, 60 kiroguramu desu.**)

A. Weight	112 lbs.	= 50 kg
B. Height	5 ft. 7 in.	= 170 cm
C. Temperature	98.6 degrees	= 37 degrees
D. Blood pressure	110/78	

Signs & Symptoms I
(Shōjyō)

Basic Vocabulary (CD 8-1)

Listen to the CD and repeat the vocabulary.

1.	cough	**seki**	咳
2.	phlegm	**tan**	痰
3.	headache	**zu-tsū**	頭痛
4.	stiff shoulder	**kata-kori**	肩こり
5.	eczema	**shisshin**	湿疹
6.	runny nose/nasal mucus	**hana-mizu**	鼻水
7.	tonsillitis	**hentōsen-en**	扁桃腺炎
8.	sneeze	**kushami**	くしゃみ
9.	hiccup	**shakkuri**	しゃっくり
10.	nausea	**hakike**	吐き気
11.	belching	**geppu**	げっぷ
12.	discomfort	**fukai(kan)**	不快感
13.	anorexia/loss of appetite	**shoku-yoku fushin**	食欲不振
14.	diarrhea	**geri**	下痢
15.	constipation	**benpi**	便秘
16.	vomiting	**ōto**	嘔吐
17.	tinnitus/ringing or buzzing in the ears	**mimi-nari**	耳鳴り
18.	bleeding	**shu-kketsu**	出血
19.	nosebleeds	**hana-ji**	鼻血
20.	bloody stool	**ketsu-ben**	血便
21.	bloody urine	**ketsu-nyō**	血尿
22.	bloody phlegm	**ke-ttan**	血痰
23.	lung hemorrhage	**kakketsu**	喀血
24.	anemia	**hin-ketsu**	貧血
25.	wound	**kizu**	傷
26.	burn	**yakedo**	火傷
27.	inflammation	**enshō/-en**	炎症/炎
28.	eruption	**fuki-demono**	吹き出物
29.	rash/exanthema	**hasshin**	発疹
30.	obesity	**himan(shō)**	肥満(症)

Dialogue (CD 8-2)

Listen to the CD and repeat the dialogue.

In the Consultation Room

| Kris (nurse): | **Suzuki-san, dō shimashita ka.** |
| | Is anything the matter, Mr. Suzuki? |

| Mr. Suzuki (patient): | **Saikin, miminari ga suru(n) desu.** |
| | Recently, my ears have been ringing. |

| | **Soshite, netsu-ppoi(n) desu.** |
| | And I have a somewhat low-grade fever. |

| | **Sorekara, hinketsu-gimi desu.** |
| | And I also feel anemic. |

| Kris: | **Shōjyō wa itsu kara desu ka.** |
| | When did the symptoms begin? |

| Mr. Suzuki: | **Kinō kara dato omoimasu.** |
| | I think they started yesterday. |

| Kris: | **Hoka-ni nani-ka shōjyō ga arimasu ka.** |
| | Do you have any other symptoms? |

| Mr. Suzuki: | **Hai, geri o shite, koko ni shisshin ga arimasu.** |
| | Yes, I have diarrhea and a skin rash here. |

| Kris: | **Geri wa itsu kara desu ka.** |
| | When did the diarrhea begin? |

| Mr. Suzuki: | **Mikka mae kara desu.** |
| | It started three days ago. |

Grammar

1. Connecting two sentences using the **te**-form

   To join two sentences, the verb in the first sentence must be changed to the **te**-form, which translates as "and."

Geri o shimasu. Onaka ga itai(n) desu.	I have diarrhea. My stomach is sore.
Geri o shite, onakaga itai(n) desu.	I have diarrhea, and my stomach is sore.
Miminari ga shimasu. Hinketsu desu.	My ear is ringing. I feel anemic.
Miminari ga shite, hinketsu desu.	My ear is ringing, and I feel anemic.

Seki ga demasu. Tan mo demasu.	I have a cough. I have phlegm.
Seki ga dete tan mo demasu.	I have a cough and phlegm.

2. The suffix **-ppoi**

The suffix **-ppoi** emphasizes some distinctive feature or characteristic, or an attribute identified by a noun, adjective, or verb to which the suffix is attached. It may be translated as "tend to; somewhat *or* somehow; look like; apt to; easy to; -ish; *or* -like."

Sukoshi, netsu-ppoi(n) desu.	I'm feeling somewhat feverish.
Kanjya-ppoi desu ka.	Do I look like a patient?
Otoko-ppoi desu ne.	You are boyish, aren't you?
Kodomo-ppoi desu.	You are childish.
Iro-ppoi desu.	You are sexy.

3. The suffix **-gimi**

The suffix **-gimi** means "feel (like)." It can sometimes be replaced by the suffixes **-gachi** (apt to/likely), **(no)yōna** (kind of/sort of), or **-rashii** (seem/just like).

Kaze-gimi desu.	I feel like I have a cold.
Tsukare-gimi desu.	I feel like I'm always tired.
Benpi-gimi desu.	I feel like I'm constipated.
Hinketsu-gimi desu.	I feel anemic.
Shokuyoku fushin-gachi desu ka.	Are you feeling a loss of appetite?

4. The time expressions **saikin**, **chikagoro**, and **konogoro**

Japanese has three expressions for the recent past, **saikin** (recently), **chikagoro** (lately), and **konogoro** (these days), which can be used to express recent health conditions.

Saikin yoku shakkuri ga demasu.	Recently, I have been hiccupping a lot.
Chikagoro hakike o kanjimasu ka.	Are you feeling nauseous lately?
Konogoro yoku tan ga demasu.	I often have phlegm these days.

5. The conjunctions **soshite**, **sorekara**, **shikashi**, and **demo**

The conjunction **soshite** means "and." **Sorekara** means "and then." **Shikashi** is a formal word for "but," while **demo** is informal.

Soshite, kushami mo demasu ka.
And are you sneezing, too?

Shikashi, (anata wa) ōto ga tsuzuite imasu.
But you are still continuing to vomit.

6. The location words **ko-so-a-do**

In Lesson 4, we studied the location words **koko** (here/this place), **soko** (there/that place), **asoko** (over there/that place over there), and **doko** (where), along with the corresponding polite forms **kochira, sochira, achira,** and **dochira.** The demonstrative pronouns **kore, sore,** and **are** designate objects with reference to location. **Kore** refers to objects near the speaker, **sore** to objects a little farther away, and are to object the farthest away. Study the following chart.

LOCATION/PLACE	SUBJECT (PRONOUN)	PRE-NOUN ADJECTIVE
koko (here)	**kore** (this one)	**kono** (this)
soko (there)	**sore** (that one)	**sono** (that)
asoko (over there)	**are** (that one over there)	**ano** (that over there)
doko (where)	**dore** (which one)	**dono** (which)
dochira (where) polite	**dochira** (which one) polite	**dochira no** (which) polite

Kono yakedo wa itsu dekimashita ka.   When did this burn happen?
Sono kizu wa dō shimashita ka.   What happened to that wound?
Dono fuki-demono ga itai(n) desu ka.   Which eruptions are painful?
Dochira no kizu ga itai(n) desu ka.   Which wounds hurt?

7. An interrogative followed by **ka** makes an adverb meaning "some."

An interrogative followed by **ka** forms an adverb and changes the meaning of both words: **nani-ka** (some, something), **dare-ka** (someone), **itsu-ka** (sometimes), **dore-ka** (one of them), and **doko-ka** (somewhere).

Nani-ka mondai no toki wa renraku shite kudasai.
If you have some problems, please inform us.

Dare-ka shōkai-sha wa imasu ka.
Do you have someone who is a reference?

Itsu-ka itami ga deru to omoimasu.
I think you may be in pain sometimes. (*lit.*, I think pain is coming out sometime.)

Useful Expressions (CD 8-3)

Listen to the CD and repeat the sentences.

1. **Nani-ka shōjyō wa arimasu ka.** Do you have any symptoms?
2. **Kibun ga warui(n) desu.** I feel bad.
3. **Seki ga deru(n) desu.** I have a cough.
4. **Zutsū ga arimasu ka.** Do you have a headache?
5. **Memai ga shimasu.** I have some dizziness./I feel dizzy.
6. **Benpi o shite imasu ka.** Have you been constipated?
7. **Hana-mizu ga demasu. Soshite, memai ga shimasu.** I have a runny nose. And I feel dizzy.
8. **Hana-mizu ga dete, memai ga shimasu.** I have a runny nose and dizziness.
9. **Hoka ni nani-ka shōjyō wa arimasu ka.** Do you have any other symptoms?
10. **Koko ni fuki-demono ga arimasu.** I/You have an eruption here.

Key Sentences (CD 8-4)

Listen to the CD and repeat the sentences.

1. **Nani-ka fukai-kan ga arimasu ka.** Do you have any discomfort?
2. **Shisshin ga arimasu ka.** Do you have eczema?
3. **Hinketsu gimi desu.** I feel slightly anemic.
4. **Itsu geri ga hajimari mashita ka.** When did the diarrhea begin?
5. **Hokani nani-ka shōjyō ga arimasu ka.** Do you have any other symptoms?

Additional Words

atsui hot	**samui** cold	**ketsu-eki** blood
chi blood	**saikin** recently	**chikagoro** lately
konogoro these days	**shoshite** and	**shikashi** but/however
sorekara and then	**demo** but (informal)	**iro** color
iro-ppoi sexy	**mondai** problem	**(o)tomodachi** friend
hoka other	**mae** ago/before/front	**ato** later/behind
ōkī big	**chīsai** small	**surudoi** sharp
nibui dull	**gen-in** cause	**kekka** result
hedo spew	**tsuba(ki)** spit	**kabure** skin irritation

hirogaru/hirogarimasu spread **omou/omoimasu** think
sasu/sashimasu point out/pierce/sting **hajimaru/hajimarimasu** begin

Language Notes

1. The adverbs of duration **mae kara/mae ni** are the equivalent of *since*, *for*, *ago*, *before*, or *in the past* in English.

   Ni-shū-kan mae kara, hana-mizu ga dete imashita.
   I have had a runny nose for two weeks. (*lit.*, I have had a runny nose since two weeks ago.)

   San shū kan mae ni, te ni yakedo o shimashita.
   I burned my hand three weeks ago.

	DAY AGO	WEEK AGO	MONTH AGO	YEAR AGO
1	kinō	i sshū kan mae	i kka getsu mae*	ichi nen mae
2	futsu-ka mae	ni shū kan mae	ni ka getsu mae*	ni nen mae
3	mikka mae	san shū kan mae	san ka getsu mae	san nen mae
4	yokka mae	yon shū kan mae	yon ka getsu mae	yo nen mae
5	itsuka mae	go shū kan mae	go ka getsu mae	go nen mae
6	muika mae	roku shū kan mae	ro kka getsu mae	roku nen mae
7	nanoka mae	nana shū kan mae	nana ka getsu mae	nana nen mae
8	yōka mae	ha shū kan mae	ha kka getsu mae	hachi nen mae
9	kokonoka mae	kyū shū kan mae	kyū ka getsu mae	kyū nen mae
10	tōka mae	jyu shū kan mae	jyu ka getsu mae	jyū nen mae

   * There are also the expressions **hito tsuki mae** (one month ago) and **futa tsuki mae** (two months ago).

2. Several polite commands or requests are very useful in healthcare situations: **Misete kudasai** means "Please show me"; **Akete kudasai** mean "Please open"; and **Tojite kudasai** means "Please close." These requests usually take the object marker **o**.

Shita o misete kudasai.	Please show me your tongue.
Mimi o misete kudasai.	Please show me your ear.
Kuchi o akete kudasai.	Please open your mouth.
Me o akete kudasai.	Please open your eye.
Kuchi o tojite kudasai.	Please close your mouth.
Me o tojite kudasai.	Please close your eye.

3. Japanese express color (**iro**) as follows:

black	**kuro(i)**	brown	**chairo(i)**	pink	**momo-iro**
white	**shiro(i)**	gold	**kin -iro**	orange	**mikan-iro**
blue	**ao(i)**	silver	**gin-iro**	light Blue	**mizu-iro**

red	aka(i)	green	midori-iro	gray	hai-iro
yellow	kiiro(i)	purple	murasaki-iro	colorless	tōmei

The Japanese language has six colors with **i**-adjective endings: **kuroi** (black), **shiroi** (white), **aoi** (blue), **akai** (red), **kiiroi** (yellow), and **chairoi** (brown). These words can modify a noun directly, as in **kuroi ketsu-ben** (black bloody stool). Another way to modify a noun is to use the particle **no**, which is equivalent to English *of* or *'s*, as in **kuro no ketsu-ben** (black bloody stool); **tōmei no hana-mizu** (clear runny nose)

The suffix **-ppoi** (-like) can be used to convey color as well: **kuro-ppoi** (black-like, blackish); **shiro-ppoi** (whitish). **Iro** can mean both "color" and "sex." As we have seen, **iro-ppoi** means "sexy."

4. Questions to elicit symptoms.

Doko ga itami masu ka.	Where do you feel the pain?
Yubi de sashite kudasai.	Please indicate with your finger.
Itami wa hirogari-masu ka.	Is the pain spreading?
Itai tokoro wa ōkii desu ka.	Is the area large?
[Itai tokoro wa] chiisai desu ka.	(Is the area) small?
Itami wa hoka no hō e ikimasu ka.	Does the pain go anywhere (else)?
Itami wa surudoi desu ka, nibui desu ka.	Is it a sharp or dull pain?

Language Roots

Chi (血) means "blood" and can be used as either a prefix or a suffix. **Chi** may also be pronounced **ji** or **ketsu**.

hana-ji	nosebleeds	**ji-ketsu**	hemorrhoids
shu-ketsu	bleeding	**ketsu-ben**	bloody stool
ketsu-nyō	bloody urine		

Eki (液) is used for liquids or fluids.

ketsu-eki	blood	**chūsha-eki**	injection
eki-tai	liquid	**da-eki**	saliva

Culture Notes

Atopy and allergies in Japan

In the past twenty years, atopy or allergies have become very common and a serious problem among Japanese children, who suffer from allergic symptoms such as skin disorders and asthma. Sometimes, children cannot even sleep at night because of severe itching. Current medical expertise has been unable to determine the root causes of this atopy, which can include a mixture of allergies to foods, household dust, air pollution, and so on.

Five different levels of feeling sick

Japanese patients often express their feeling of sickness in terms of several levels or degrees of discomfort. Healthcare professionals may recognize the following complaints, starting with the most severe:

Kibun ga totte mo warui(n) desu.	I feel very bad.
Kibun ga warui(n) desu.	I feel bad.
Kibun ga sukoshi warui(n) desu.	I feel a little/kind of bad.
Kibun ga yoku-nai(n) desu.	I don't feel well.
Kibun wa amari yoku-nai(n) desu.	I don't feel very well/too well.

In Japanese, the particle **ga** usually emphasizes the subject, while the particle **wa** places less emphasis on the subject and more on the object.

Comprehension

Answer the following questions.

1. Which of the following does NOT belong with the others?
    a. **Shukketsu**   b. **Nana-ji**
    c. **Ketsu-ben**   d. **Hin-ketsu**

2. Which of the following could be used to ask, "Do you have any other symptoms?"
    a. **Hoka ni nanika shōjyo wa arimasu ka.**
    b. **Koko ni shisshin ga arimasu ka.**
    c. **Koko ni kaikei ga arimasu ka.**
    d. **Hoka ni byōki ga arimasu ka.**

3. Which of the following best completes the sentence below?
    Ketsu-nyō ga (   ), kibun ga warui desu.
    a. **shite**   b. **dete**
    c. **mite**   d. **kite**

4. Which of the following is NOT a correct Japanese expression?
    a. **Shita o misete kudasai.**   b. **Kuchi o akete kudasai.**
    c. **Hakike ga shimasu ka.**   d. **Himan o torimasu ka.**

5. Use one of the following to ask when the symptom began.
   a. **Doko kara desu ka.**   b. **Dare kara desu ka.**
   c. **Itsu kara desu ka.**   d. **Naze desu ka.**

Select the correct expressions in Japanese.

---

6. 3 days ago
   a. **futsuka mae**   b. **yokka mae**   c. **mikka mae**

7. 5 days ago
   a. **itsuka ame**   b. **nanoka mae**   c. **yōka mae**

8. 2 weeks ago
   a. **yon-shū-kan ame**   b. **ni-shū-kan mae**   c. **san-shū-kan mae**

9. 4 months ago
   a. **ro-kka-getsu mae**   b. **ha-ka-getsu mae**   c. **yon-ka-getsu mae**

10. 5 years ago
    a. **go-nen mae**   b. **kyū-nen mae**   c. **ichi-nen mae**

Practice

Respond to the following in Japanese using the cues that have been provided.

---

1. Asking physical conditions:
   (Healthcare professional)   (Patient)
   1. _____ (nosebleeds)   **Sukoshi demasu.**
   2. _____ (bloody phlegm)   **Zenzen demasen.**
   3. _____ (bloody urine)   **Tokidoki demasu.**
   4. _____ (bloody stool)   **Wakarimasen.**

2. Asking when the symptom first began.
   (Patient)   (Healthcare professional)
   1. **Shoku-yoku ga arimasen.**
                                      _____
                                      (When did your anorexia start?)
   2. **Benpi-gimi desu.**
                                      _____
                                      (When did your constipation start?)
   3. **Shukketsu shite imasu.**
                                      _____
                                      (When did your bleeding start?)
   4. **Hasshin ga kayui(n) desu.**
                                      _____
                                      (When did your rash appear?)

3. Asking about a symptom.
    (Patient)   (Healthcare professional)
    1. **Fuki-demono ga arimasu.**
    _____
    (Tell me about your eruption.)
    2. **Yakedo ga arimasu.**
    _____
    (Tell me about your burn.)
    3. **Shisshin ga arimasu.**
    _____
    (Tell me about your eczema.)

4. How do you say the following points in time?
    (Questions)   (Healthcare professional)
    1. **Itsu kara hakike ga shimasu ka.**   _____ (two days ago)
    2. **Itsu kara ōto o shite imasu ka.**   _____ (three days ago)
    3. **Kono shisshin wa itsu kara desu ka.**   _____ (one week ago)
    4. **Kono kizu wa itsu kara desu ka.**   _____ (one month ago)

5. Dialogue comprehension. Based on the dialogue, answer the following questions.
    1. **Suzuki-san wa miminari ga shimasu ka.**   _____
    2. **Suzuki-san wa netsu ga arimasu ka.**   _____
    3. **Suzuki-san no miminari wa itsu kara desu ka.** _____
    4. **Kanjya-san wa benpi o shite imasu ka.**   _____
    5. **Geri wa itsu kara desu ka.**   _____

6. Free response questions.
    (Colleague)   (Answers)
    1. **Saikin himan gimi desu ka.**   _____
    2. **Chikagoro hinketsu gimi desu ka.**   _____
    3. **Konogoro dare-ka (o)tomodachi wa imasu ka.**_____
    4. **Kyō wa netsu ga arimasu ka.**   _____
    5. **Hokani nani-ka shōjyō wa arimasu ka.**   _____

Exercises

1. Say the following words in Japanese.
    A. Nausea   _____
    B. Tinnitus   _____
    C. Headache   _____
    D. Cough   _____
    E. Phlegm   _____

2. Ask the following questions in Japanese.
    A. Do you have any symptoms?   _____
    B. Do you have a headache?   _____
    C. Do you have constipation?   _____
    D. Do you have bloody urine?   _____
    E. Do you have any other symptoms?   _____

3. How do you say the following in Japanese?
    A. I have tinnitus, and I feel discomfort.   _____
    B. I have diarrhea, and I have a stomachache. _____
    C. I feel constipated.   _____
    D. I feel anemic.   _____
    E. When did the diarrhea begin?   _____

4. Respond to the following questions.

    Q. **Geri wa itsu kara desu ka.**
    A. _____ (one week ago)

    Q. **Benpi wa itsu kara desu ka.**
    B. _____ (since yesterday)

5. Ask the questions in Japanese.

    Q: _____ (When did your bleeding begin?)
    A: **Yokka mae kara desu.** (It started four days ago.)

    Q: _____ (When did your bloody urine begin?)
    A: **Itsu-ka mae kara desu.** (It started five days ago.)

LESSON 9 Signs & Symptoms II
(Shōjyō)

Basic Vocabulary (CD 9-1)

Listen to the CD and repeat the vocabulary.

1.	boil	**odeki**	おでき
2.	puffy	**muku-mi**	浮腫み
3.	pimple	**nikibi**	にきび
4.	facial furuncle	**menchō**	面疔
5.	chill	**samu-ke**	寒気
6.	migraine	**hen-zutsū**	偏頭痛
7.	stuffed nose	**hana-zumari**	鼻詰り
8.	whiplash	**muchi-uchi-shō**	むち打ち症
9.	bruising/bruise	**uchi-mi**	打身
10.	joint pain	**kansetsu-tsū**	関節痛
11.	muscular pain/myalgia	**kin-niku-tsū**	筋肉痛
12.	lower back pain/lumbago	**yō-tsū**	腰痛
13.	chest pain	**kyō-tsū**	胸痛
14.	back pain	**haibu-tsū**	背部痛
15.	jaundice	**ōdan**	黄疸
16.	shortness of breath	**iki-gire**	息切れ
17.	shaking	**furue**	震え
18.	heartburn	**mune-yake**	胸焼け
19.	attack	**hossa**	発作
20.	lump	**shikori**	しこり
21.	palpitation	**dōki**	動悸
22.	hard to breath	**iki-gurushii**	息苦しい
23.	stomachache	**fuku-tsū**	腹痛
24.	menstrual pain	**seiri-tsū**	生理痛
25.	giddiness/light-headedness	**tachi-kurami**	立眩み
26.	fester	**kanō**	化膿
27.	hot flash	**nobose**	のぼせ
28.	dizziness	**memai**	眩暈
29.	cramps	**keiren**	痙攣
30.	numbness	**shibire**	痺れ

Dialogue (CD 9-2)

Listen to the CD and repeat the dialogue.

In the Examination Room with the Doctor

Dr. Simon (male doctor): **Kyō wa don-na shojyō desu ka.**
What symptoms do you have today?

Mrs. Tanaka (patient): **Ikigire to dōki ga shimasu. Soshite, chotto iki-gurushii(n) desu.**
I have shortness of breath and palpitations. And it is hard to breathe.

Dr. Simon: **Taihen-sō desu ne. Sono-yōna shojyō ga deta nowa itsu deshita ka.**
You are having difficulty aren't you? How long have you had these symptoms?

Mrs. Tanaka: **Kinō kara desu.**
Since yesterday.

Dr. Simon: **Yoku, onaji yōna shōjyō ga arimasu ka.**
Do you have the same symptoms often?

Mrs. Tanaka: **Hai, tokidoki aru-mitai desu.**
Yes, I have them sometimes.

Dr. Simon: **Shinzō ni mondai ga aru-kamo shiremasen ne.**
You might have a problem with your heart.

Dewa, nen no tame ni shinzō no kensa o shimashō ka.
Then shall we examine your chest just in case?

Mrs. Tanaka: **Hai, onegai shimasu.**
Yes, please.

Grammar

1. The suffix -sō

The suffix -sō is added to the verb base and/or i-adjective to indicate that something "seems" or "looks like." To add it to the i-adjective, drop the suffix -i and replace it with -sō.

Shōjyō wa waru-sō desu.	The symptom seems bad.
Iki-gurushi-sō desu.	You seem like you're having difficulty breathing.
Ita-sō desu.	You seem to be in pain.

2. The suffix -yō(na)

The suffix -yō(na) added to the verb base or i-adjective also conveys the meaning of "looks like" or "appears." To add it to the i-adjective, drop the suffix -i and replace it with -yō(na).

Ashita byōin ni iku-yō desu.	It looks like he/she is going to hospital.
Sono nikibi wa itai-yō desu.	That pimple appears painful.
Memai wa onaji-yō desu.	My dizziness appears the same.
Kanjya wa onaji yō(na) shōjyō desu.	The patient looks like (she/he has) the same symptom.

3. The suffix -ta nowa

The suffix -ta nowa is used to indicate new and important information when it is placed between phrases. The sentence can usually be translated as "it is/ was . . . that; the one who; the place where; the time when."

Shōjyō ga deta nowa itsu desu ka.
When was it that the symptom first appeared? (*lit.,* The time when the symptom appeared?)

Shōjyō ga deta nowa kinō kara desu.
It was yesterday that I first had the symptom.

Hossa ga deta nowa itsu desu ka.
When was it that the attack happened?

Hossa ga deta nowa shokuji no toki deshita.
It was when I was eating that I had the attack.

4. The expression **mitai desu**

The expression **mitai desu** also indicates that something "looks (like)." **Mitai desu** works like a suffix for verbs and adjectives. This is a useful expression for discussing the diagnosis of symptoms with patients.

Shōjyō wa warui mitai desu.	Your symptoms look serious.
Iki-gurushii mitai desu.	You look like it's hard to breathe.
Itai mitai desu ne.	You look like you have pain, don't you?

5. The expression **kamo shiremasen**

The expression **kamo shiremasen** indicates the possibility or potential of something, as conveyed by the English word *might*.

Muchiuchi-shō kamo shiremasen.
You might have whiplash.

Hossa kamo shiremasen.
This might be a heart attack.

Kono byōki wa kurushii kamo shiremasen.
You might be suffering from this disease (*lit.*, This disease might be the cause of your suffering).

6. The adverb **nen-no-tame (ni)**

The adverb **nen-no-tame (ni)** is a common way to convey the sense of "making sure, just to be certain, just in case" and may be handy when discussing a diagnosis or the reason for a test or exam. Sometimes the particle **ni** is omitted. **Anzen** and **shinpai** may be substituted for **nen** to make the adverbial phrases **anzen no tame** (for safety's sake) and **shinpai no tame** (from/due to worry(ing)).

Nen-no-tame (ni), mō ichido kensa shimasu.
Just to be sure, I would like to examine it one more time.

Nen-no-tame (ni) onaka no sai-kensa o shimasu.
I would like to re-examine your stomach just in case.

Nen-no-tame (ni) shikori ni natte inaika mimashō.
I would like to make sure and check whether you have a lump or not.

Anzen no tame (ni), muchiuchi-shō no sai-kensa o shite mimasu.
I would like to try re-examining your whiplash for safety's sake.

Shinpai no tame (ni) henzutsū ga shimasu.
I have a migraine from worrying.

7. The verb ending **-mashō + ka**

The verb ending **-mashō** with the question maker **ka** requests or invites someone to do something together with the speaker and is used when making a suggestion or seeking permission. It can be translated by "Shall we."

Ketsu-atsu no kensa o shimashō ka.
Shall we examine your blood pressure?

Keiren o mimashō ka.
Shall I look at your muscle cramps?

Tokidoki onaji kensa o shimashō ka.
Shall we have the same test you sometimes have?

Useful Expressions (CD 9-3)

Listen to the CD and repeat the sentences.

1. **Don-na shojyō ga arimasu ka.** What symptoms do you have?
2. **Yoku onaji shōjyō ga demasu ka.** Do you have the same symptom often?
3. **Kono shōjyō ga deta nowa hajimete desu ka.** Is this the first time you've had this symptom?
4. **Kono shōjyō ga deta nowa itsu desu ka.** When did this symptom begin/manifest?
5. **Genin wa nani-ka wakari masu ka.** Can you think of any cause?
6. **Shinpai wa nai desu.** Don't worry./There's nothing to worry about.
7. **Shōjyō wa karu-sō desu.** Your symptoms seem mild.
8. **Warui tokoro wa arimasen.** There isn't anything wrong.
9. **Warui kamo shiremasen.** It might be serious.
10. **Onaji nenrei no hito ni yoku aru shōjyō desu.** People of your age often have this symptom.

Key Sentences (CD 9-4)

Listen to the CD and repeat the sentences.

1. **Chō no enshō mitai desu.** It looks like a stomach inflammation.
2. **Kono shōjyō ga deta nowa hajimete desu ka.** Is this the first time you've had this symptom?
3. **Nen no tame (ni) onaji shōjyōwa yoku demasu ka.** Just to be sure, do you have the same symptom often?
4. **Warui kamo shiremasen.** It might be serious.
5. **Shinsatsu o shimashō ka.** Shall I examine you?

Additional Words

ugoku/ugokimasu move	**muku/mukimasu** peel off
tomeru/tomemasu stop	**hashiru/hashirimasu** run
tsuzuku/tsuzukimasu continue	**koru/korimasu** stiff
onaji same	**chigau** different
shinpai worry	**anzen** safe
daijyōbu all right	**kurushii** suffering
karui mild/light	**hajimete** first time
muki direction	**hō** toward (direction)
kyūsei acute	**mansei** chronic
mada not yet	**donokurai** how much/how long

fukaku deeply	**asaku** shallowly
nochi later/after	**hō(gaku)** direction
gan cancer	**umi** pus

Language Notes

1. The following instructions or requests are used often in the examination room.

Ugoka-nai de kudasai.	Don't move, please./Please hold still.
Mae o mite kudasai.	Look straight, please.
Migi o muite kudasai.	Turn to the right, please.
Hidari o muite kudasai.	Turn to the left, please.
Ushiro o muite kudasai.	Turn around, please
Watakushi no hō o muite kudasai.	Turn toward me, please
Watakushi no yubi o mite kudasai.	Look at my finger, please

2. The following expressions are used when chest X-rays are administered.

Iki o sutte kudasai.	Take a breath, please.
Iki o fukaku suttee kudasai.	Take a deep breath, please.
Iki o tomete kudasai.	Hold your breath, please.
Iki o haite kudasai.	Exhale, please.
Iki o su-tari, hai-tari shite kudasai.	Breathe deeply in and out, please.

3. The Japanese term for chronic symptoms is **mansei**. Japanese usually express chronic symptoms as follows:

mansei byō	chronic disease
mansei byō kanjya	chronic patients
mansei i-en	chronic gastritis
mansei shikkan	chronic malady

4. The Japanese term for acute symptoms is **kyūsei**. Japanese usually express acute symptom as follows:

kyūsei chūdoku	acute poisoning
kyūsei kansen-shō	acute infection
kyūsei kan-en	acute hepatitis
kyūsei mochō-en	acute appendicitis
kyūsei hakketsu-byō	acute leukemia
Koko ni kyūsei no itami ga arimasu.	I have an acute pain here.

5. When Japanese have no conversation topic, they usually talk about recent weather conditions by using **mitai desu** (looks like, seems to). By cultural training, Japanese tend not to express their answers clearly during ordinary conversation. For example, if Japanese are asked what kind of weather it is today, they tend to answer, **Hare mitai desu.** "It's look like a clear day." Japanese also favor **kamo shiremasen** (might, might be) for speaking about future weather. The word **nochi** means "after" or "later." The following are other weather-related expressions.

Hare desu.	**Hare mitai desu.**
It's a clear day	It looks like a clear day.
Kumori desu.	**Kumori mitai desu.**
It's a cloudy day.	It looks like it will be cloudy.
Ame desu.	**Ame mitai desu.**
It's a rainy day.	It looks like rain.
Yuki desu.	**Yuki mitai desu.**
It's a snowy day.	It looks like snow.
Kaze desu.	**Kaze mitai desu.**
It's windy.	It looks like it will be windy.
Arashi desu.	**Arashi kamo shiremasen.**
It's stormy.	It might be stormy.
Hyō desu.	**Hyō kamo shiremasen.**
It's hailing.	It might hail.
Shimo desu.	**Shimo kamo shiremasen.**
There's frost.	There might be frost.

Hare nochi ame deshō.
It is clear now but may rain later. (*lit.*, It seems clear and later may rain.)

Kyō wa kumori nochi yuki deshō.
It is cloudy but may snow later today (*lit.*, It seems cloudy and later may snow today).

6. When giving a medical opinion about a bad result or a negative prognosis, the healthcare professional can use **mitai desu** (look like, seems to) instead of **desu** (it is) to attenuate the effect and help patients accept their medical condition with hope.

Kaze no shōjyō wa warui mitai desu.
It looks like a bad cold symptom.

Kensa no kekka wa yoku nai mitai desu.
The results of your test do not seem very good.

Gan mitai desu.
It looks like you have cancer.

7. Several useful expressions incorporate **shinsatsu** (medical examination).

shinsatsu	medical examination
shinstau-bi	day of medical examination/consultation
shinsatsu-ken	patient's registration card
shinsatsu-shitsu	examining or examination room
shinsatsu-dai	examination table (in a doctor's office)
shinsatsu-hiyō/he/dai	examination fee/consultation or doctor's fee

8. Questions to elicit symptoms:

Soko ga itsumo itai(n) desu ka.	Is the pain there all the time?
Chi o hakimashita ka.	Did you spit blood?
Donokurai hakimashita ka.	How much did you vomit?
Oshiete kudadsai.	Tell me, please.
Misete kudasai.	Show me, please.
Donokurai tsuzuki-mashita ka.	How long did it last?
Jikan ga tatsu to yoku narimashita ka.	Did it get better with time?
Jikan ga tatsu to waruku narimashita ka.	Did it get worse with time?
Doko kara itami ga hajimari-mashita ka.	Where did the pain start?
Hoka ni don-na shōjyō ga arimashita ka.	What other symptom occurred/ were there?

Language Roots

The prefix **kō-** (高) means "high."

kō-ketsu-atsu	high blood pressure
kō-netsu	high fever
kō-rei	advanced/old age
kō-kō-sei	high school student

The prefix **tei-** (低) means "low."

tei-ketsu-atsu	low blood pressure
tei-shibō	low fat
tei-on	low temperature, or low tone/voice
tei-soku	low speed

Culture Notes

Hay fever in Japan

From February to May, many Japanese suffer from hay fever (**kafun-shō**) caused by the pollen from cedar trees. Japanese often wear white masks made of gauze when they go out to shop or commute. Some even wear eyeglasses and hats to protect them from the pollen, which causes various symptoms such as a runny nose, headache, and itchy eyes.

Health-related Japanese proverbs II

Anxiety is poison to the body.
Shinpai wa mi no doku.
心配は身の毒

Prevention is better than cure.
(Note the similarity to: An ounce of prevention is worth a pound of cure.)
Korobanu saki no tsue.
転ばぬ先の杖

Comprehension

Answer the following questions.

1. Which of the following does NOT belong with the others?
   a. **Hossa**   b. **Haremono**
   c. **Mukumi**   d. **Menchō**

2. Which of the following could be used to say, "Your condition isn't serious"?
   a. **Shojyō wa omoi desu.**   b. **Shojyō wa karui desu.**
   c. **Shojyō wa wakarimasu.**   d. **Shojyō wa mansei desu.**

3. Which of the following best completes the sentence below?
   Kono shojyo (   ) deta nowa itsu desu ka. (When did this symptom start?)
   a. **o**   b. **ni**
   c. **ga**   d. **to**

4. Which of the following does NOT belong with the others?
   a. **Shojyō wa warui mitai desu.**
   b. **Shojyō wa warui kamo shiremasen.**
   c. **Shojyō wa warui desu.**
   d. **Shojyō wa waru sō desu.**

5. You are saying there is no major problem. Which of the following is correct?
   a. **Mansei desu.**   b. **Kyūsei desu.**
   c. **Shinpai wa arimasen.**   d. **Shinpai ga arimasu.**

Select the correct meaning in Japanese.

---

6. Little, few
   a. **tokidoki**   b. **tottemo**   c. **sukoshi**

7. Sometimes
   a. **hontōni**   b. **tokidoki**   c. **yoku**

8. Always
   a. **sukoshi**   b. **tottemo**   c. **itsumo**

9. Often
   a. **yoku**   b. **sukoshi**   c. **tottemo**

10. Really
    a. **tottemo**   b. **itsumo**   c. **hontōni**

Match the expressions in Column A and Column B.

Column A	Column B
11. ( ) **Ushiro o muite kudasai.**	a. Look straight, please.
12. ( ) **Migi o muite kudasai.**	b. Turn around, please.
13. ( ) **Ugoka nai de kudasai.**	c. Don't move, please.
14. ( ) **Hidair o muite kudasai.**	d. Turn to the left, please.
15. ( ) **Mae o mite kudasai.**	e. Turn to the right, please.

Practice

Respond to the following in Japanese using the cues that have been provided.

1. Asking about physical conditions.
   (Healthcare professional)   (Patient)
   1. _____ (lower back pain)   **Mada itami masu.**
   2. _____ (joint pain)   **Tokidoki shibire masu.**
   3. _____ (pimple)   **Tokidoki kayui desu.**
   4. _____ (chill)   **Netsu ga aru mitai desu.**

2. Telling what kind of symptoms.
   (Patient)   (Healthcare professional)
   1. **Nodo ga tottemo itai(n) desu.**   _____ (inflammation)
   2. **Hiza ga tottemo itai(n) desu.**   _____ (bruising)
   3. **Kubi ga itai(n) desu.**   _____ (whiplash)
   4. **Atama ga itain(n) desu.**   _____ (migraine)

3. Give the following directions.
   (Questions)   (Healthcare professional)
   1. Turn toward me, please.   _____
   2. Don't move, please.   _____
   3. Look at my finger, please.   _____

4. How do you say the following symptoms?
   (Questions)   (Healthcare professional)
   1. **Don-na shōjyō desu ka.**   _____ (giddiness)
   2. **Don-na shōjyō ga arimasu ka.**   _____ (palpitation)
   3. **Onaka ni don-na itami ga arimasu ka.** _____ (menstrual pain)
   4. **Kibun wa dōdesu ka.**   _____ (heartburn)

5. Dialogue comprehension. Based on the dialogue, answer the following questions.
   1. **Tanaka-san wa karada no doko ga itai(n) desu ka.** _____
   2. **Itsu-kara itai(n) desu ka.**   _____
   3. **Onaji-yōna shōjyō wa arimasu ka.**   _____
   4. **Don-na shōjyō desu ka.**   _____
   5. **Karada no doko ga warui(n) desu ka.**   _____

6. Free response questions.
   (Questions)   (Answers)
   1. **Muneyake o shita koto ga arimasu ka.**   _____
   2. **Shinzō-hossa wa itai(n) desu ka.**   _____
   3. **Dokoka itai tokoro ga arimasu ka.**   _____
   4. **Hashiru to ikigire ga shimasu ka.**   _____
   5. **Karada no chōshi wa dō desu ka.**   _____

Exercises

1. Say the following words in Japanese.
   A. Swelling   _____
   B. Chill   _____
   C. Puffy   _____
   D. Bruising   _____
   E. Lump   _____

2. How do you ask the following questions?
   A. What symptoms do you have?   _____
   B. When did this symptom happen?   _____
   C. Is this the first time you've had this symptom?_____
   D. Do you have the same symptom often?   _____
   E. Can you think of any cause?   _____

3. How do you say the following?
   A. Don't worry.   _____
   B. Your condition isn't serious.   _____
   C. There isn't anything wrong.   _____
   D. It might be serious.   _____
   E. It might need to be examined.   _____

4. Answer the following questions in Japanese.

   Q: **Don-na shōjyō ga arimasu ka.**
   A: _____ (I have a palpitation.)

   Q: **Kono shōjyō ga deta-nowa itsu desuka.**
   B: _____ (It's been three days since it began.)

   Q: **Yoku, onaji shōjyō ga arimasu ka.**
   C: _____ (Yes, I have it sometimes.)

   Q: **Kensa o shimashō ka.**
   D: _____ (Yes, please.)

Discharge
(Tai-in)

Basic Vocabulary (CD 10-1)

Listen to the CD and repeat the vocabulary.

1.	discharge	**tai-in**	退院
2.	attending doctor	**tantō-i(shi)**	担当医(師)
3.	preparation	**junbi**	準備
4.	recovery	**kaifuku**	回復
5.	bill/invoice	**seikyū-sho**	請求書
6.	payment	**shiharai**	支払い
7.	confirmation	**kakunin**	確認
8.	stay quiet	**ansei**	安静
9.	school	**gakkō**	学校
10.	workplace	**shigoto-ba**	仕事場
11.	medical rest	**seiyō**	静養
12.	normal	**seijyō**	正常
13.	abnormal	**ijyō**	異常
14.	fluid	**suibun**	水分
15.	nutrition	**eiyō**	栄養
16.	medical treatment	**ryōyō**	療養
17.	gargle	**ugai**	嗽
18.	sleep	**suimin**	睡眠
19.	question	**shitsumon**	質問
20.	wash hand	**te-arai**	手洗い
21.	go out	**gai-shutsu**	外出
22.	return to home	**kitaku**	帰宅
23.	malnutrition	**eiyō-busoku**	栄養不足
24.	plenty/enough	**jyūbun**	十分
25.	lie on your back	**aomuke**	仰向け
26.	lie on your stomach	**utsubuse**	うつ伏せ
27.	lifestyle disease	**seikatsu-shūkan-byō**	生活習慣病
28.	insufficient exercise	**undō-busoku**	運動不足
29.	lack of sleep	**suimin-busoku**	睡眠不足
30.	examination table	**shinsatsu-dai**	診察台

Dialogue (CD 10-2)

Listen to the CD and repeat the dialogue.

Dr. Simon:	**Shinzō kensa no kekka wa waruku-nai mitai desu.**
	Your chest test result seems to show no problem.
Mrs. Tanaka:	**Yokatta desu. Arigatō-gozaimasu. Ashita Shigoto ni ittemo ii desu ka.**
	I'm glad. Thank you very much. Can I go to work tomorrow?
Dr. Simon:	**Iie. Shigoto wa yasunda-hō ga ii desu. Mushiro, mada uchi de ansei-ni shite-ite kudasai.**
	No. You shouldn't go to work. Instead, please rest quietly at home still.
Mrs. Tanaka:	**Hai, wakari mashita. Nani-ka tabete mo ii desu ka.**
	Yes, I understand. Can I eat some food? (*lit.*, Can I eat something?)
Dr. Simon:	**Hai, ii desu yo. Suibun mo jyūbun totte kudasai.**
	Yes, you should also drink plenty of liquids.
Mrs. Tanaka:	**Wakari mashita. Nani-ka kusuri o nonda hō ga ii desu ka.**
	I understand. Is it better to take medicine?
Dr. Simon:	**Hai, shohōsen o dashimasu. Sugu-ni naorimasu yo. Odaiji ni.**
	Yes, I will give you a prescription. You should be well soon. Take care of yourself.
Mrs. Tanaka:	**Dōmo arigatō-gozaimashita.**
	Thank you very much.

Grammar

1. **A noun followed by the particle no may modify another noun.**

In Lesson 1, we saw that the particle **no** may be used to indicate someone's affiliation. The particle **no** also allows a noun to modify another noun. Thus, in the first example below, the noun **kekka** (result) is modified by **kensa** (examination, test) plus **no** to form the expression **kensa no kekka** "the examination result."

Kensa no kekka wa seijyō desu.	The result of the examination is normal.
Test no kekka wa yoku-nai desu.	The test result is not good.

2. The expression **-te mo ii desu ka**

In Japanese, requesting or asking permission is expressed by the **te**-form followed by the particle **mo** plus **ii desu ka**. The literal meaning of **-itte mo ii desu ka** is "May I?; Can I?"

Shigoto ni itte mo ii desu ka.	May I go to work?
Gakkō ni itte mo ii desu ka.	May I go to school?
Futsū ni shokuji o tabete mo ii desu ka.	Can I eat normally?
Ocha o nonde mo ii desu ka.	Can I drink tea?
Yasunde mo ii desu ka.	May I rest?

3. The expressions **hō ga ii** and **nai hō ga ii**

The idiomatic expression **hō ga ii** is a comparative and means "better to do (something)" in the sense of "should." The opposite is expressed by **nai hō ga ii**, which means "better not to do (something)" or "shouldn't."

Shigoto wa yasunda hō ga ii desu.
You better/should stay home (*lit.*, be absent) from work.

Suimin o jyūbun totta hō ga ii desu.
You better/should get a lot of sleep.

Kazoku ni renraku o totta hō ga ii desu.
You better/should inform your family.

Suibun o takusan totta hō ga ii desu.
You better/should drink a lot of liquid.

Gaishutsu o shinai hō ga ii desu.
You better not/shouldn't go out.

Ashita wa gakkō ni ikanai hō ga ii desu.
You better not/shouldn't go to school.

Kyō wa shigoto ni ikanai hō ga ii desu.
You shouldn't go to work today.

4. The adverb **mushiro**

The adverb **mushiro** expresses a recommendation or suggestion and translates as "instead, rather, better." It may be used to suggest when something is better or preferable to another.

Mushiro, uchi de yasunde kudasai.
You should rest at home instead.

Mushiro, suibun o jyūbun totte kudasai.
Rather, you should drink plenty of liquids.

Mushiro, undō-busoku wa seikatsu-shūkan-byō no genin ni narimasu.
Insufficient exercise is causing a lifestyle disease in you instead.

5. The verb in the te-form + iru/imasu expresses a present condition.

In Lesson 6, we saw that the **te**-form plus **iru/imasu** expresses the present progress of an action (is doing). The **te**-form plus **iru/imasu** may also express a present condition or state.

Uchi de ansei ni shite ite kudasai.
Please rest quietly at home. (*lit.*, Please you should be quietly resting at home.)

Sensei wa shinsatsu o owatte imasu.
The doctor has finished with the examination.

Kanjya wa mō fuku o kigaete imasu.
The patient has changed his/her clothes.

Kanjya wa byōin o taiin shite imasu.
The patient has been discharged from the hospital.

Note that in the last two examples, the emphasis in Japanese is not on the past action, as it is in English, but on the ongoing condition that results from the action of changing clothes or being discharged from the hospital.

6. The sentence-final particle yo

The sentence-final particle **yo** indicates the speaker's conviction, assertion, or suggestion. It may be translated into English as "you should, I tell you, you know," etc.

Kusuri o nonda hō ga ii desu yo.	You should take your medicine.
Sugu ni naori masu yo.	I tell you, you will be cured/get well soon.
Shibaraku shie, yoku narimasu yo.	I'm telling you, you will be cured after a short while.
Mō byōki ga naotte imasu yo.	You know, you're already cured of your illness.

Useful Expressions (CD 10-3)

Listen to the CD and repeat the sentences.

1. **Kaze mitai desu.** It seems like a cold.

2. **Sugu ni naorimasu.** It will be cured soon.
3. **Shinpai wa nai desu yo.** I'm telling you, don't worry.
4. **Mushiro ansei ni shite kudasai.** Rather, please stay quiet/rest quietly.
5. **Gakkō wa yasunde kudasai.** You shouldn't go to school.
6. **Suibun o jyūbun totte kudasai.** You should drink a lot of liquids.
7. **Shohōsen o dashimasu.** I will give you a prescription.
8. **Senmon-i o shōkai shiamsu.** I will refer you to a specialist.
9. **Shitsumon ga arimasu ka.** Do you have a question/any questions?
10. **Mondai ga attara sugu ni renraku shite kudasai.** If you have any problems, please inform us immediately.

Key Sentences (CD 10-4)

Listen to the CD and repeat the sentences.

1. **Shigoto ni ittemo ii desu ka.** Can I go to work?
2. **Mushiro shigoto wa yasunda hō ga ii desu.** You better not go to work.
3. **Kensa no kekka wa seijyō deshita yo.** I tell you, the test result was normal.
4. **Nani-ka shitsumon ga arimasu ka.** Do you have any questions?
5. **Kanjya-san wa shinsatsu-dai ni agatte imasu.** The patient is on (*lit.*, has gotten up on) the examination table.

Additional Words

agaru/agarimasu go up	**oriru/orimasu** get off/step down
owaru/owarimasu end/finish/complete	**shitagau/shitagaimasu** follow
hone bone	**shiji** instruction
busoku lack/insufficient	**sugu(ni)** soon
shohōsen prescription	**shita-gi** underwear
mushiro instead	**su-ashi** bare feet
waki-bara flank	**eikyō** influence
bitamin vitamins	**botsu-botsu** pimple
karushūmu calcium	**shorui** document
dairi-nin representative/agent	**shibarak** a while
nyūin hiyō hospital charge	**yoko ni naru/narimasu** lie down

Language Notes

1. **Jyūbun** means "plenty, enough, sufficient, in full."

Suimin o jyūbun totte kudasai.	Please get plenty of sleep.
Suibun o jyūbun totte kudasai.	Please drink plenty of water.
Jyūbun eiyō o totte kudasai.	Please get enough nutrition.

Jyūbun desu means "it's enough." It is also a set expression corresponding to "No, thank you."

Mō jyūbun itadakimashita.	I have had plenty./That's plenty./No, thank you.
Jyūbun kusuri o nomimashita.	I have had a lot of/enough medicine.
Mō jūbun kensa o shimashita.	I have had enough tests. No more, please.

2. **Odaiji ni** is a common Japanese expression for "Take care" or "Take care of yourself." It is the abbreviation of **Odaiji ni (shite kudasai)**.

Odaiji ni shite kudasai.	Please take care of yourself.
Odaiji ni.	Take care.

3. The following are additional useful commands:

Jō-han-shin hadaka ni natte kudasai.	Please undress from the waist up.
Botan o hazushite kudasai.	Please undo your button.

Shitagi wa tsuketa mama de ii desu yo.
You know, you can keep your undershirt on (*lit.*, wear your undershirt).

Shatsu o agete kudasai.	Please lift your shirt up.
Gaun ni kigaete kudasai.	Please change into this gown.
Aomuke ni natte kudasai.	Lie on your back.
Utsubuse ni natte kudasai.	Lie on your stomach.
Muki o kaete kudasai.	Please turn over.
Yoko ni natte kudasai.	Please lie down.

Shinsatsu-dai de (On the Examination Table)

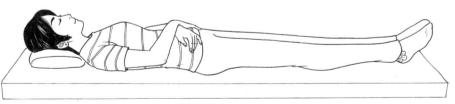

Ao make (Lie on your back).

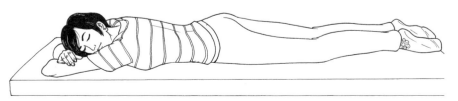

Utsu-buse (Lie on your stomach).

Migi-waki-bara o shita ni shite, yoko ni natte kudasai.
Lie on your right side.

Hidai-waki-bara o shita ni shite, yoko ni natte kudasai.
Lie on your left side.

Shinsatsu-dai kara orite kudasai.
You can get off the examination table.

4. To say, "I will give you a prescription," Japanese doctors does not use the verb **agemasu** (give) but rather **dashimasu** (submit, turn in).

    *****Shohōsen o agemasu.** (not a proper Japanese expression)
    Shohōsen o dashimasu. (the correct Japanese expression)

5. When a medical professional conveys the diagnosis of something wrong or abnormal (**ijyō**) in Japanese, the following two expressions are often used. It is recommended that you not say, **Ijyō ga arimasu.** "You have an abnormal . . ." to a Japanese patient, who is not accustomed to this kind of directness and consequently may be unduly shocked or upset. Recall that **mitai desu** may be used to attenuate bad news.

Ijyō ga aru mitai desu.	It seems there is something abnormal.
Yoku nai mitai desu.	It seems that there is something not good.

6. The verb base plus the suffix **-sugi** expresses "too much, excessive, over- (*as in* overeating)."

    Tabako no sui-sugi ni kiotsukete kudasai.
    Please be careful about smoking too much/excessively.

    Osake no nomi-sugi wa dame desu.
    Don't drink too much alcohol.

    Niku no tabe-sugi wa karada ni yokunai desu.
    Overeating/Eating too much meat is not good for your body.

    Supōtsu no shi-sugi de karada ga itai(n) desu ka.
    Does your body hurt from overexercising? (*lit.*, Do you have pain in your body from overexercising?)

7. The suffix **-fusoku/-busoku** is used to express a lack or shortage of things.

    Undō-busoku de genki ga arimasen.
    Lack of exercise whittled away my energy.

Konogoro, bitamin-busoko desu.
I haven't had enough vitamins lately.

Eiyō-busoku no eikyō ga dete kita.
Lack of nutrition began to tell on me.

Saikin, suimin-busoku de kao ni botsu-botsu ga dekite imasu.
I am getting little pimples on my face because I have not had enough sleep lately.

Karushūmu-busoku de hone ga itai(n) desu ka.
Do you have pain in your bones because of lack of calcium?

Language Roots

The negative prefix **fu-/bu-** (不) means "irregularity" and often translates as "un-, non-, dis-, *or* a-."

fu-kaikan	discomfort
shokuyoku-fu-shin	anorexia
fu-sei-myaku	arrhythmia/irregular pulse
fu-kisoku	irregularity, disorderly
eiyō-bu-soku	malnutrition

The suffix **-yō** (養) indicates support or treatment.

sei-yō	rest
ryō-yō	medical treatment
fu-yō	support

Culture Notes

The leading causes of death in Japan

The leading causes of death in Japan are cancer, which accounts for 30 percent, followed by heart disease at 15 percent, cerebral hemorrhage at 15 percent, and other forms of stroke at 15 percent. These last three used to be called adult diseases (**seijin-byō**) but now are called life-habit or lifestyle diseases (**seikatsu-shūkan-byō**) because they are caused by habits such as smoking (**tabako**), drinking (**osake**), and not getting enoug physical exercise (**undō-busoku**).

Health-related Japanese proverbs III

Cure the disease and kill the patient.
Byōki o naoshite byō-nin o korosu.
病気を治して病人を殺す

Out of one difficulty, another one awaits.

Ichi-nan satte, mata ichi nan.

一難去ってまた一難

Comprehension

Answer the following questions.

1. Which of the following does NOT belong with the others?
    a. **Suibun**
    b. **Shohōsen**
    c. **Eiyō**
    d. **Seiyō**

2. Which of the following could be used to say, "You should drink plenty of liquids?"
    a. **Suibun o sukoshi totte kudasai.**
    b. **Eiyō o jyūbun totte kudasai.**
    c. **Suibun o jyūbun totte kudasai.**
    d. **Eiyō o takusan totte kudasai.**

3. Which of the following best completes the sentence below?
    Mondai ga attara sugu (   ) renraku shite kudasai.
    (If you have any problems, please inform us immediately.)
    a. **o**
    b. **ni**
    c. **ga**
    d. **to**

4. Which of the following does NOT belong with the others?
    a. **Gaishutsu shite kudasai.**
    b. **Ansei ni shite kudasai.**
    c. **Yasun de kudasai.**
    d. **Ryoyō shite kudasai.**

5. You are talking about the patient being cured soon.
    a. **Sugu ni naori masu.**
    b. **Sugu ni shōkai shimasu.**
    c. **Sugu ni kensa shimasu.**
    d. **Sugu ni renraku shimasu.**

Select the correct meaning in Japanese.

6. Nutrition
    a. **ijyō**
    b. **eiyō**
    c. **shojyō**

7. Gargle
    a. **ugai**
    b. **shikori**
    c. **dōki**

8. Sleep
   a. **shitsumon**   b. **kesuben**   c. **suimin**

9. Liquid
   a. **hossa**   b. **suibun**   c. **shikori**

10. Medicine
    a. **mansei**   b. **kyūsei**   c. **kusuri**

Match the expressions in Column A and Column B.

Column A   Column B

11. (   ) **Aomuke ni natte kudasai.**   a. Please put your shirt on.
12. (   ) **Utsubuse ni natte kudasai.**   b. Lie on your back.
13. (   ) **Muki o kaete kudasai.**   c. Please turn over.
14. (   ) **Shatsu o agete kudasai.**   d. Please lift your shirt up
15. (   ) **Fuku o kite kudasai.**   e. Lie on your stomach

Practice

Respond to the following in Japanese using the cues that have been provided.

1. Express your observations about the patient's condition.
   (Patient)   (Healthcare professional)
   1. Lack of adequate nutrition.   _____
   2. Lack of exercise.   _____
   3. Overeating.   _____
   4. Overdrinking.   _____
   5. Excess medication.   _____

2. Giving advice when the patients are being discharged.
   (Patient)   (Healthcare professional)
   1. **Gaishitsu shite mo ii desu ka.**   _____ (no)
   2. **Shitsumon o shite mo ii desu ka.**   _____ (yes)
   3. **Renraku wa dō shimasu ka.**   _____ (telephone)
   4. **Ugai o shimasu ka.**   _____ (yes)
   5. **Uchi de ryōyō no hō ga ii desu ka.** _____ (yes)

3. Before the examination: What shall I do? (**Dō shimasu ka.**)

   (Patient)   (Healthcare professional)

   1. **Fuku wa dō shimasu ka.**

      _____
      (Please change into this gown.)

   2. **Shinsatsu-dai de dō shimasu ka.**

      _____
      (Lie on your back.)

   3. **Shatsu wa dō shimasu ka.**

      _____
      (Please lift your shirt up.)

   4. **Kore kara dō shimasu ka.**

      _____
      (Please turn over.)

   5. **Shinsatsu ga owari-mashita.
      Dō shimasu ka.**

      _____
      (Please get down from the examination table.)

4. At the time of discharge: Respond to the following.

   (Patient)   (Healthcare professional)

   1. **Nyūin hiyō wa dō shimasu ka.**

      _____
      (Pay at the casher.)

   2. **Kusuri wa dō shimasu ka.**

      _____
      (Get a prescription.)

   3. **Mata, itsu byōin e kimasu ka.**

      _____
      (Please come next month.)

   4. **Osewa ni narimashita.**

      _____
      (Please take care of yourself.)

5. Dialogue comprehension. Based on the contents of the dialogue, answer the following questions.

   1. **Kensa no kekka wa ijyō deshita ka, seijō deshita ka.** _____

   2. **Nani-ka tabete mo ii desu ka.** _____

   3. **Suibun o totta hō ga ii desu ka.** _____

   4. **Itsu byōki wa naorimasu ka.** _____

6. Free response questions.

   (Questions)   (Answers)

   1. **Suimin to totta hō ga ii desu ka.** _____

   2. **Kusuri o nonda hō ga ii desu ka.** _____

   3. **Mada nyūin shite ita hō ga ii desu ka.** _____

   4. **Taiin shite mo ii desu ka.** _____

Exercises

1. Say the following words in Japanese.
    A. Stay quiet./Rest quietly. _____
    B. Result _____
    C. Attending doctor _____
    D. Liquid _____
    E. Medical treatment _____

2. Say the following in Japanese.
    A. It will be cured soon. _____
    B. Please stay quiet. _____
    C. You should not go to school. _____
    D. The result of the examination is normal. _____
    E. Do you have any questions? _____

3. What are the meanings in English of the following advice to patients?
    A. **Suibun o jyūbun totte kudasai.** _____
    B. **Senmon-i o shōkai shiamsu.** _____
    C. **Shinpai wa nai desu.** _____
    D. **Gakkō wa yasunde kudasai.** _____
    E. **Mondai ga attara sugu ni renraku shite kudasai.** _____

4. Answer the following questions.

    Q: **Shigoto ni itte mo ii desu ka.**
    A: _____ (No, you should not to go work.)

    Q: **Uchi ni ita hō ga ii desu ka.**
    B: _____ (Yes, you should get a lot of sleep.)

    Q: **Shokuji o shite mo ii desu ka.**
    C: _____ (Yes, you should drink lots of fluids.)

    Q: **Shiharai o shita hō ga ii desu ka.**
    D: _____ (Yes, I will give you an invoice.)

Internal Organs
(Naizō)

Basic Vocabulary (CD 11-1)

Listen to the CD and repeat the vocabulary.

	English	Rōmaji	Japanese
1.	esophagus	**shokudō**	食道
2.	windpipe/trachea	**ki-kan**	気管
3.	bronchus	**ki-kan-shi**	気管支
4.	lung	**hai**	肺
5.	heart	**shin-zō**	心臓
6.	kidney	**jin-zō**	腎臓
7.	liver	**kan-zō**	肝臓
8.	spleen	**hi-zō**	脾臓
9.	adrenal glands	**fuku-jin**	副腎
10.	pancreas	**sui-zō**	膵臓
11.	gall bladder	**tan-nō**	胆囊
12.	small bowel/intestine	**shō-chō**	小腸
13.	duodenum	**jyūnishi-chō**	十二指腸
14.	jejunum	**kū-chō**	腔腸
15.	ileum	**kai-chō**	回腸
16.	large bowel/colon	**dai-chō**	大腸
17.	cecum	**mō-chō**	盲腸
18.	appendix	**chū-sui**	虫垂
19.	ascending colon	**jyōkō-dai-chō**	上行大腸
20.	transverse colon	**ōkō-dai-chō**	横行大腸
21.	descending colon	**kakō-dai-chō**	下行大腸
22.	sigmoid colon	**esu-jyō-kkechō**	S状結腸
23.	rectum	**choku-chō**	直腸
24.	uterus/womb	**shikyū**	子宮
25.	urinary bladder	**bōkō**	膀胱
26.	anus	**kōmon**	肛門
27.	cancer	**gan**	癌
28.	ulcer	**kaiyō**	潰瘍
29.	tumor	**shuyō**	腫瘍
30.	suspect/doubt	**utagai**	疑い

Naizō, Mae
(Internal Organs, Front)

Naizō, Ushiro
(Internal Organs, Back)

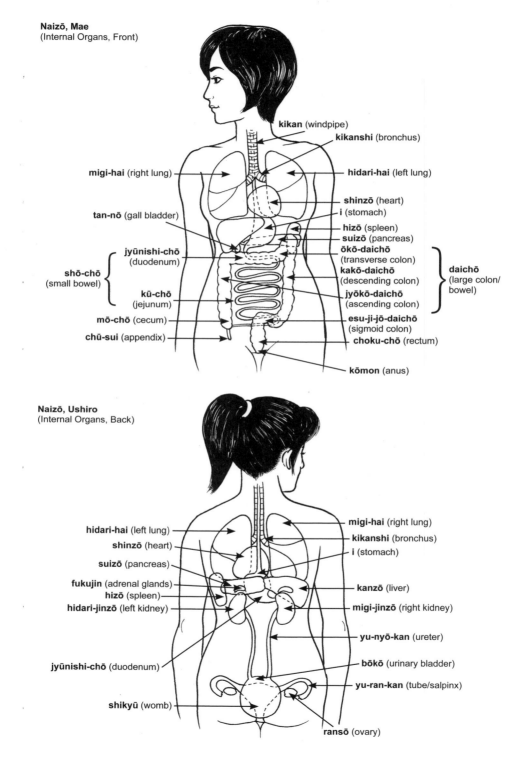

kikan (windpipe)

kikanshi (bronchus)

migi-hai (right lung)

hidari-hai (left lung)

shinzō (heart)

i (stomach)

tan-nō (gall bladder)

hizō (spleen)

suizō (pancreas)

jyūnishi-chō
(duodenum)

ōkō-daichō
(transverse colon)

shō-chō
(small bowel)

kakō-daichō
(descending colon)

daichō
(large colon/
bowel)

kū-chō
(jejunum)

jyōkō-daichō
(ascending colon)

mō-chō (cecum)

esu-ji-jō-daichō
(sigmoid colon)

chū-sui (appendix)

choku-chō (rectum)

kōmon (anus)

hidari-hai (left lung)

migi-hai (right lung)

shinzō (heart)

kikanshi (bronchus)

suizō (pancreas)

i (stomach)

fukujin (adrenal glands)

hizō (spleen)

kanzō (liver)

hidari-jinzō (left kidney)

migi-jinzō (right kidney)

yu-nyō-kan (ureter)

jyūnishi-chō (duodenum)

bōkō (urinary bladder)

yu-ran-kan (tube/salpinx)

shikyū (womb)

ransō (ovary)

Dialogue (CD 11-2)

Listen to the CD and repeat the dialogue.

At the Family Doctor's Office

Dr. Simon:	**Kon-nichi wa. Kyō wa dō shimashita ka.**
	Hello, how are you feeling today?
Miss Yamada:	**I no atari ga motare-te iru mitai desu.**
	I seem to have a heavy feeling around my stomach.
Dr. Simon:	**Shoku-go, i ga itami masu ka.**
	Does your stomach hurt after meals?
Miss Yamada:	**Iie, onaka ga suku-to, i ga kiri-kiri shimasu.**
	No, when my stomach is empty, it begins to hurt sharply.
Dr. Simon:	**I-kaiyō dato omoimasu. I no kensa o shita koto ga arimasu ka.**
	I think you may have a peptic ulcer. Have you ever had your stomach examined?
Miss Yamada:	**Iie, mada (kensa o) shita koto wa arimasen.**
	No, I haven't had one (an examination) yet.
Dr. Simon:	**Soredewa, i-eki no kensa kara hajime mashō.**
	Well then, let's do a test to examine your gastric juices first.
Miss Yamada:	**Hai, onegai shimasu.**
	Yes, please.

Grammar

1. The construction PLACE/BODY + **no atari/no tokoro**

   The phrases **no atari** and **no tokoro** are used to indicate the area around a place on the body or a part of the body. Often patients aren't able to locate the exact place or source of pain, so they will frequently use one of these expressions.

   Shinzō no atari ga itai(n) desu.
   I have a pain around my heart.

   I no atari ga itai(n) desu ka.
   Do you have a pain in your stomach area?

   I no tokoro ga warui(n) desu ka.
   Is something wrong in the area around your stomach?

2. The **te**-form + **iru mitai**

We studied the **te**-form plus **iru/imasu** in Lessons 6 and 10, and in Lesson 10 we saw that this construction expresses a present condition. The **te**-form plus **iru mitai** may also be used to express an observation about a present condition. In this construction, **yō-da/yō-desu** may be substituted for **mitai**.

Bōkō ga harete iru mitai desu.
Your (urinary) bladder looks like it's swollen.

I ga mukatsuite iru mitai desu.
My stomach seems to be upset.

Yume o mite iru mitai desu.
It feels like I'm in a dream.

Kanjya wa kōmon ni enshō o okoshite iru yō-da.
The patient looks like he may have an inflammation on his anus. (informal)

3. NOUN or **na**-ADJECTIVE + **dato omoimasu**

The construction NOUN or **na**-ADJECTIVE plus **dato omoimasu** expresses a firm opinion or statement and translates as "I think (that)."

Kaze dato omoimasu.	I think you have cold.
Hai-en dato omoimasu.	I think that you have pneumonia.
Shizuka dato omoimasu.	I think it's quiet.

4. VERB or **i**-ADJECTIVE + **to omoimasu**

For **i**-adjectives and verbs, the construction becomes VERB or **i**-ADJECTIVE plus **to omoimasu**. The meaning is the same, "I think (that)."

Netsu ga takai to omoimasu.	I think your fever is high.
Kanzō ga warui to omoimasu.	I think that your liver is diseased.
Netsu ga aru to omoimasu.	I think you have a fever.

5. Questions of the form **shita koto ga arimasu ka**

A past-tense verb plus **koto** in questions of the form **shita koto ga arimasu ka** asks whether you did something or something happened at an earlier time and translates as "Have you ever?" The verb should be the stem form past tense. Some verbs in the past tense of the stem form are as follows: for **suru** (do), the past is **shita** (done); for **yomu** (read), **yonda** (read); for **nomu** (drink), **nonda** (drunk), etc. To learn more about stem verbs, see Lesson 13, Language Notes 2.

Kanzō no kensa o shita koto ga arimasu ka.
Have you ever had your liver examined?

Mōchō no shujyutsu o shita koto ga arimasu ka.
Have you ever had an appendix operation?

Kikanshi-en no kusuri o nonda koto ga arimasu ka.
Have you ever taken medicine for bronchitis?

6. The expression **sore-dewa**

Lesson 7 introduced the interjection **dewa** (then). The expression **sore-dewa** is used in the sentence's initial position and means "in that case." In informal speech, **sore-dewa** is contracted to **sore jā**. **Sore-dewa** is also often shortened to **dewa**, which is further contracted to the informal **jaa**.

Koko wa itaku-nai desu.	**Sore-dewa, koko wa dō desu ka.**
There is no pain here.	In that case, how about here?
Koko wa kayuku-nai desu.	**Dewa, kōmon wa dō desu ka.**
There is no itch here.	In that case, how about the anus?
Shoku-yoku ga arimasen.	**(Sore) Jā, mite mimashō.**
I don't have an appetite.	In that case, let's take a look.

Useful Expressions (CD 11-3)

Listen to the CD and repeat the sentences.

1. **Shinzō o kensa shimashō.** I will examine your heart.
2. **Hai o shirabete mimashō ka.** Shall we try to check your lungs?
3. **Mōchō-en kamo shiremasen.** It's probably appendicitis.
4. **I no atari ga itai(n) desu ka.** Do you have pain around your stomach?
5. **Kikanshi-en dato omoimasu.** I think that you have bronchitis.
6. **Kōmon kara shukketsu shite imasu ka.** Do you have a bloody discharge from the anus?
7. **Choku-chō-gan no utagai ga arimasu.** I suspect it may be rectal cancer.
8. **Hai-en mitai desu.** It may be pneumonia.
9. **Jyūnishi-cho ga warui mitai desu.** It looks like something is wrong with your duodenum. (*lit.*, Your duodenum looks like something is wrong.)
10. **Jyūnishi-cho-kaiyō no yō desu.** It seems to be a duodenal ulcer.

Key Sentences (CD 11-4)

Listen to the CD and repeat the sentences.

1. **I no atari ga itai(n) desu ka.** Do you have pain around your stomach?
2. **Jyūnishi-cho-kaiyō no yō desu.** It seems to be a duodenal ulcer.
3. **Hai-en dato omoimasu.** I think that you have pneumonia.
4. **Kanzō no kensa o shita koto ga arimasu ka.** Have you ever had your liver examined?
5. **Kikanshi ga enshō o okoshite iru mitai desu.** Your bronchus seems to be inflamed.

Additional Words

shiraberu/shirabemasu investigate
kikanshi-en bronchitis
atari around
shoku-go after meals
i-eki gastric juice
hai-en pneumonia
takai high
shujyutsu operation
chō-kan digestive tract

mukatsuku/mukatsukimasu upset
motareru/motaremasu heavy feeling
tokoro place/area
shoku-zen before meals
yume dream
shizuka quiet
hikui low
ji-ketsu bloody discharge from anus
i-kaiyō peptic ulcer

Language Notes

1. The expressions **motareru/motaremasu** (feel heavy) and **muka-muka** (upset, queasy) are used only for the stomach (**i** and **onaka**).

I ga motarete imasu.	I have a heavy feeling in my stomach.
Onakga ga motarete imasu.	I have a heavy feeling in my stomach.
I ga muka-muka shite imasu.	I feel sick to my stomach.

    The verb **mukatsuku/mukatsuki-masu** (be upset) is used both to express feelings and for an upset stomach that is much more serious than **motareru/muka-muka**.

    I ga mukatsuite imasu.
    My stomach feels really queasy.

    (Watakushi wa) onaka ga mukatsuki masu.
    I have a really upset stomach.

    (Watakushi wa) ano kanjya ni mukatsuki masu.
    I feel very upset about that patient.

2. The following Japanese expressions are used to convey uncertainty about the statements that contain them and may also be used to blunt or attenuate the meaning of the statements:

Hai-en mitai desu.	It looks like pneumonia.
Kikanshi-en mitai desu.	It looks like bronchitis.
Jyūnishi-cho-kaiyō no yō desu.	It seems to be a duodenal ulcer.
Mōchō-en kamo shiremasen.	You may have appendicitis.
Jyūnishi-cho ga warui mitai desu.	Your duodenum looks like something is wrong.

In particular, when healthcare professionals want to soften an opinion in consideration of a patient's feelings, these expressions may be useful.

Kanzō-gan no yō desu.
It seems to be liver cancer.

Daichō-en kamo shiremasen.
It may be an inflammation of the large intestine.

Choku-chō gan no utagai ga arimasu.
I suspect it may be rectal cancer.

Suizō ga warui mitai desu.
Your pancreas looks like it is diseased (*lit.*, something is wrong).

Hai-gan no utagai ga arimasu.
I suspect it may be lung cancer.

3. There are many expressions for the different kinds of pains relating to the internal organs:

man-sei no itami	chronic pain
kyū-sei no itami	acute pain
taema-nai itami	continuous pain
shitsukoi itami	persistent pain
hiri-hiri suru itami	stinging pain
zuki-zuki suru itami	throbbing pain
chiku-chiku suru itami	prickling pain
yakeru itami	burning pain
sashikomu itami	squeezing pain
shimetsuke-rareru itami	gripping pain

4. Lessons 5 and 6 explained that most Japanese adjectives end in **-i** and are called **i**-adjectives. **i**-adjectives can modify nouns. The sentence structure is **i**-ADJECTIVE plus NOUN **desu**.

Shōchō no chōkan wa nagai desu.
The digestive tract of small bowel is long.

Nagai shōchō no chōkan desu.
It's the long digestive tract of small bowel.

Daichō no chōkan wa mijikai desu.
The digestive tract of large bowel is short.

Mijikai daichō no chōkan desu.
It's the short digestive tract of large bowel.

The following **i**-adjectives modify things.

large/big	**ōkii**	light	**karui**	slim/ slender	**hosoi**
small	**chiisai**	heavy	**omoi**	wide	**hiroi**
long	**nagai**	high/ expensive	**takai**	narrow	**semai**
short	**mijikai**	low	**hikui**	slow/late	**osoi**
bright	**akarui**	cheap	**yasui**	many	**ōi**
dark	**kurai**	new	**atarashii**	few	**sukunai**
nearby	**chikai**	old	**furui**	correct	**tadashii**
far away	**tōi**	fat	**futoi**	young	**wakai**
strong	**tsuyoi**	weak	**yowai**	wise/clever	**kashikoi**

The following **i**-adjectives describe feelings (**kimochi**).

good	**yoi/ii**	interesting	**omoshiroi**
busy	**isogashii**	bad	**warui**
easy/gentle	**yasashii**	dangerous	**abunai**
enjoyable	**tanoshii**	difficult	**muzukashii**
sad	**kanashii**	dirty	**kitanai**
boring	**tsumaranai**	lonely	**sabishii**
wonderful	**subarashii**	beautiful	**utsukushii**
happy	**ureshii**	severe/terrible	**hidoi**
intense/violent	**hageshii**	persistent	**shitsukoi**
scary	**kowai**	dazzling/radiant	**mabushii**
sly	**zurui**	soft	**yawarakai**
hard	**katai**	sharp	**surudoi**
disgusting	**iyarashii**	depressing	**uttōshii**

cute	**kawaii**	envy	**urayamashii**
innocent/pitiful	**iji-rashii**	correct	**tadashii**
careless	**sosokkashii**	annoying	**wazurawashii**
confusing	**magirawashii**	pitiful/pathetic	**itaitashii**

The following six **i**-adjectives describe temperature (**ondo**).

hot	**atsui**	cold (touch)	**tsumetai**
warm	**atatakai**	cold (weather)	**samui**
moderate	**hodo-yoi**	cool	**suzushii**

Note: Japanese has two words for cold: **tsumetai** and **samui**. **Tsumetai** is used to express touching cold, and **samui** is used to express weather cold.

The following are ten **i**-adjectives that describe taste (**aji**).

delicious	**oishii**	salty	**shoppai**
flavorful	**umai***	bitter	**nigai**
bad tasting	**mazui**	sour	**suppai**
sweet	**amai**	hot/spicy	**karai**
astringent	**shibui**	harsh	**egui**

* This adjective also means "skillful."

5. In addition, Japanese has **na**-adjectives that modify nouns. The difference between **i**-adjectives and **na**-adjectives is that **na**-adjectives require that the particle **na** be inserted between the adjective and the noun they precede.

Hai wa kirei desu.
The lung is clean

kirei na hai desu.
clean lung

Sensei wa yūmei desu
The doctor is famous.

yūmei na sensei desu.
famous doctor

Na-adjectives

beautiful/clean	**kirei(na)**	unskillful	**heta(na)**
various	**iro-iro(na)**	famous	**yūmei(na)**
favorite, liked/ preferred	**suki(na)**	quite	**shizuka(na)**

important	**taisetsu(na)**	disliked, hated	**kirai(na)**
not good	**dame(na)**	valuable	**daiji(na)**
convenient	**benri(na)**	free time	**hima(na)**
safe	**anzaen(na)**	inconvenient	**fuben(na)**
kind	**shinsetsu(na)**	healthy/well	**genki(na)**
polite	**teinei(na)**	unkind	**fushinsetsu(na)**
skillful	**jōzu(na)**	rude	**shitsurei(na)**
lively (noise)	**nigiyaka(na)**	miserable	**mijime(na)**
insensitive	**donkan(na)**	abnormal	**hentai(na)**

Language Roots

The suffix **-zō** (臓) indicates internal organs, intestines, and viscera.

shin-zō	heart
kan-zō	liver
hi-zō	spleen
sui-zō	pancreas
jin-zō	kidney

The word **chō** (腸) is also used for internal organs and indicates guts, bowels, and intestines.

shō-chō	small bowel/intestine
jūnishi-chō	duodenum
dai-chō	large bowel
mō-chō	cecum/appendicitis
chō-kan	digestive tract

Culture Notes

The Japanese educational system

The Japanese educational system is described as the 6-3-3-4-year system: six years in elementary school (**shō-gakkō**), from the age of six; three years in junior middle school (**chū-gakkō**); three years in high school (**kōtō gakkō** or **kōkō**); and four years in college/university (**daigaku**). Attending elementary and middle school is compulsory. The school term starts in April and ends the following March. Before enrollment at elementary school, children between three and five years of age may go to kindergarten (**yōchi-en**) or nursery school (**hoiku-en**). The child's age is counted in full as of April 1. Children are referred to as children up to the age of five (**go-sai-ji**) or six (**roku-sai-ji**). **Ji** is the abbreviation for **ji-dō** (schoolchildren). Elementary school students are called **shō-gaku-sei**, Middle school students are **chū-gaku-sei**, High school students are **kōkō-sei**, and college or university students are **dai-gaku-sei**. Japanese makes no distinction between college and university. Community college is called **tanki-daigaku**, and community college students are called **tan-dai-sei**. Graduate school is called **dai-gaku-in**, and grad students are called **dai-gaku-in-sei**. Vocational school is called **senmon-gakkō**, and their students are called **senmon-gakkō-sei**.

Comprehension

Answer the following questions.

1. Which of the following does NOT belong with the others?
   a. **Mōchō**
   b. **Kikanshi**
   c. **Shokudō**
   d. **Kikan**

2. Which of the following could be used to say, "I think that you probably have appendicitis?"
   a. **Hai-gan no utagai ga arimasu.**
   b. **Mōchō-en dato omoimasu.**
   c. **Jūnishi-chō kaiyō no yō desu.**
   d. **Kikanshi-en mitai desu.**

3. Which of the following best completes the sentence below?
   Choku-chō gan (   ) utagai ga arimasu.
   (I suspect it may be rectal cancer.)
   a. **o**
   b. **ni**
   c. **no**
   d. **to**

4. Which of the following does NOT belong with the others?
   a. **Kai-chō**
   b. **Dai-chō**
   c. **Shō-chō**
   d. **Shin-chō**

5. You are giving a STRONG opinion.
   a. **Kaze dato omoimasu.**
   b. **Hai-en mitai desu.**
   c. **I-gan no yō desu.**
   d. **Mōchō-en kamo shiremasen.**

Select the correct meaning for the Japanese term.

6. **Kōmon**
   a. lung
   b. heart
   c. anus

7. **Shokudō**
   a. liver   b. esophagus   c. duodenum

8. **Mōchō**
   a. spleen   b. pancreas   c. appendix

9. **Kikanshi**
   a. bronchus   b. ascending colon   c. ileum

10. **Daichō**
    a. rectum   b. transverse colon   c. large bowel

Match the expressions in Column A and Column B.

Column A	Column B
11. ( ) **Hai-en mitai desu.**	a. I suspect it may be rectal cancer.
12. ( ) **Jūnishi-chō ga warui mitai desu.**	b. I think that you have bronchitis.
13. ( ) **I no atari ga itai desu ka.**	c. Do you have pain around your stomach?
14. ( ) **Choku-chō gan no utagai ga arimasu.**	d. It may be pneumonia.
15. ( ) **Kikanshi-en dato omoimasu.**	e. Your duodenum looks like something is wrong.

Practice

Respond to the following in Japanese using the cues that have been provided.

1. Asking about physical condition.

   (Healthcare professional)   (Patient)

   1. _____ (lung)   **Daijyōbu desu.**
   2. _____ (stomach)   **Motarete imasu.**
   3. _____ (heart)   **Sukoshi itai(n) desu.**
   4. _____ (bronchus)   **Zensoku gimi desu.**

2. Responding to the patient's complaints.

   (Patient)   (Healthcare professional)

   1. **Kōmon ni zuki-zuki suru**   _____
      itami ga arimasu.   (Let's examine/take a look at your anus.)

2. **Shinzō ni shimetsuke-rareru itami ga arimasu.**

_____

(Let's have a blood test done.)

3. **Bōkō ni yakeru itami ga arimasu.**

_____

(Let's have a urine test done/Let's test your urine.)

4. **I ga kiri-kiri shimasu.**

_____

(Let's have X-rays done.)

3. Give your medical opinion.

(Patient)   (Healthcare professional)

1. **I ga itai(n) desu.**   _____ (**i-en**/gastritis)
2. **Onaka ga itai(n) desu.**   _____ (**mōchō-en**/appendicitis)
3. **Bōkō ga itai(n) desu.**   _____ (**bōkō-en**/cystitis)

4. Say "Let's examine . . ." the following organs.

(Internal organ)   (Healthcare professional)

1. Heart _____
2. Uterus _____
3. Liver _____
4. Pancreas _____
5. Large bowel _____

5. Dialogue comprehension. Based on the dialogue, answer the following questions.

1. **Yamada-san wa karada no doko ga itai(n) desu ka.** _____
2. **Don-na itami desu ka.** _____
3. **Itsu itaku narimasu ka.** _____
4. **Yamada-san wa i no kensa o shita koto ga arimasu ka.** _____
5. **Byōmei wa nan-desu ka.** _____

6. Free response questions.

(Questions)   (Answers)

1. **Shinzō no kensa o shita koto ga arimasu ka.** _____
2. **I ga itai(n) desu ka.** _____
3. **Dokoka warui tokoro ga arimasu ka.** _____
4. **Hai wa daijyōbu desu ka.** _____
5. **Nani-ka kusuri o nonde imasu ka.** _____

Exercises

1. Say the following words in Japanese.

A. Appendix _____

      B. Heart   _____

      C. Liver   _____

      D. Large bowel/colon   _____

      E. Lung   _____

2. Ask the following questions in Japanese.   _____

    A. Do you have pain around your stomach?   _____

    B. Do you have a bloody discharge from your anus? _____

    C. Have you ever had your gall bladder examined? _____

    D. Does your stomach hurt before meals?   _____

    E. Shall I try to examine your windpipe?   _____

3. What do the following diagnoses mean in English?

    A. **Mōchō-en kamo shiremasen.**   _____

    B. **Hai-en mitai desu.**   _____

    C. **Choku-chō gan no utagai ga arimasu.**   _____

    D. **Jūnishi-chō ga warui mitai desu.**   _____

    E. **Kikanshi-en dato omoimasu.**   _____

4. Select the correct expressions of pain from the right column.

A. **Man-sei no itami**	(	)	gripping pain
B. **Kyū-sei no itami**	(	)	stinging pain
C. **Taema nai itami**	(	)	prickling pain
D. **Shitsukoi itami**	(	)	burning pain
E. **Hiri-Hiri suru itami**	(	)	continuous pain
F. **Zuki-Zuki suru itami**	(	)	persistent pain
G. **Chiku-Chiku suru itami**	(	)	acute pain
H. **Yakeru itami**	(	)	squeezing pain
I. **Sashikomu itami**	(	)	chronic pain
J. **Shimetsuke-rareru itami**	(	)	throbbing pain

5. Answer (or ask) the questions in Japanese.

    Q: **Kensa no kekka wa dō deshita ka.**

    A: _____. (I suspect it may be pneumonia.)

    Q: _____. (Where do you have pain?)

    A: **Shinzō no atari ga itai(n) desu.**

    Q: **Sensei, nodo ga itai(n) desu ga.**

    A: _____. (Your bronchus seems to be inflamed.)

LESSON 12 Examination
(Kensa)

Basic Vocabulary (CD 12-1)

Listen to the CD and repeat the vocabulary.

1.	clinical history	**byōreki**	<ruby>病<rt>びょう</rt></ruby><ruby>歴<rt>れき</rt></ruby>
2.	diagnosis	**shindan**	<ruby>診<rt>しん</rt></ruby><ruby>断<rt>だん</rt></ruby>
3.	medical checkup	**ken-shin**	<ruby>検<rt>けん</rt></ruby><ruby>診<rt>しん</rt></ruby>
4.	palpation	**shoku-shin**	<ruby>触<rt>しょく</rt></ruby><ruby>診<rt>しん</rt></ruby>
5.	rectal examination	**choku-chō-shin**	<ruby>直<rt>ちょく</rt></ruby><ruby>腸<rt>ちょう</rt></ruby><ruby>診<rt>しん</rt></ruby>
6.	pelvic examination	**nai-shin**	<ruby>内<rt>ない</rt></ruby><ruby>診<rt>しん</rt></ruby>
7.	clinical test	**rinshō kensa**	<ruby>臨<rt>りん</rt></ruby><ruby>床<rt>しょう</rt></ruby><ruby>検<rt>けん</rt></ruby><ruby>査<rt>さ</rt></ruby>
8.	reference ranges	**kijyun-chi**	<ruby>基<rt>き</rt></ruby><ruby>準<rt>じゅん</rt></ruby><ruby>値<rt>ち</rt></ruby>
9.	electrocardiogram/ ECG or EKG	**shin-den-zu**	<ruby>心<rt>しん</rt></ruby><ruby>電<rt>でん</rt></ruby><ruby>図<rt>ず</rt></ruby>
10.	electroencephalogram/EEG	**nōha**	<ruby>脳<rt>のう</rt></ruby><ruby>波<rt>は</rt></ruby>
11.	urine test	**nyō kensa**	<ruby>尿<rt>にょう</rt></ruby><ruby>検<rt>けん</rt></ruby><ruby>査<rt>さ</rt></ruby>
12.	blood test	**ketsueki-kensa**	<ruby>血<rt>けつ</rt></ruby><ruby>液<rt>えき</rt></ruby><ruby>検<rt>けん</rt></ruby><ruby>査<rt>さ</rt></ruby>
13.	cholesterol test	**koresuterōru-kensa**	コレステロール<ruby>検<rt>けん</rt></ruby><ruby>査<rt>さ</rt></ruby>
14.	HDL cholesterol	**zendama koresuterōru**	<ruby>善<rt>ぜん</rt></ruby><ruby>玉<rt>だま</rt></ruby>コレステロール
15.	LDL cholesterol	**akudama koresuterōru**	<ruby>悪<rt>あく</rt></ruby><ruby>玉<rt>だま</rt></ruby>コレステロール
16.	collecting a blood sample	**sai-ketsu**	<ruby>採<rt>さい</rt></ruby><ruby>血<rt>けつ</rt></ruby>
17.	red blood cell	**sekkekkyū**	<ruby>赤<rt>せっ</rt></ruby><ruby>血<rt>けっ</rt></ruby><ruby>球<rt>きゅう</rt></ruby>
18.	white blood cell	**hakkekkyū**	<ruby>白<rt>はっ</rt></ruby><ruby>血<rt>けっ</rt></ruby><ruby>球<rt>きゅう</rt></ruby>
19.	lymphocyte	**rinpa-kyū**	リンパ<ruby>球<rt>きゅう</rt></ruby>
20.	blood sugar level test	**kettōchi-kensa**	<ruby>血<rt>けっ</rt></ruby><ruby>糖<rt>とう</rt></ruby><ruby>値<rt>ち</rt></ruby><ruby>検<rt>けん</rt></ruby><ruby>査<rt>さ</rt></ruby>
21.	eye examination	**shi-ryoku-kensa**	<ruby>視<rt>し</rt></ruby><ruby>力<rt>りょく</rt></ruby><ruby>検<rt>けん</rt></ruby><ruby>査<rt>さ</rt></ruby>
22.	hearing test	**chō-ryoku-kensa**	<ruby>聴<rt>ちょう</rt></ruby><ruby>力<rt>りょく</rt></ruby><ruby>検<rt>けん</rt></ruby><ruby>査<rt>さ</rt></ruby>
23.	funduscopy	**gantei-kensa**	<ruby>眼<rt>がん</rt></ruby><ruby>底<rt>てい</rt></ruby><ruby>検<rt>けん</rt></ruby><ruby>査<rt>さ</rt></ruby>
24.	X-rays	**rentogen kensa**	レントゲン<ruby>検<rt>けん</rt></ruby><ruby>査<rt>さ</rt></ruby>
25.	gastro camera	**i-kamera**	<ruby>胃<rt>い</rt></ruby>カメラ
26.	endoscope	**naishi-kyō**	<ruby>内<rt>ない</rt></ruby><ruby>視<rt>し</rt></ruby><ruby>鏡<rt>きょう</rt></ruby>
27.	endoscopy	**naishi-kyō kensa**	<ruby>内<rt>ない</rt></ruby><ruby>視<rt>し</rt></ruby><ruby>鏡<rt>きょう</rt></ruby><ruby>検<rt>けん</rt></ruby><ruby>査<rt>さ</rt></ruby>
28.	first-aid treatment/first aid	**ōkyū shochi**	<ruby>応<rt>おう</rt></ruby><ruby>急<rt>きゅう</rt></ruby><ruby>処<rt>しょ</rt></ruby><ruby>置<rt>ち</rt></ruby>

| 29. | operation/surgery | **shujyutsu** | <ruby>手<rt>しゅ</rt></ruby><ruby>術<rt>じゅつ</rt></ruby> |
| 30. | intensive care unit/ICU | **shūchū chiryō-shitsu** | <ruby>集<rt>しゅう</rt></ruby><ruby>中<rt>ちゅう</rt></ruby><ruby>治<rt>ち</rt></ruby><ruby>療<rt>りょう</rt></ruby><ruby>室<rt>しつ</rt></ruby> |

Dialogue (CD 12-2)

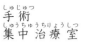 Listen to the CD and repeat the dialogue.

At the Family Doctor's Office

Dr. Simon: **Dō shimashita ka. Saikin, kenkō-shindan o mō ukemashita ka.**
Is anything the matter? Have you had already a checkup recently?

Miss Yamada: **Iie, (Kenkō shindan wa) mada ukete imasen.**
No, I have not had a checkup yet.

Dr. Simon: **Nani-ka karada ni mondai ga arimasu ka.**
Do you have any complaints?

Miss Yamada: **Hai, nani-yorimo maiban no yōni hidoi nease ga demasu.**
Yes, more than anything, I sweat heavily almost every night.

Dr. Simon: **Chi o haitari, kettan ga detari shimasu ka.**
Have you ever coughed up blood or had bloody phlegm?

Miss Yamada: **Hai, saikin tokidoki kettan ga deta koto ga sukoshi arimasu.**
Yes, I have sometimes had a little bloody phlegm recently.

Dr. Simon: **Hontō desu ka. Soredewa suguni kensa o shinai-wake-niwa ikimasen ne.**
Really? I can't help, but you should have a test immediately.

Mazu saisho-ni, rentogen o toritai desu ne.
First of all, I want to have an X-ray done.

Miss Yamada: **Hai, (wakarimashita.) Yoroshiku onegai shimasu.**
Yes, (I understand.) Please. (*lit.*, Please treat me well.)

Grammar

1. The adverb **mō**

The adverb **mō** means "already" and is used in affirmative sentences for actions that have already happened.

Kensa o mō oemashita ka.
Have you already had an examination?

Shinden-zu o mō torimashita.
I already had an electrocardiogram/EKG.

Kensa no kekka ga mō wakarimashia.
The result of the exam is already known.

Gohan o mō tabemashita ka.
Did you already eat?

2. The adverb **mada**

The adverb **mada** means "yet" and is used in negative sentences for an action that has not yet been taken.

Kensa o mada shite imasen.
I have not yet had a test. (*lit.*, The test has not been done yet.)

Shinden-zu o mada totte imasen.
I haven't had an electrocardiogram/EKG yet.

Kensa no kekka ga mada wakari-masen.
The test results are not yet known.

Gohan o mada tabete imasen.
I haven't eaten any meals yet. (*lit.*, The meal is not eaten yet.)

3. The adverb **nani-yorimo**

The adverb **nani-yorimo** expresses the notion of "more important than; above all; first of all; before anything else." The comparative **yorimo** can be used with the interrogatives **dare** (who), **doko** (where), and **itsu** (when) to indicate an urgent best choice.

Nani-yorimo kenkō ga taisetsu desu.
Health is more important than anything else.

Nani-yorimo ketsueki-kensa o shite kudasai.
Above all, please have a blood test done.

Nani-yorimo shinden-zu o torimashō.
Let's have an EKG done before anything else.

Dare-yorimo, kanjya no nyō-kensa o shimasu.
I will test this patient's urine before anyone else's.

Kono byōin wa doko-yorimo atarashii kensa-ki ga arimasu.
This hospital has more new lab equipment than anywhere else.

Itsu-yorimo, kensa ga hayaku owarimashita.
The test was done earlier than usual.

4. The construction DAY/WEEK/MONTH/FREQUENCY + **no yōni**

The construction DAY/WEEK/MONTH/FREQUENCY plus **no yōni** is used for re-curring actions and means "hoping or wishing for (something) every (time); take care to do (something) every (time)." Some time expressions used in this construction are **mai-nichi** (every day); **mai-shū** (every week); **mai-tsuki** (every month); **mai-nen** (every year); and **mai-kai** (every time). The prefix **mai-** means "every."

> **Mai-nichi no yōni kettochi no kensa o shite kudasai.**
> I hope you have a blood sugar (level) test every day.
>
> **Mai-kai no yōni kagaku-ryōhō ga hitsu-yō desu.**
> I hope you have chemotherapy every time.
>
> **Kanjya wa mai-tsuki no yōni hōsha-sen chiryō o ukete imasu.**
> The patient has had maintenance radiotherapy every month.

5. The suffix **-tari**

The **te**-form can express two or more sequential actions in one sentence. However, expressions using the verb suffix **-tari** indicate two actions that are simultaneous or in the same time frame.

> **Kangoshi wa kanjya no taion o hakattari, myaku-haku o tottari shimashita.**
> The nurse took the patient's temperature and at the same time checked his pulse rate.
>
> **Shinryō-shitsu de ōkyū shochi o shitari, kensa no kekka o mattari shimasu.**
> They are giving first aid and waiting for the test result in sick bay.

To change from the **te-** to the **tari** form, drop the -te/-de ending and replace it with -tari/-dari. Whether the new ending is -tari or -dari depends on the **te**-form. If the **te**-form ends with -te/-ite/-tte, the **tari** form ending is -tari. If the **te**-form ends with -nde or -ide, the **tari** form ending is -dari.

ENGLISH	MASU FORM (VERB BASE)	TE-FORM	TARI FOM
think	omoi-masu	omo-tte-kudasai	omo-ttari
point out/pierce/ sting	sashi-masu	sashi-te-kudasai	sashi-tari
begin	hajime-masu	hajime-te-kudsai	hajime-tari
move	ugoki-masu	ugoi-te-kudasai	ugoi-tari
turn/peel off	muki-masu	mu-ite-kudasai	mui-tari
stop	tome-masu	tome-te-kudasai	tome-tari

ENGLISH	MASU FORM (VERB BASE)	TE-FORM	TARI FOM
spread/open	hiroge-masu	hiroge-te-kudasai	hiroge-tari
run	hashiri-masu	hashi-tte-kudasai	hashi-ttari
continue	tsuzuke-masu	tsuzuke-te kudasai	tsuzuke-tari
go up	age-masu	age-te-kudasai	age-tari
get off/step down	ori-masu	ori-te-kudasai	ori-tari
end/finish	owari-masu	owa-tte-kudasai	owa-ttari
change clothes	kigae-masu	kigae-te-kudasai	kigae-tari
investigate	shirabe-masu	shibire-te-kudasai	shibire-tari
upset mind	mukatsuki-masu	mukatsui-ite-kudasai	mukatsui-tari
empty/be hungry	suki-masu	su-ite-kudasai	sui-tari
have a heavy stomach feeling	motare-masu	motare-te kudasai	motare-tari
throw up	hakidashi-masu	hakidashi-te-kudasai	hakidashi-tari
complete/end	owari-masu	owa-tte-kudasai	owa-ttari
receive	uke-masu	uke-te-kudasai	uke-tari
measure	hakari-masu	haka-tte-kudasai	haka-ttari
swallow	nomikomi-masu	nomiko-nde-kudasai	nomiko-ndari
drink	nomi-masu	no-nde-kudasai	no-ndari
massage	momi-masu	mo-nde-kudasai	mo-ndari
die	shini-masu	shi-nde kudasai	shi-ndari
take off clothes	nugi-masu	nu-ide kudasai	nu-idari

6. The adverb **sugu (ni)**

The adverb **sugu (ni)** is used for immediate action and proximity and translates as "immediately, instantly, right away." The expression **mō sugu (ni)** is used for actions that take more time, are slower, or more distant than those **sugu (ni)** would be used for, and translates as "soon." The particle **ni** can be dropped.

Sugu ni nōha kensa o shimashō.
You need to have an electroencephalogram immediately.

Sugu(ni) hakidashite (kudasai).
Throw up right away.

Mō sugu ōkyū-shochi o shimasu.
We will give you first aid soon.

Sugu soko ni shujyutsu-dai ga arimasu.
There is an operating table near here.

7. The construction NEGATIVE VERB + **wake-ni(wa) ikanai**

A negative verb plus **wake-ni(wa) ikanai/ikimasen** indicates that one does not have any other choice and is usually translated as "cannot help; cannot help but do." In contrast, an affirmative verb plus **wake-ni(wa) ikani** is used when the speaker can't do certain things for some reason.

Kanjya no byōreki o shiranai wake ni(wa) ikanai desu.
I can't help without knowing the patient's clinical history.

Kanjya no byōreki o shiru wake ni(wa) ikanai desu.
I can't know the patient's clinical history.

Koresuterōru ga takai node, niku o taberu wake-niwa ikanai desu.
I have high cholesterol, so I can't eat meat.

Koresuterōru ga takai desuga, niku o tabenai wake-niwa ikimasen.
I have high cholesterol, but I can't help but eat meat.

Rinshō-kensa o shinai wake-ni(wa) ikimasen.
I can't help without the clinical test.

Suguni kanjya o shūchū-chiryō-shitsu ni ireru wake-niwa ikanai desu.
I can't put the patient into the Intensive Care Unit immediately.

8. The expression **mazu saisho ni**

Mazu saisho ni means "first of all." **Mazu** or **saisho ni** by themselves mean "first." The use of either of these expressions tells the order of doing things and indicates that another step or other steps will follow.

Mazu saisho ni i-kamera de i o shirabemashō ka.
First of all, shall we check out your stomach using the gastro camera?

Mazu, nyō-kensa o shimasu. First, we will have a urine test done.
Saisho ni, ketsu-eki-kensa o shimasu. First, we'll test your blood.

9. The verb suffix **-tai**

The verb suffix **-tai** adds the idea of "wish" and "want" to the verb's meaning. To make the **tai** form, first drop -**masu** from the **masu** form to identify the verb base, and then add the suffix -**tai**.

ENGLISH	MASU FORM (VERB BASE)	TAI FORM (WISH/WANT)
see/look/watch	mi-masu	mi-tai
do/play	shi-masu	shi-tai
speak	hanashi-masu	hanashi-tai
drink	nomi-masu	nomi-tai
move	ugoki-masu	ugoki-tai
listen/hear	kiki-masu	kiki-tai
inform/teach	oshie-masu	oshie-tai

Kanzō no kensa o shitai(n) desu.
I want to examine your liver.

Mizu ga nomitai(n) desu ka.
Do you want to have water?/Would you like water?

Kanjya-san ni naishikyō-kensa o oshietai(n) desu.
I wish to inform the patients about endoscopy.

Useful Expressions (CD 12-3)

Listen to the CD and repeat the sentences.

1. **Byōreki o oshiete kudasai.** Please tell me your medical history.
2. **Kenkō-shindan o shita-koto ga arimasu ka.** Have you had a checkup?
3. **Kagaku-ryōhō o shite mimashō.** Let's try chemotherapy.
4. **Rentogen-kensa to shinden-zu kensa ga hitsuyō desu.** You need to have an X-ray and an electrocardiogram/ECG.
5. **Nyō-kensa o shimasu kara, kono kappu ni 3 bun no 1 gurai totte kudasai.** You're here for a urine test, so please fill about one-third of this cup.
6. **Rentogen kensa o shimasu kara, rentogen-shitsu ni itte kudasai.** We will take an X-ray, so please go to the X-ray room.
7. **Shujyutsu o shimasu kara beddo ni aomuke ni natte kudasai.** You are going to have an operation, so please lie down on your back.
8. **Kensa no ato-ni chūsha o shimasu.** You will have an injection after the examination.
9. **Tenteki o shimasu kara sode o makutte kudasai.** Please roll up your sleeve, because you will be having an intravenous drip.
10. **Chiryō o shimasu kara, beddo ni utusbuse ni natte kudasai.** Please lie face down for your treatment.

Key Sentences (CD 12-4)

Listen to the CD and repeat the sentences.

1. **Mazu saisho ni byōreki o oshiete kudasai.** Please tell me your medical history.
2. **Kensa no kekka ga mada wakarimasen.** The results of the test are not known yet.
3. **Naniyorimo shiryoku-kensa o shita hō ga ii to omoimasu.** I think you should have an eye examination more than anything else.
4. **Ashita kettō-chi (no) kensa ga arimasu kara, amai-mono wa taberu wake-ni(wa) ikimasen.** I can't eat sweets because I have a blood sugar-level test tomorrow.
5. **Ōkyū-shochi o shitari, kensa o shitari shimasu.** I do things like give first aid and examine patients.

Additional Words

hakidasu/hakidashimasu throw up
ukeru/ukemasu receive
sokutei measurement
taisetsu important
tei-ketsu-atsu low blood pressure
jyumyō life span
jyōmyaku-chūsha intravenous injection
shujyutsu-dai operating table
chiryō treatment
shinryō-shitsu sick bay
hoken-shitsu school infirmary
amai-mono sweet

oeru/oemasu finish
nomikomu/nomikomimasu swallow
kenkō healthy
kō-ketsu-atsu high blood pressure
ne-ase sweat/perspire while sleeping
hika-chūsha hypodermic injection
kesshō-ban platelet
shujyutsu-shitsu operating room
rinshō-kensa-gishi clinical laboratory technician
hōshasen chiryō radiotheraphy
shoppai-mono salty foods

Language Notes

1. In the Languge Notes in Lesson 9, we studied basic X-ray-related expressions. X-ray examinations often use patterned expressions, in other words, expressions that recur in a similar form because the situation is similar.

Jyō-han-shin [o] hadaka ni natte kudasai. Please undress from the waist up.
Kono kensa-gi o kite kudasai. Please put this examination gown on.

Akusessarī o totte kudasai. Please take your accessories off.
Kono dai ni mune o tsuke te kudasai. Please press your chest against this board.

Ago o dai ni tsuke te kudasai.	Please put your chin on this board.
Iki o fukaku suttari haitari shite kudasai.	Take a deep breath in and out, please.
Hai, Iki o ōkiku sutte kudasai.	Okay, please take a deep breath.
Hai, Iki o tomete ugokanai de kudasai.	Okay, please hold your breath and don't move.
Hai, Iki o haite kudasai.	Okay, please breathe out.
Hai, Iki o suttemo ii desu yo.	Okay, you can breathe now.
Hai, owarimashita.	Okay, that's all.

2. Fractions are expressed using **bun no** as follows:

ni bun no ichi	½	or **han bun** (half)
san bun no ichi	⅓	
yon bun no ichi	¼	
go bun no ichi	⅕	
san bun no ni	⅔	
yon bun no san	¾	
go bun no ni	⅖	
go bun no san	⅗	
go bun no yon	⅘	

3. In Lesson 9, we studied some basic instructions or requests that are useful in the examination room. Here is a more complete list of expressions that may come in handy:

Kuchi o akete kudasai.	Please open your mouth.
Kuchi o tojite kudasai.	Please close your mouth.
Me o akete kudasai.	Please open your eyes.
Me o tojite kudasai.	Please close your eyes.
Shita o misete/dashite kudasai.	Please show me your tongue.
Mae o mite kudasai.	Please look forward.
Ue o mite kudasai.	Please look up.
Chikara o nuite kudasai.	Please relax.
Shita o mite kudasai.	Please look down.
Ushiro muki ni natte kudasai.	Please turn around.
Migi o muite kudasai.	Please turn to the right.
Hidari o muite kudasai.	Please turn to the left.
Ugokanai de kudasai.	Please do not move.
Muki o kaete kudasai.	Please turn over.
Ashi o nobashite kudasai	Please stretch your legs.
Hiza o magete kudasai.	Please bend your knees.

Watakushi no hō o muite kudasai.	Turn toward me, please.
Watakushi no yubi o mite kudasai.	Look at my finger, please.

Shinsatsu-dai ni aomuke ni natte kudasai.
Please lie on your back on the examining table.

Shinsatsu-dai ni utsubuse ni natte kudasai.
Please lie on your stomach on the examination table.

Shinsatsu-dai ni agatte kudasai.
Please get up on the examination table.

Shinsatsu-dai kara orite kudasai.
Please step down from the examination table.

Migi-waki o shita ni shite, yoko ni natte kudasai.
Please lie on your right side.

Hidari-waki o shita ni shite, yoko ni natte kudasai.
Please lie on your left side.

4. To ask a favor, make a request, or express a wish, Japanese use the polite form **onegai shimasu**.

Yoyaku o onegai shimasu.	I would like to request an appointment.
Mizu o onegai shimasu.	Please give me some water.
Kensa o onegai shimasu.	I would like to have a physical.

5. Japanese might use the more formal polite expression **Yoroshiku onegai shimasu** to express their gratitude to a doctor or nurse or other healthcare professional. **Yoroshiku onegai shimasu** may be translated variously as "please treat me well; please take care of me; please remember me; please help me; I look forward to working with you; best regards," though these English translations don't really convey the level of extreme politeness that the idiom does in Japanese.

Language Roots

The suffix **-hō** (法) indicates a principle or method.

kagaku-ryō-hō	chemotherapy
meneki-ryō-hō	immunotherapy
kensa no hō-hō	method of examination
chiryō-hō-hō	method of treatment

The word **ken** (検) indicates an examination, inspection, or investigation. A similar meaning of "examination" is conveyed by the **ken** reading of a different character, 験, and by **sa** (査).

nyō ken-sa	urine test
ken-eki	quarantine
ten-ken	check/inspection
shi-ken	examination/test
ken-sa	checkup/test/exam

Culture Notes

X-rays and the name Rentogen in Japan

Japanese medicine has been strongly influenced by Germany since the Meiji Period, beginning in 1868. Wilhelm Conrad Röntgen (1845–1923) of Germany discovered X-rays and was awarded the first Nobel Prize in Physics in 1901. Based on his name, Japanese call X-rays Rentogen (Röntgen).

Health-related Japanese proverbs IV

Poverty is mother of health.
Binbō wa kenkō no haha.
貧乏は健康の母

Health is better than wealth.
Kenkō wa tomi ni masaru.
健康は富にまさる

Comprehension

Answer the following questions.

1. Which of the following does NOT belong with the others?
   a. **Hōsha-sen ryōhō**
   b. **Meneki ryōhō**
   c. **Ōkyū-shochi**
   d. **Kagaku ryōhō**

2. Which of the following could be used to say, "I suspect that . . ."
   a. **Hai-gan no utagai ga arimasu.**
   b. **Ōkyū shochi o shite, kensa no kekka o machimasu.**
   c. **Kyō kensa ga arimasu kara, yasu-nde kudasai.**
   d. **Kikanshi-en dato omoimasu.**

3. Which of the following best completes the sentence below?
    Monshin-hyō ni kinyū (   ), kensa o shi-tari shimasu.
    You do things such as fill in the physical questionnaire and have an examination.

    a. **o**   b. **shi-tari**
    c. **no**   d. **to**

4. Which of the following does NOT belong with the others?
    a. **Nyō kensa**   b. **Ketsu-eki kensa**
    c. **Kettōchi**   d. **Naishi-kyō**

5. You are suggesting that a patient have an injection.
    a. **Chūsha o mimashō.**
    b. **Hika-shūsha wa mada desu.**
    c. **Chūsha o shita hō ga ii desu yo.**
    d. **Chūsha no hitsuyō ga arimasen.**

Select the correct instructions from the right column.

---

6. **Me o ake te kudasai.**	( )	a. Please look forward.
7. **Mae o mite kudasai.**	( )	b. Please lie on your back.
8. **Ushiro muki ni natte kudasai.**	( )	c. Please turn around.
9. **Ugokanai de kudasai.**	( )	d. Please turn over.
10. **Aomuke ni natte kudasai.**	( )	e. Please do not move.
11. **Utsubuse ni natte kudasai.**	( )	f. Please lie on your stomach.
12. **Muki o kaete kudasai.**	( )	g. Please open your eyes.

Practice

Respond to the following in Japanese using the cues that have been provided.

---

1. What kinds of examinations are required for the following conditions:
    (Conditions)   (Healthcare professional)
    1. **Kō-ketsuatsu desu.**   _____
    2. **Mune ga itai(n) desu.**   _____
    3. **Atama ga itai(n) desu.**   _____
    4. **I ga itai(n) desu.**   _____
    5. **Hone ga oremashita.**   _____

2. Give the patient the proper instruction for the examination or test.

(Examination or test)   (Healthcare professional)

1. **Nyō-kensa**   _____

(Provide a urine sample of one-third of the cup.)

2. **Tenteki**   _____

(Roll up your sleeve.)

3. **Rentogen-kensa**   _____

(Take off your shirt.)

4. **Shinsatsu-dai de**   _____

(Please lie face down.)

5. **Shinsatsu-dai de**   _____

(Please lie down on your back.)

3. Say the correct instruction in Japanese.

(Patient)   (Healthcare professional)

1. Look to the left.   _____
2. Look to the right.   _____
3. Open your mouth.   _____
4. Relax.   _____
5. Show or stick out your tongue.   _____

4. Say the following to the patient.

(Patient)   (Healthcare professional)

1. You need to provide a half cup of urine   _____
2. You need to provide a third of a cup of urine.   _____
3. You need to eat and drink.   _____
4. You need to rest and sleep.   _____

5. Dialogue comprehension. Based on the dialogue, answer the following.

1. **Yamada-san wa maiban no yō ni nani ga demasu ka.**

_____

2. **Yamada-san wa kettan ga demasu ka.**

_____

3. **Itsu kara kettan ga dete imasu ka.**

_____

4. **Mazu saisho ni don-na kensa o shimasu ka.**

_____

6. Free response questions.

(Questions)   (Answers)

1. **Rentogen kensa o shita koto ga arimasu ka.**   _____

2. **Itsu Rentogen kensa o shimashita ka.** _____

3. **Koresuterōru no kensa o shite imasu ka.** _____

4. **Koresuterōru kensa no kekka wa dō deshita ka.** _____

Exercises

1. Say the following words in Japanese.
   A. Clinical history _____
   B. Urine test _____
   C. Operation/surgery _____
   D. Hearing test _____
   E. Palpation _____

2. Say the following expressions in Japanese.
   A. Please tell me your clinical history. _____
   B. I do such things as test urine and _____
      give electrocardiograms.
   C. Do you have pain in your chest? _____
   D. Please do not eat anything, because _____
      you have an examination today.
   E. The X-ray results are not known yet. _____

3. When speaking to a patient, how do you say the following in Japanese?
   A. Are you having a checkup today? _____
   B. Let's try chemotherapy. _____
   C. We will take an X-ray, so please go _____
      to the X-ray room.
   D. Please roll up your sleeve so you can _____
      have an IV drip.
   E. Please lie face down so you can have _____
      a treatment.

4. Answer the following questions in Japanese.

   Q: Do you have the results of the electrocardiogram/ECG?
   A: _____
      (No, the test results are not known yet.)

   Q: What is the result of the examination?
   B: _____
      (I think the result is good.)

After the Examination
(Shinsatsu-go)

Basic Vocabulary (CD 13-1)

Listen to the CD and repeat the vocabulary.

No.	English	Romaji	Japanese
1.	commute to the hospital	**tsū-in**	通院
2.	stress	**sutoresu**	ストレス
3.	absolute rest	**zettai-ansei**	絶対安静
4.	poor health (condition)	**taichō-furyō**	体調不良
5.	rest (for physical reasons)	**kyūyō**	休養
6.	liquid food	**ryūdō-shoku**	流動食
7.	infectious disease	**kansen-shō**	感染症
8.	possibility	**kanō-sei**	可能性
9.	danger	**kiken-sei**	危険性
10.	side effect	**fuku-sayō**	副作用
11.	fasting	**zesshoku**	絶食
12.	overdo/overwork	**muri**	無理
13.	permission	**kyoka**	許可
14.	positive	**yō-sei**	陽性
15.	negative	**in-sei**	陰性
16.	pseudo/false positive	**giji-yōsei**	擬似陽性
17.	recurrence	**sai-hatsu**	再発
18.	chronic disease	**ji-byō/mansei-byō**	持病 /慢性病
19.	prevention	**yobō**	予防
20.	early detection	**sōki-hakken**	早期発見
21.	periodical check up	**teiki-kenshin**	定期健診
22.	medical record/chart	**karute**	カルテ
23.	complete recovery	**kanchi**	完治
24.	immunotherapy	**meneki-ryōhō**	免疫療法
25.	chemotherapy	**kagaku ryōhō**	化学療法
26.	radiotherapy	**hōsha-sen ryōhō**	放射線療法
27.	hormone therapy	**horumon-ryōhō**	ホルモン療法
28.	diet therapy	**shokuji-ryōhō**	食事療法
29.	complications	**gappei-shō**	合併症
30.	metastasis/spread	**ten-i**	転移

Dialogue (CD 13-2)

Listen to the CD and repeat the dialogue.

At the Primary Care Physician's Office

Dr. Simon: **Shinsatsu wa ijō desu. Shibaraku yōsu o mimashō.**
We finished the examination. Let's see if your condition improves.

Miss Yamada: **Gakkō ni ikanai-tsumori desu ga, shindan-sho o kudasai.**
I intend not to go to school, but please give me a doctor's note.

Dr. Simon: **Hai, ii desu yo. Gakkō wa yasunda-hō ga ii deshō. Muri wa shinai de kudasai.**
Yes, sure. You would do better not go to school. Please don't overdo.

Miss Yamada: **Hai, (wakarimashita). Itsu goro naorimasu ka. Gakkō ni ikitai(n) desu.**
Yes, (I understand). When will I be well again? I want go to school.

Dr. Simon: **Ni-shū kan mo sureba yoku narimasu yo.**
You should be better in about two weeks.

              Shikashi, tsūin suru hitsuyō ga arimasu.
But you need to check in with us regularly.

Miss Yamada: **Hai, (wakarimashita). Sai-hatsu ga shinpai desu ga.**
Yes, (I understand). I am worried about a recurrence.

Dr. Simon: **Sō desu ne. Nani-ka attara suguni renraku shite kudasai. Odaiji-ni.**
I agree. If you have any problems, please contact us immediately. Take care of yourself.

Miss Yamada: **Hai. Osewa ni narimashita.**
Yes. Thank you very much for your help.

Grammar

1. ### The construction STEM VERB PRESENT TENSE + tsumori

    The construction STEM VERB PRESENT TENSE plus **tsumori** is used to express intentions or plans for the future. The negative form of this construction uses **nai tsumori** to describe what one doesn't intend to do or intends not to do.

Kansen-shō no yobō o suru tsumori desu.
I intend to prevent an infection.

Kyō kensa o suru tsumori desu.
I'm scheduled to have a test today.

Kensa o shi-nai tsumori desu.
I do not intend to examine you.

In order to make verbs negative, you need first to change the stem verb. The following charts show stem verbs and their negative forms for two different groups or conjugations of verbs. Almost all Japanese verbs are classified as **ru**-verbs or **u**-verbs. The only exceptions, which you will see in the first chart, are **shimasu** (to do) and **kimasu** (to come), which are irregular and change form irregularly. For a detailed explanation of **ru**-verbs and **u**-verbs, see the Language Notes in this lesson. The Language Notes will also explain about the **masu** form and the verb base.

To make the negative form of **ru**-verbs, first drop -**ru** from the stem verb and replace it with the negative ending -**nai**. When verb base ends in -**ri**, change the -**ri** to -**ra** and add -**nai** for the negative form.

Ru-verbs

ENGLISH	MASU FORM	VERB BASE	STEM VERB	NEGATIVE
sleep	ne-masu	ne	ne-ru	ne-nai
eat	tabe-masu	tabe	tabe-ru	tabe-nai
teach/tell	oshie-masu	oshie	oshie-ru	oshie-nai
open	ake-masu	ake	ake-ru	ake-nai
close	shime-masu	shime	shime-ru	shime-nai
exhaust	tsukare-masu	tsukare	tsukare-ru	tsukae-nai
investigate	shirabe-masu	shirabe	shirabe-ru	shirabe-nai
roll up/give	age-masu	age	age-ru	age-nai
attach/connect/ turn on	tsuke-masu	tsuke	tsuke-ru	tsuke-nai
warm	atatame-masu	atatame	atatame-ru	atatame-nai
bend	mage-masu	mage	mage-ru	mage-nai
suppress/ keep down	osae-masu	osae	osae-ru	osae-nai
measure	hakari-masu	haka-ri	haka-ru	hakara-nai
sit down	suwari-masu	suwa-ri	suwa-ru	suwara-nai

ENGLISH	MASU FORM	VERB BASE	STEM VERB	NEGATIVE
do/play*	shi-masu	shi	su-ru	shi-nai
come*	ki-masu	ki	ku-ru	ko-nai

* Irregular

To make the negative form of **u**-verbs, 1) first drop the -**u** from the stem verb, replace it with -**a**, then add the -**nai** ending. 2) If the stem verb end with -**tsu**, replace it -**ta** and add the -**nai** ending, 3) If the stem verb ends with -**u**, replace it with -**wa** and add the -**nai** ending.

U-verbs

ENGLISH	MASU FORM	VERB BASE	STEM VERB	NEGATIVE
drink	nomi-masu	nomi	nomu	noma-nai
read	yomi-masu	yomi	yomu	yoma-nai
go	iki-masu	iki	iku	ika-nai
listen	kiki-masu	kiki	kiku	kika-nai
smell/sniff	kagi-masu	kagi	kagu	kaga-nai
rub	momi-masu	momi	momu	moma-nai
speak	hanashi-masu	hanashi	hanasu	hanasa-nai
pull down	oroshi-masu	oroshi	orosu	orosa-nai
cooling	hiyashi-masu	hiyashi	hiyasu	hiyasa-nai
send out/ prescribe	dashi-masu	dashi	dasu	dasa-nai
stretch	nobashi-masu	nobashi	nobasu	nobasa-nai
wait	machi-masu	machi	matsu	mata-nai
stand up	tachi-masu	tachi	tatsu	tata-nai
buy	kai-masu	kai	kau	kawa-nai
wash	arai-masu	arai	arau	arawa-nai
say	ii-masu	ii	iu	iwa-nai
follow/obey	shitagai-masu	shitagai	shitagau	shitagawa-nai

2. **The constructions** STEM VERB-**deshō** and STEM VERB-**nai-deshō**

The suffix -**deshō** (probably) and its negative -**nai-deshō** (probably not) can be used when making a guess or prediction. Both of these expressions are also used with the stem verbs, which we will study in the Language Notes.

Ashita yoku naru-deshō.
You will probably be well by tomorrow.

Ashita kensa no kekka ga deru-deshō.
You probably will receive the test results tomorrow.

Ashita made yoku naranai-deshō.
You probably will not be well by tomorrow.

3. Mo sureba . . . narimasu

The particle **mo** conveys the notion of an upper or outside limit in the expression **mo sureba . . . nari-masu**, which means "as much as, within, no more than."

Ni shū-kan mo sureba yoku narimasu.
It will get better in as much as two weeks.

San-yokka mo sureba narimasu.
It will be cured within three to four days.

Shi-go nich mo sureba shizen ni narimasu.
It will heal/be better itself in no more than four to five days.

4. The construction STEM VERB + hitsuyō ga arimasu

The construction STEM VERB plus **hitsuyō ga arimasu** means "it's necessary to."

Sugu ni kensa o suru hitsuyō ga airmasu.
You need to be examined immediately (*lit.*, It's necessary to examine you immediately).

Sugu, ōkyū shochi o suru hitsuyō ga arimasu.
You need to have temporary treatment immediately.

Sugu, nyūin suru hitsuyō ga arimasu.
You need to be hospitalized immediately.

5. VERB + ga combines two sentences while expressing a contrast.

In Lesson 2, we studied the particle **ga** as a subject marker in the pattern NOUN plus **ga**. However, the particle **ga** can convey the sense of English *but* in the pattern VERB plus **ga** and can combine two sentences while expressing contrast.

Karui kaze no yō desu ga, shigoto wa yasunde kudasai.
It's only a slight cold, but you shouldn't go to work (*lit.*, You have a slight cold, but please take a day off from work).

Shōjyō wa karui desu ga, naoru no ni shibaraku jikan ga kakarimasu yo.
I'm telling you that your condition isn't serious, but it will take a while to get better.

Shinsatsu wa owarimasu ga, zettai ni kyūyō shite kudasai.
This medical examination is over, but you must get absolute rest.

6. VERB + **ga** also expresses when the speaker trails off.

Ga in the pattern VERB plus **ga** can also be used to abbreviate a thought or a sentence or to trail off, for example when the speaker feels that the meaning is clear from the context or chooses not to enunciate it.

Shōjō wa karui-to omoimasu ga.	I think the symptom is not serious, but . . .
Taishita koto wa nai-yō desu ga.	It does not seem to be serious, but . . .
Shizen ni naoru-to omoimasu ga.	I think it will cure itself, but . . .

Useful Expressions (CD 13-3)

Listen to the CD and repeat the sentences.

1. **Shinsatsu wa ijyō desu.** We're finished with your checkup/examination.
2. **Shibaraku yōsu o mimashō.** Let's wait for a while and see how your condition is.
3. **Zettai-ansei ga hitsuyō desu.** You should get absolute rest.
4. **Kizuguchi o sawaranai de kudasai.** Don't touch the wound/sore/injury.
5. **Shokuji ryōhō ni sitagatte kudasai.** Please follow a strict diet.
6. **Tsumetai mono wa sakete kudasai.** You shouldn't have anything cold.
7. **Sutoresu o sakeru koto ga hitsuyō desu.** It's necessary to avoid stress.
8. **Nyūin shinakute mo ii desu.** You don't have to be hospitalized.
9. **Shibaraku tsūin suru hitsuyō ga arimasu.** You'll have to visit us regularly for a while.
10. **Kensa no kekka ga detara denwa o shimasu.** I'll call you when I get the results of the test.

Key Sentences (CD 13-4)

Listen to the CD and repeat the sentences.

1. **Kensa o suru tsumori desu.** I intend to examine you.
2. **Ashita yoku naru-deshō.** You will probably be well by tomorrow.
3. **San-yokka mo sureba narimasu.** You will heal within three to four days.
4. **Sugu ni kensa o suru hitsuyō ga arimasu.** We need to examine it right away.

5. **Karui kaze no yō desu ga, shigoto wa yasunde kudasai.** It's only a slight cold, but you shouldn't go to work.

Additional Words

osaeru/osaemasu suppress/keep down
modoru/modorimasu return
hikaeru/hikaemasu avoid
okiru/okimasu wake up/rise
hitsuyō necessary
karui mild/light
tsumetai-mono a thing that's cold
ryō quantity/amount
eiyō-ka food value
eiyō-shicchō malnutrition

momu/momimasu rub
sakeru/sakemasu tear off
zettai(ni) absolute (as in rest)
shizen(ni) naturally
(o)sewa care/assistance
omoi serious/weighty
ijyō that's it/that's all
ten-in transfer to a different hospital
machiai-shitsu waiting room
kansen-shō taisaku infection control measures

Language Notes

1. The following are some useful phrases for the completion of the examination:

> **Hai, owarimashita.**
> That's all./That's it./You are done./We're all finished.

> **Okite kudasai.**
> Wake up, please.

> **Oki-agatte kudasai.**
> Please get up.

> **Fuku o kite kudasai.**
> Please put on your clothes/dress.

> **Koko o osaete-ite kudasai.**
> Please hold (that position).

> **Shinsatsu-dai kara orite kudasai.**
> Please get down from the examination table.

> **Omatase shimashita.**
> Sorry to have kept you waiting.

> **Chotto matte kudasai.**
> Please wait a moment.

> **Yoku monde kudasai.**
> Please rub it well.

(Koko o) moma-naide osaete kudasai.
Please do not rub, but press here.

Chi ga tomattara bando-eido o totte kudasai.
When it stops bleeding, remove the Band-aid.

Machiai-sitsu ni modotte kudasai.
Please go back to the waiting room.

Kaikei ni itte kudasai./Kaikei de shiharai o shite kudasai.
Please go pay at the cashier.

2. Stem verbs (dictionary form)

The three main forms of Japanese verb are the **masu** form, **te**-form, and stem verb (also known as the dictionary form). The **masu** form is used for general polite conversation. The **te**-form is used 1) to make a request or issue polite instructions, as in, "Please (do something)"; 2) to express more than one action in a sentence; and 3) to form the present progressive (-**te imasu**) and in certain constructions, such as -**te mimasu** (try to do something), as explained in Lessons 3 and 4. The stem verb is the core Japanese verb and can be conjugated in many different types of sentences. The following are some examples using the stem verb of **shimasu** (to do). **Shimasu** is the **masu** form of the verb. As we saw in the chart above, the stem verb form is **suru**.

Kanjya o shinsatsu suru to omoimasu.
I think I will examine the patient.

Kanjya o shinsatsu suru tsumori desu.
I intend to examine the patient.

Kanjya o shinsatsu suru hitsuyō ga arimasu.
It's necessary to examine the patient.

As mentioned in the Grammar section, there are two types of stem verbs: **u**-verbs and **ru**-verbs. It's easy to identify which verbs are which. The **u**-verbs always end with the vowel -**i**, -**shi**, or -**chi** in the verb base. The **ru**-verbs end in a vowel other than -**i** or in -**shi**, or -**chi** in the verb base, or they end in -**ri**, as shown in the chart below. The verb base is the part of the verb that remains when the -**masu** ending is dropped from the **masu** form.

The **u**-verbs use the suffix -**u**. There are three types of **u**-verb, according to how the stem verb is formed from the **masu** form. 1) For verbs ending in -**i** in the verb base, first drop -**masu** and replace final vowel -**i** with -**u**. 2) For verbs ending in -**shi** in the base, first drop -**shi-masu** and replace it with -**su**. 3) For verbs ending in -**chi** in the base, first drop -**chi-masu** and replace it with -**tsu**.

ENGLISH	**MASU** FORM	VERB BASE	STEM VERB (PRESENT)
drink	**nomi-masu**	**nomi(masu)**	**nomu**
read	**yomi-masu**	**yomi(masu)**	**yomu**
go	**iki-masu**	**iki(masu)**	**iku**
listen	**kiki-masu**	**kiki(masu)**	**kiku**
buy	**kai-masu**	**kai(masu)**	**kau**
wash	**arai-masu**	**arai(masu)**	**arau**
say	**ii-masu**	**ii(masu)**	**iu**
smell/sniff	**kagi-masu**	**kagi(masu)**	**kagu**
follow/obey	**shitagai-masu**	**shitagai(masu)**	**shitagau**
rub	**momi-masu**	**momi(masu)**	**momu**
speak	**hanashi-masu**	**hanashi(masu)**	**hanasu**
pull down	**oroshi-masu**	**oroshi (masu)**	**orosu**
cool	**hiyashi-masu**	**hiyashi (masu)**	**hiyasu**
send out/prescribe	**dashi-masu**	**dashi(masu)**	**dasu**
stretch	**nobashi-masu**	**nobashi(masu)**	**nobasu**
wait	**machi-masu**	**machi(masu)**	**matsu**
stand up	**tachi-masu**	**tachi(masu)**	**tatsu**

The **ru**-verbs all add the suffix -**ru**. There are three types of **ru**-verbs, again according to how the stem verb is formed from the **masu** form. 1) For the first type, to form the stem verb you drop -**masu** and replace it with -**ru**.

ENGLISH	**MASU** FORM	VERB BASE	STEM VERB
sleep	**ne-masu**	**ne(masu)**	**ne-ru**
eat	**tabe-masu**	**tabe(masu)**	**tabe-ru**
teach/tell	**oshie-masu**	**oshie(masu)**	**oshie-ru**
open	**ake-masu**	**ake(masu)**	**ake-ru**
close	**shime-masu**	**shime(masu)**	**shime-ru**
exhaust	**tsukare-masu**	**tsukare(masu)**	**tsukare-ru**
investigate	**shirabe-masu**	**shirabe(masu)**	**shirabe-ru**
roll up/give	**age-masu**	**age(masu)**	**age-ru**
attach/connect/turn on	**tsuke-masu**	**tsuke(masu)**	**tsuke-ru**
warm	**atatame-masu**	**atatame(masu)**	**atatame-ru**
bend	**mage-masu**	**mage(masu)**	**mage-ru**

ENGLISH	MASU FORM	VERB BASE	STEM VERB
avoid	**sake-masu**	**sake(masu)**	**sake-ru**
suppress/keep down	**osae-masu**	**osae(masu)**	**osae-ru**
finish/complete	**oe-masu**	**oe(masu)**	**oe-ru**

The second type ends has a **-ri** just before **-masu**. For this type, drop the -**masu** and then replace the -**ri** with -**ru**.

ENGLISH	MASU FORM	VERB BASE	STEM VERB
become	**nari-masu**	**na-ri(masu)**	**na-ru**
measure	**hakari-masu**	**haka-ri(masu)**	**haka-ru**
sit down	**suwari-masu**	**suwa-ri(masu)**	**suwa-ru**
return	**kaeri-masu**	**kae-ri(masu)**	**kae-ru**
paint/apply	**nuri-masu**	**nu-ri(masu)**	**nu-ru**
cut	**kiri-masu**	**ki-ri(masu)**	**ki-ru**
roll up	**makuri-masu**	**maku-ri(masu)**	**maku-ru**
return	**modori-masu**	**modo-ri(masu)**	**modo-ru**

The third type includes the irregular verbs **mimasu, okimasu, shimasu**, and **kimasu**. The verb **mimasu** and **okimasu** have an **-i** before the **-masu**, but they behave like **ru**-verbs rather than **u**-verbs. As we saw above, **shimasu** and **kimasu** are the only generally irregular verbs in the Japanese language.

ENGLISH	MASU FORM	VERB BASE	STEM VERB
see/look/watch/examine	**mi-masu**	**mi(masu)***	**mi-ru**
wake up	**oki-masu**	**oki(masu)***	**oki-ru**
do/play*	**shi-masu**	**shi(masu)***	**su-ru***
come*	**ki-masu**	**ki(masu)***	**ku-ru***

* Irregular

3. We studied the conjunction **ga** (but/however) placed just after the verb. **Shikashi** and **shikashi-nagara** express the same contrastive idea as **ga** but are more formal.

> **Kyō wa kensa o shimasu ga, kekka wa ashita wakarimasu.**
> I will examine you today, but the result will be available tomorrow.

> **Kyō kensa o shimasu. Shikashi, kensa no kekka wa ashita wakarimasu.**
> I will examine you today. But the result won't be in until tomorrow.

Suguni yoku nari-masu. Shikashi-nagara, kyō wa nani mo shinaide kudasai.
You will be cured soon. However, you would do better to refrain from activity today.

The informal words of opposition or contrast are **demo**, **daga**, and **dakeredo (mo)**.

Shinsatsu wa ijyō desu. Demo, muri o shinai yō ni (shite kudasai).
We finished the checkup. But (please) don't overdo it.

Chiryō wa owarimashita. Dakeredomo, sai-hatsu no kanō-sei ga arimasu.
I finished your treatment. However, there is the possibility of a recurrence.

4. Other common statements after a physical examination are:

Shibaraku yōsu o mimashō.
Let's see if your condition improves.

Sukoshi netsu ga deru kamo shiremasen.
You may have a slight fever.

Eiyō o jyūbun totte kudasai.
You need to get enough nutrients.

Senmon-i o goshōkai shimasu.
I will give you the name of a specialist.

Arukōru wa hikaete kudasai.
You should not drink any alcohol, please.

Tabako no ryō o herashita hō ga iidesu.
You should smoke less.

Kyō wa nyū-yoku o hikaete kudasai.
You should not take a bath or shower today, please.

Nyūin ga hitsuyō desu.
You need to be hospitalized.

Nyūin shita hō ga ii desu.
You should/had better check into a hospital.

Nyūin shinakute mo ii desu.
You don't have to stay in the hospital.

Shibaraku tsūin suru hitsuyō ga arimasu.
You will have to visit the clinic regularly for a while.

5. The prefix **giji-** means "suspected, pseudo, false." The following are some medicine-related examples:

giji-korera	para-cholera, a suspected case of cholera
giji-shojyō	a suspected case
giji-iden-shi	a pseudo gene

Language Roots

The word **sei** (性) indicates nature, gender, sex, quality, or condition. There are four homophones for **sei** that all have different meanings: **sei** (生) "birth," **sei** (正) "truth," and **sei** (制) "system," and **sei** (精) "energy."

jyo-sei	female	**dan-sei**	male
in-sei	negative	**yō-sei**	positive
kanō-sei	possibility	**sei-kaku**	personality
sei-yoku	sexual appetite	**sei-nen-gappi**	birth date
shussei-chi	birthplace	**sei-to**	student
sei-jyō	normal	**kōtai-sei**	shift system
sei-shi	sperm/semen	**sei-shin**	spirit

The word **hatsu** (発) conveys the sense of "start, departure, emit."

hatsu-netsu	become feverish (*lit.*, start fever)
ha-sshin	rash/eruption
hatsu-byō	onset of a disease
sai-hatsu	recurrence

Culture Notes

New name for Japanese nurses

Japanese nurses used to be called **kango-fu** for women and **kango-shi** for men. However, In 2002, the Japanese government passed a law that required both male and female nurses to be called **kango-shi**.

Some traditional Japanese expressions that remain in use today

When a doctor gives a prescription to a patient, one might expect the doctor to say, "**Shohōsen o agemasu**" "I'm giving you a prescription." However, Japanese doctors express this as "**Shohōsen o dashimasu**," which literally means, "I'm submitting a prescription." **Dashimasu** means "turn in, submit." The reason for this curious choice of words is that, in the past, prescriptions were not given directly to patients but were instead submitted to the pharmacy. Another example of traditional language is when you make a telephone call. Japanese do not use the verb **yobimasu** (call) for this but rather **kakemasu** (hail, call, spur), as in "**Denwa o kakemasu** (call on the telephone)." **Kakemasu** is used for an action that influences another person. When Japanese use the telephone, they consider the telephone to be influencing the other party through the call. Another example is that the verb for both telephone dialing and TV channel changing is **mawashimasu**. **Mawashimasu** means "turn." When telephones were introduced to Japan, they used a dial system, and televisions used to have dials for changing channels. The same is true in the United States, of course, where "dial a number" refers to the dial on old telephones.

Comprehension

Answer the following questions.

1. Which of the following does NOT belong with the others?
   a. **Insei**   b. **Fukusayō**
   c. **Yōsei**   d. **Giji yōsei**

2. Which of the following could be used to express "probably"?
   a. **Ikka getsu mo sureba yoku narimasu.**
   b. **Nyūin shinaide kudasai.**
   c. **Ashita wa yoku narimasen.**
   d. **Nyū-in suru hitsuyō ga arimasu.**

3. Which of the following best completes the sentence below?
   Shōjyō wa waruku nai desu (   ), naoru no ni shibaraku kakarimasu.
   (Your condition isn't serious, but it will take a while to cure.)
   a. **o**   b. **ga**
   c. **wa**   d. **ni**

4. You are suggesting the patient not touch the wound. How do you say it in Japanese?
   a. **Muri wa shinaide kudasai.**
   b. **Shitsumon ga arimasu ka.**
   c. **Kizuguchi ni sawara-naide kudasai.**
   d. **Tsumetai-mono wa sakete kudasai.**

Match the following sentence with those in the column below.

5. **Shibaraku yōsu o mimashō.**   (   )
6. **Suimin o jyūbun totte kudasai.**   (   )
7. **Senmon-i o shōkai shimasu.**   (   )
8. **Tabako no ryō o herashite kudasai.** (   )
9. **Nyūin ga hitsuyō desu.**   (   )
10. **Tsūin suru hitsuyō ga arimasu.** (   )

a. You had better enter the hospital.
b. I will give you the name of a specialist.
c. You should smoke less.
d. You will have to visit the clinic regularly.
e. Let's wait and see how your condition improves.
f. You should have a good sleep.

Practice

Respond to the following in Japanese using the cues that have been provided.

1. Give the patient advice in the following situations.
   (Situations)   (Healthcare professional)
   1. Need absolute rest.   _____
   2. Need to improve diet/regimen. _____
   3. Need to avoid cold drinks.   _____
   4. Need hospitalization.   _____
   5. Need to visit clinic regularly. _____
   6. Be careful of a recurrence.   _____
   7. The result is positive.   _____
   8. The results are negative.   _____
   9. The result is a false positive. _____
   10. The medicine has side effects. _____

2. After the examination, how do you respond to the patient?
   (Patient)   (Healthcare professional)
   1. I want to put my clothes on. _____
                        (Yes, please put them on.)
   2. I want to get up.   _____
                        (Please stay there for a while.)
   3. I feel pain after the injection. _____
                        (It will go away soon.)

4. I've been waiting for a while. _____

(You're next.)

5. Where do I pay the fee. _____

(Please pay at the cashier.)

3. After the examination, give advice to the patient.
   (Patient)   (Healthcare professional)
   1. **Shigoto ni ittemo ii desu ka.** _____

   (need absolute rest)

   2. **Nyūin ga hitsuyō desu ka.** _____

   (no need to be hospitalized)

   3. **Itsu kekka ga wakarimasu ka.** _____

   (I will call you when I get the result.)

4. Dialogue comprehension. Based on the dialogue contents, answer the following.
   1. **Yamada-san wa gakkō ni ikimasu ka.** _____
   2. **Yamada-san wa gakkō ni nani ga hitsuyō desu ka.** _____
   3. **Itsu-goro yoku narimasuka.** _____
   4. **Yamada-san wa nani ga hitsuyō desu ka.** _____
   5. **Yamada-san wa nani ga shinpai desu ka.** _____

5. Free response questions.
   (Questions)   (Answers)
   1. **Shokuji-ryōhō o shite imasu ka.** _____
   2. **Sutoresu ga arimasu ka.** _____
   3. **Saikin kyūyō o shite imasu ka.** _____
   4. **Zesshoku o shita koto ga arimasu ka.** _____
   5. **Nani-ka jibyō ga arimasu ka.** _____

Exercises

1. Say the following words in Japanese.
   A. Prevention _____
   B. Infection/contagion _____
   C. Recurrence _____
   D. Side effect _____
   E. Positive _____

2. Say the following in Japanese.
   A. You should get absolute rest. _____
   B. It will go away by itself in four to five days. _____
   C. It's necessary to have periodic checkups. _____
   D. Your condition isn't serious, but it will _____
   take a while to get better.
   E. I think it will heal itself. _____

3. When you speak with patients, how do you say the following in Japanese?
   A. Do you have have an examination _____
   scheduled today?
   B. You need to maintain a better diet. _____
   C. I will give you the name of a specialist. _____
   D. You need to be hospitalized immediately. _____
   E. You will have to visit the clinic regularly _____
   for a while.

4. Answer the following questions in Japanese.

   Q: **Itsu yoku narimasu ka.**
   A: _____
   (You'll probably be well by tomorrow.)

   Q: **Ashita gakkō e ittemo ii desu ka.**
   B: _____
   (It's only a slight cold, but you shouldn't go to school tomorrow).

   Q: **Onakaga itai(n) desu ga.**
   C: _____
   (You need to be examined immediately.)

At the Pharmacy I
(Yakkyoku de)

Basic Vocabulary (CD 14-1)

Listen to the CD and repeat the vocabulary.

1.	pharmacy/drugstore	**yakkyoku**	薬局
2.	prescription	**sohōsen**	処方箋
3.	over-the-counter drug	**shihan-yaku**	市販薬
4.	ID card	**mibun-shōmei-sho**	身分証明書
5.	compress	**shippu-yaku**	湿布薬
6.	preparation/compound drug	**chōgō-zai**	調合剤
7.	household medicine	**jyōbi-yaku**	常備薬
8.	ointment	**nankō**	軟膏
9.	oral medicine	**nomi-gusuri/**	飲み薬／内服薬
		naifuku-yaku	
10.	medicine for external application	**nuri-gusuri**	塗り薬
11.	powdered medicine	**kona-gusuri/**	粉薬／粉末剤
		funmatsu-zai	
12.	tablet	**jyō-zai**	錠剤
13.	capsule	**kapuseru-zai**	カプセル剤
14.	inhaler	**kyūnyū-yaku**	吸入薬
15.	orally dispensed drug	**kōkūyō-yaku**	口腔用薬
16.	suppository	**za-yaku**	座薬
17.	granulated	**karyū**	顆粒
18.	vaccine	**wakuchin**	ワクチン
19.	aspirin	**asupirin**	アスピリン
20.	stomach medicine	**i-gusuri**	胃薬
21.	gargle medicine	**ugai-gusuri**	嗽薬
22.	cold medicine	**kaze-gusuri**	風邪薬
23.	vitamin pill/tablet	**bitamin-zai**	ビタミン剤
24.	sleeping pill/tablet	**suimin-dōnyū-zai**	睡眠導入剤
25.	eyedrops	**me-gusuri**	目薬
26.	analgesic/pain reliever	**chintsū-zai**	鎮痛剤
27.	antacid tablet/digestive	**shōka-zai**	消化剤
28.	antipyretic	**genetsu-zai**	解熱剤
29.	expiration date	**yūkō-kigen**	有効期限
30.	effectiveness	**kōka/yūkō-sei**	効果／有効性

Dialogue (CD 14-2)

Listen to the CD and repeat the dialogue.

At the Pharmacy

Ann (pharmacist):	**Shohōsen o omochi desu ka.**
	Do you have a prescription?
Mr. Suzuki (patient):	**Hai, arimasu. Dōzo.**
	Yes, I do. Here you are (please).
Ann:	**Onamae to denwa-bangō o oshiete kudasai.**
	Please tell me your name and phone number.
Mr. Suzuki:	**Namae wa Suzuki Kenji desu. Denwa-bangō wa 808 no 509 no 8349 desu.**
	My name is Suzuki Kenji. My phone number is 808-509-8349.
Ann:	**Arigatō gozaimasu. Kusuri ni (wa) nani-ka arerugī ga arimasu ka.**
	Thank you. Do you have any medication allergies?
Mr. Suzuki:	**Iie, nanimo (arerugī wa) arimasen.**
	No, I don't have any.
	Kono kusuri wa don-na fukusayō ga arimasu ka.
	What kind of side effects does this medication have?
Ann:	**Sukoshi nemuku-naru kamo (shiremasen).**
	(This medicine) might make you a little drowsy.
	Ni-jyu-ppun goni tori ni kite kudasai.
	Please come back to pick it up in twenty minutes.
Mr. Suzuki:	**Hai, wakarimashita. Dō mo.**
	I understand. Thanks.

Grammar

1. The polite expression **omochi-desu ka**

Omochi-desu ka is a polite form of **arimasu ka**, and both expressions mean "Do you have . . . ?" The particle **o** is required before **omochi-desu ka**.

ID ga arimasu ka.	Do you have an ID?
Mibun-shōmei-sho o omochi desu ka.	
Hoken-shō ga arimasu ka.	Do you have an insurance card?
Hoken-shō o omochi-desu ka.	

Shohōsen ga arimasu ka?	Do you have a prescription?
Shohōsen o omochi desu ka.	

2. Nani-ka

In Lesson 7, we studied the adverb **nani-ka** (something). **Nani-ka** has two meanings, depending on the grammatical context: "something" in affirmative declarative sentences and "any, anything" in questions.

Nani-ka tabemasu.	I will eat something.
Nani-ka nomi-mono o kudasai.	Please give me something to drink.
Nani-ka nomimasu ka.	Would you like anything to drink?
Nani-ka kusuri o nonde imasu ka.	Are you taking any medication?

3. Nani-mo . . . masen

Nani-mo . . . masen means "not anything, any . . . at all" in negative sentences and questions.

Nani-mo tabe masen.
I haven't eaten anything./I'm not eating anything at all.

Nani-mo amai-mono o tabete imasen.
I am not eating any sweets (at all).

Nani-mo kusuri o nonde imasen ka.
Aren't you taking any medication?

The interrogatives **dare** (who/person) and **doko** (where/location) express the similar idea of "no, not any at all" when used with **mo** plus the negative ending **masen**.

Dare-mo yakuzai-shi wa imasen.
There are no pharmacists./There aren't any pharmacists at all.

Doko-mo yakkyoku wa aite imasen.
There is no pharmacy open (at all).

4. The construction NOUN + ni(wa)

A noun phrase consisting of NOUN plus **ni(wa)** places emphasis on the noun and topic. **Ni(wa)** is demonstrative and usually is associated with the particle **ga**, as in the following sentences.

Kaze-gusuri niwa genetsu-zai ga haitte imasu.
This cold medicine includes an antipyretic.

Watakushi niwa kono kusuri ga nomemasen.
I can't take this medicine (*lit.*, As for me, I can't drink this medicine).

Kenkō ni(wa) undō ga taisetsu desu.
It's important to exercise for your health.

5. STEM VERB **+ niwa**

The construction STEM VERB plus **niwa** means "in order to; to; for the purpose of; for."

Kono suimin-dōnyū-zai o uru niwa, shohō-sen ga hitsuyō desu.
In order to sell (you) this sleeping pill, I need to see a prescription (*lit.*, To sell this sleeping pill, I need a prescription).

Kusuri o kenkyū suru niwa jikan to okane ga kakarimasu.
To research and develop medicines takes time and money.

Za-yaku o tsukau niwa, kōmon kara iremasu.
As for the suppository, it has to used anally.

Kaze o naosu niwa, kono genetsu-zai ga kikimasu.
For (the purpose of) curing a cold, this antipyretic medicine is effective.

6. The interrogative pronoun **don-na**

The interrogative **don-na** means "What kind of " and is always associated with the question marker **ka**. (See Lesson 6, Grammar point 8.)

Don-na tabemono ga arimasu ka.	What kind of food do you have?
Don-na kusuri ga arimasu ka.	What kind of medicine do you have?
Don-na nomimono ga hoshii desu ka.	What kind of drinks do you want?

7. STEM VERB **+ kamo**

In Lesson 9, we studied the construction STEM VERB plus **kamo shiremasen** (might). In informal conversation, **kamo shiremasen** can be shortened to **kamo** and convey the same meaning.

Fukusayō ga aru kamo.	You might be feeling a side effect.
Nemuku naru kamo.	You might feel drowsy.

Kono kusuri wa i ni futan ga kakaru kamo.
This medicine might upset your stomach.

The following expressions are ranked in decreasing order of certainty:

A. **Nemuku-naru ni chigai arimasen.**	You will become drowsy.
B. **Nemuku-naru deshō.**	You will probably become drowsy.
C. **Nemuku-naru kamo shiremasen.**	You may become drowsy.

8. The constructions TIME + **goni** + VERB BASE + **ni kite kudasai;** and TIME + **goni** + PLACE + **ni kite kudasai**

The construction TIME plus **goni** plus VERB BASE plus **ni kite kudasai** is used to request that a certain action be taken after a certain interval of time.

San-jyu-ppun goni torini kite kudasai.
Please come to pick it up after thirty minutes.

Ni-ji-kan goni mō ichido torini kite kudasai.
Please come again after two hours.

The construction TIME plus **goni** plus PLACE plus **ni kite kudasai** is also used to request that a person go to a certain place after certain interval of time.

Sūjitsu goni mō ichido koko ni kite kudasai.
Please come here again after a few days.

Mikka goni yakkyoku ni kite kudasai.
Please visit the pharmacy after three days.

9. The interrogative pronoun **dono-kurai**

The interrogative **dono-kurai** is used to ask "How long?; How many?; or "How much?" The context determines which meaning is applicable.

Dono-kurai kakarimasu ka.	How long will it take? (asking about time)
	How much will it be? (asking about cost)
Dono-kurai nomimasu ka.	How many will it take?
Dono-kurai tsukai masu ka.	How much use is it?

Useful Expressions (CD 14-3)

Listen to the CD and repeat the sentences.

1. **Shohōsen o misete kudasai.** Please show me your prescription.
2. **Nani-ka kusuri o nonde imasu ka.** Are you taking any medication?
3. **Kono kusuri wa yoku kikimasu.** This medicine works well/is effective.

4. **Kono kusuri wa itami ni yoku kikimasu.** This medicine is effective against pain.

5. **Kono kusuri wa netsu o sageru kōka ga arimasu.** This medicine is effective in reducing fever.

6. **Sugu (ni) kusuri ga demasu. Shōshō omachi kudasai.** It will be ready soon. Please wait a moment.

7. **Jyu-ppun omachi kudasai.** Please wait ten minutes.

8. **Fukusayō no shinpai wa naidesu yo.** There is no need to worry about side effects.

9. **Kono kusuri o nomu to, hakike ga suru-kamo shiremasen.** This medicine makes you sick to your stomach.

10. **Nyō no iro ga kawaru kamo shiremasen ga, shinpai (wa) shinaide kudasai.** The color of your urine might change, but that is nothing to worry about.

Key Sentences (CD 14-4)

Listen to the CD and repeat the sentences.

1. **Chintsū-zai ga arimasu ka.** Do you have a pain reliever?

2. **Nani-ka genetsu-zai o nonde imasu ka.** Are you taking any antipyretic medicine?

3. **Don-na ugai-gusuri ga arimasu ka.** What kind of gargle medicine do you have?

4. **Nemuku naru kamo shiremasen.** You might feel drowsy.

5. **Go-fun goni torini kite kudasai.** Please come back to pick it up after five minutes.

Additional Words

tsukaikiru/tsukaikirimasu use up
oshieru/oshiemasu teach
sageru/sagemasu decrease
fujin women
kakasu/kakashimasu lack/miss
undō exercise
kusuri-ya drugstore
kenkyū research
jiken incident
kōreisha elderly person
rōjin old person
seinen young person

kiku/kikimasu effect
hairu/hairimasu enter/include
ageru/agemasu increase
sasu/sashimasu apply (eyedrops)
mō ichido once more/again
unten drive
hoshii wish/want
futan burden
-hodo (for verbs or adjectives) about, used for extent/limit/degree/measure
soshō lawsuit
anzen-sei safety

fuhei complaining

on-shippu hot compress

rei-shippu cold compress

yūkō-seibun active ingredient

Language Notes

1. In Lesson 3, we studied studied the expression **dō-desu ka** (how about), which is used to ask someone how things are going. **Dō-yatte** is used to ask questions of the form "Do you know how to . . . ?"

   Kono nankō wa dō-yatte tsukai masu ka.
   Do you know how to use this ointment?

   Kono shippu-yaku wa dō-yatte tsukai maus ka.
   Do you know how to use this compress?

   Kono funmatsu-zai wa dō-yatte nomimasu ka.
   Do you know how to take this medicine that's in a powder?

   Kono kapuseru-zai wa dō-yatte nomimasu ka.
   Do you know how to take this medicine that's in capsules?

   Kono za-yaku wa dō-yatte tsukai masu ka.
   Do you know how to use this suppository medicine?

   The following are some possible answers.

Hifu ni nutte kudasai.	You apply it to the skin.
Itai tokoro ni hatte kudasai.	Place the compress against the areas where the pain is (*lit.*, Please put the compress to the pain area).
Mizu to (issho ni) nonde kudasai.	You just swallow it with water.
Oshiri ni irete kudasai.	You insert it into the anus.

2. Questions from patients for pharmacists. (**Kanjya kara yakuzai-shi ni shitsumon.**)

Q1:	**Shohōsen ga naku-temo kusuti ga kaemasu ka.**	
	Can I buy medicine without a prescription?	
A1:	**Hai, kaemasu yo.**	
	Yes, you can (buy it).	
	Iie, Shohōsen ga nakute wa dame desu.	
	No, you can't without a prescription.	
Q2:	**Kusuri ga deru made, dono-kurai jikan ga kakari masu ka.**	
	How long will it take to prepare the medicine?	

A2: **Suguni demasu.**
It will be done soon.

Shōshō omachi kudasai.
Please wait a moment.

Jyū-go-fun hodo kakarimasu.
It will take about fifteen minutes.

Q3: **Kaze ni kiku, nani-ka ii kusuri wa arimasen ka.**
Don't you have any good medicine for colds?

A3: **Kore wa dō-desu ka.**
What do you think about this one?

Kochira wa ikaga desu ka.
What do you think about this one? (polite)

Q4: **Ge-zai o kudasai.**
Please give me a laxative.

A4: **Hai, wakarimashita.**
Yes, of course. (I understand.)

Q5: **Chinsei-zai ga arimasu ka.**
Do you have a sedative?

A5: **Hai, arimasu.**
Yes, we do (have one).

Q6: **Zutsū ni kiku kusuri ga arimasu ka.**
Do you have a good medicine for headaches?

A6: **Hai, gozaimasu.**
Yes, we do (have one). (polite)

Q7: **Kanpō yaku wa oite arimasu ka.**
Do you carry Chinese herbal medicine?

A7: **Hai, oite arimasu.**
Yes, we do (we carry it).

Q8: **Hifu no kayumi o tomeru kusuri ga hoshii(n) desu.**
I need medicine for itchy skin.

A8: **Kore wa ikaga desu ka.**
How about this one? (polite)

Q9: **Nani-ka ii kusuri o oshiete kudasai.**
Is there any medicine you recommend for me?

A9: **Kore wa dō-desu ka.**
What do you think about this one?

Q10:   **Kono kusuri wa itsu dono-kurai ii desu ka.**
       How often do I take the medicine?

A10:   **Maiasa kakasazu nonde kudasai.**
       Please take it every morning without skipping.

Q11:   **Kono kusuri wa dono-kurai nomeba ii desu ka.**
       What dose should I take?

A11:   **Nakunaru made (kusuri o) nonde kudasai.**
       Please keep taking it (the medicine) until it is used up.

Q12:   **Kono kusuri wa dono-kurai nomeba ii desu ka.**
       How long should I take this medicine?

A12:   **Nakunaru made (kusuri o) nonde kudasai.**
       Please continue taking it (the medicine) until it's finished.

Q 13: **(O) ikura desu ka.** How much is it?
A 13: **Nijyū doru de gozaimasu.** It costs twenty dollars. (polite)

3. There are many expressions about allergies.

arerugī tesuto	allergy testing
arerugī-sei	allergenic; allergic
arerugī taishitsu	allergic diathesis, predisposition to be allergic
arerugī-sei bien	allergic rhinitis
arerugī-shōjyō	allergy symptoms
arerugī-sei enshō	allergic inflammation
arerugī-sei shikkan	allergic disease

4. When asking someone to recommend (**suisen**) something, Japanese do not say **Nani-ka ii kusuri o suisen shite kudasai**. Rather, they use the verb **aru** (have) or **oshieru** (teach). Expressions with **arimasu ka** (do you have one?) and **oshiete kudasai** (please teach) include the notion of "recommend" as well as "introduce." When asking a person to recommend someone, however, Japanese use **Dare-ka ii hito o suisen shite kudasai** "Please recommend a good person."

Zutsū ni nani-ka ii kusuri ga arimasu ka.
Do you have some good medicine for a headache?

Yōtsū ni nani-ka ii kusuri o oshiete kudasai.
Please tell me which medicine is good for a backache.

I-in ni dare-ka ii hito o suisen shite kudasai.
Please recommend a good doctor at the clinic.

5. **Nani(ka)** (what/something) is used in many important Japanese expressions. The following are some examples.

> **nanika-to** (one way or another)
> **Kangoshi-san ga inai to nakika-to fuben desu.**
> I am inconvenienced one way or another when the nurse is away.

> **nani-kashira** (somewhat) (informal)
> **Kanjya wa nani-kashira fuhei o itte imasu.**
> The patient has somewhat vague complaints.

> **nani-kashira** (wonder) (informal)
> **Kono kusuri wa nani-kashira.**
> I am wondering what kind of medicine.

> **nanika-kanika** (this and that)
> **Byōin wa nanika kanika isogashii desu.**
> The hospital is busy because of this and that.

> **nani-kara nani-made** (in every way; from tip to toe; from A to Z)
> **Kango-shi wa nani-kara nani-made shinsetsu desu.**
> The nurse is very kind in every way.

> **nanika betsu no** (different; something else; another)
> **Nanika betsu no kusuri ga arimasu ka.**
> Do you have a different medicine?

Language Roots

The suffix **-kusuri/-gusuri** (薬) refers to medicine. The character is also pronounced **yaku**.

ugai-gusuri	gargle medicine
kaze-gusuri	cold medicine
me-gusuri	eyedrops
i-gusuri	stomach medicine
za-yaku	suppository

The suffix **-zai** (剤) also refers to medicine or a tablet.

jyō-zai	tablet
chintsū-zai	analgesic/pain reliever
genetsu-zai	antipyretic
shōka-zai	anti-acid tablet/digestive
bitamin-zai	vitamin pill/tablet
eiyō-zai	nutrient

Culture Notes

Japanese sensitivity about environmental pollution and the harmful side effects of medicine on humans and animals

Japanese have a special sensitivity about environmental pollution and the harmful side effects of medicine as well as the radiation sickness caused by atomic bombs. There have been lawsuits in Japan over pollution at the Ashio mine (**Ashio kōdoku jiken**), radiation sickness (**genbaku-shō**), Minamata disease (**Minamata byō**), blood products contaminated with AIDS (**eizu soshō**), and type B and type C hepatitis infections from contaminated drugs (**A-gata, B-gata kanen soshō**). When Japanese need a blood transfusion, they are sometimes fearful of the possibility that unscreened viruses might be transmitted to them. Healthcare professionals need to be aware of this fear and communicate effectively with the patients about the blood product in order to allay their concern.

Health-related Japanese proverbs V

Good medicine tastes bitter.
Ryō-yaku wa kuchi ni nigashi.
良薬口に苦し

Too much medicine turns into poison.
Kusuri mo sugire-ba doku to naru.
薬も過ぎれば毒となる

Comprehension

Answer the following questions.

1. Which of the following does NOT belong with the others?
   a. **Shōka-zai**   b. **Genetsu-zai**
   c. **Jō-zai**   d. **Chintsū-zai**

2. Which of the following could be used to express "might"?
   a. **Nemuku naru ni chigai arimasen.**
   b. **Nemuku naru kamo shiremasen.**
   c. **Nemuku naru desu.**
   d. **Nemuku naru hitsuyō ga arimasu.**

3. Which of the following best completes the sentence below?
   Kusuri ga deru (   ), donokurai jikan ga kakari masu ka.
   How long will it take to prepare the medicine?
   a. **kamo**   b. **made**
   c. **kara**   d. **ii**

4. You are suggesting how many tablets an adult must take. How do you say this in Japanese?
   a. **Otona wa san jyō nonde kudasai.**
   b. **Kodomo wa ni jyō nonde kudasai.**
   c. **Mizu to issho ni nonde kudasai.**
   d. **Jyū-ni sai ika wa nomanaide kudasai.**

Select the following matching words from the list below.

---

5. **Arerugī-sei bien**   (   )
6. **Arerugī-sei enshō**   (   )
7. **Arerugī-sei shikkan**   (   )
8. **Arerugī taishitsu**   (   )
9. **Arerugī shōjyō**   (   )

a. allergic diathesis, predisposition to be allergic
b. allergic rhinitis
c. allergy symptoms
d. allergic inflammation
e. allergic disease

Practice

Respond to the following in Japanese using the cues that have been provided.

---

1. Explain how to use the medicine:
   (Patients)   (Healthcare professionals)
   1. **Kono nankō wa dōyatte tsukai masu ka.**   _____
                                                  (apply it to the skin)
   2. **Kono shippu-yaku wa dōyatte tsukai maus ka.** _____
                                                  (put it on your back)
   3. **Kono funmatsu-zai wa dōyatte nomimasu ka.** _____
                                                  (take with water)
   4. **Kono kapuseru-zai wa dōyatte nomimasu ka.** _____
                                                  (take with juice)

5. **Kono za-yaku wa dōyatte tsukaimasu ka.** _____

(insert into the anus)

2. Give the correct term in Japanese for the following medicines?
(Name of medicines)   (Healthcare professionals)
1. Analgesic/pain reliever   _____
2. Antacid tablet/digestive   _____
3. Antipyretic   _____
4. Cold medicine   _____

3. Reply to the questions in parenthesis.
(Patient)   (Healthcare professionals)
1. **Kusuri o kudasai.**   _____
   (Show me your prescription.)
2. **Kusuri wa yoku kikimasu ka.** _____
   (Yes, it works well.)
3. **Donokurai machimasu ka.**   _____
   (It will be ready soon.)
4. **Fukusayō ga arimasu ka.**   _____
   (There is no need to worry.)
5. **Donokurai nomimasu ka.**   _____
   (until used up/finished)

4. How do you respond to the following questions?
(Patient)   (Healthcare professional)
1. **Nani-ka ii kusuri o oshiete kudasai.** _____
   (How about this one?)
2. **Kono kusuri wa itsu nomeba iidesu ka.** _____
   (Take it every day without inter-
   ruption.)
3. **Zutsū no kusuri ga arimasu ka.** _____
   (Yes, we do. (polite))

5. Dialogue comprehension. Based on the dialogue, answer the following questions.
1. **Shohōsen ga arimasu ka.**   _____
2. **Suzuki-san no denwa-bangō wa nan desu ka.** _____
3. **Suzuki-san wa kusuri ni arerugii ga arimasu ka.** _____
4. **Don-na fukusayō ga arimasu ka.**   _____
5. **Itsu kusuri o torini ikimasu ka.**   _____

6. Free response questions.

(Questions) (Answers)
1. **Jōbiyaku wa arimasu ka.** _____
2. **Funmatsu-zai to kapuseru-zai no** _____
   dochira ga suki desu ka.
3. **Ugai-gusuri ga arimasu ka.** _____
4. **Bitaminzai o nonde imasu ka.** _____
5. **Me-gusuri o sashite imasuka.** _____

Exercises

1. Say the following words in Japanese.
   A. Cold medicine _____
   B. Antipyretic _____
   C. Vaccine _____
   D. Prescription _____
   E. Stomach medicine _____

2. Say the following in Japanese.
   A. What kind of medicine do you want? _____
   B. Do you have a prescription? _____
   C. You might feel drowsy. _____
   D. Please come back after fifteen minutes to _____
      pick it up.
   E. It will be ready soon. Please wait a moment. _____

3. How do you say the following expressions in Japanese?
   A. Please take (the medicine) until finish. _____
   B. Please take three tablets for an adult and _____
      one tablet for children.
   C. Please take it every day without skipping. _____
   D. This medicine makes you sick to your stomach. _____
   E. This medicine is effective against colds. _____

At the Pharmacy II
(Yakkyoku de)

Basic Vocabulary (CD 15-1)

Listen to the CD and repeat the vocabulary.

#	English	Rōmaji	Japanese
1.	antibiotic	**kōsei-bushitsu**	抗生物質
2.	painkiller	**itami-dome**	痛み止め
3.	anticancer drug	**kōgan-zai**	抗癌剤
4.	contraceptive/pill	**hinin-yaku**	避妊薬
5.	intestinal medicine	**ichō-yaku**	胃腸薬
6.	AZT/azidothymidine	**eizu-yaku**	エイズ薬
7.	itch lotion/medicine	**kayumi-dome**	痒み止め
8.	Chinese herbal medicine	**kanpō-yaku**	漢方薬
9.	cardio tonic	**kyōshin-zai**	強心剤
10.	restorative	**kyōsō-zai**	強壮剤
11.	laxative	**ge-zai**	下剤
12.	antidiarrheal/ binding medicine	**geri-dome**	下痢止め
13.	hematopoietic drugs	**ketsueki sei-zai**	血液製剤
14.	stimulants	**kōfun-zai**	興奮剤
15.	disinfectant	**sakkin-zai**	殺菌剤
16.	ataractic/tranquilizer	**seishin antei-zai**	精神安定剤
17.	sedative/tranquilizer	**chinsei-zai**	鎮静剤
18.	antihistamine	**kō-hisutamin-zai**	抗ヒスタミン剤
19.	anesthetic	**masui-yaku**	麻酔薬
20.	drug/crack/narcotic	**ma-yaku**	麻薬
21.	preventative medicine	**yobō-yaku**	予防薬
22.	antidiabetic drug	**tōnyō-byō-yaku**	糖尿病薬
23.	antidote/remedy against poison	**gedoku-zai**	解毒剤
24.	antihypertensive drug	**kōatsu-zai**	降圧剤
25.	directions/directions for use	**shiyō-hōhō**	使用方法
26.	dose/dosage	**yōryō**	用量
27.	generic drug	**jenerikku iyaku-hin/ kōhatsu iyaku-hin**	ジェネリック医薬品/ 後発医薬品
28.	drug facts (labeling)	**tenpu bunsho**	添付文書
29.	printed instructions for use	**setsumei-sho**	説明書
30.	warnings	**chūi-jikō**	注意事項

Dialogue (CD 15-2)

Listen to the CD and repeat the dialogue.

At the Pharmacy

Ann: **Suzuki-san. (Kono kusuri no) nomi-kata o setsumei shimasu.**
              Mr. Suzuki, I'll explain how to take this (medicine).

              **(Kono kusuri wa) shoku-go sanjyu-pun inai ni ichi-nichi san-kai
              fukuyō shite kudasai.**
              You should take it (this medicine) within thirty minutes after every
              meal three times a day.

              Otona wa ichi-nichi (ni) roku-jyō ga gendo desu.
              Six tablets is the maximum daily dosage for an adult.

              Otona wa ikkai ni-jyō, kodomo wa ichi-jyō desu.
              Take two tablets for an adult and one tablet for children.

              Nana-sai ika wa noma-naide kudasai.
              Please, this medicine is not for under seven years old.

Mr. Suzuki: **Hai, wakarimashita.**
              Yes, I understand.

Ann: **Kono kusuri-dai wa hoken ga kikimasu kara jiko-futan kihon-
              ryōkin no ni-jyū doru desu.**
              The medicine is twenty dollars for the copayment, because your in-
              surance covers it.

Mr. Suzuki: **Hai. (Shiharai wa) kurejito-kādo demo ii desu ka.**
              Yes. May I pay for it by credit card?

Ann: **Hai, kekko desu. (Koko ni) Shomei o onegai shimasu.**
              Yes, that's fine. Please sign here.

Mr. Suzuki: **Hai, ii desu yo. Ryōshū-sho o kudasai.**
              Okay. Please give me a receipt.

Ann: **Hai dōzo. Soredewa, odaiji-ni.**
              Here you are. Well then, take care of yourself.

Mr. Suzuki: **Dōmo arigatō gozaimashita.**
              Thank you very much.

Grammar

1. The suffix **-kata**

-kata is a noun-forming suffix that indicates a way, manner, or method. The construction VERB BASE plus **-kata** means "how to (do something)" or expresses the notion of a method.

Ge-zai no nomi-kata o oshiete kudasai.
Please tell me how (I'm supposed) to take the laxative.

Nankō no nuri-kata ga taisetsu desu.
It's important to know how to apply it (the ointment) properly.

Karada no hiyashi-kata o shitte imasu ka.
Do you know how to cool the body?

Kensa no shi-kata ga wakarimasu ka.
Do you know how to do the test?

The following are some verb bases with the **-kata** ending added.

ENGLISH	MASU-FORM	METHOD (HOW TO)	VERB BASE + KATA
do/play	**shi-masu**	how to do/play	**shi-kata**
cool	**hiyashi-masu**	how to cool	**hiyashi-kata**
warm up, heat	**atatame-masu**	how to warm	**atatame-kata**
read	**yomi-masu**	how to read	**yomi-kata**
drink	**nomi-masu**	how to drink	**nomi-kata**
rest/be absent	**yasumi-masu**	how to rest/take a sick day	**yasumi-kata**
sit down	**suwari-masu**	how to sit down	**suwari-kata**
turn/roll up	**makuri-masu**	how to turn/roll up	**makuri-kata**
cut	**kiri-masu**	how to cut	**kiri-kata**
wash	**arai-masu**	how to wash	**arai-kata**
apply/plaster	**nuri-masu**	how to spread/plaster	**nuri-kata**
bend	**mage-masu**	how to bend	**mage-kata**
stretch/spread	**nobashi-masu**	how to stretch	**nobashi-kata**
mix	**maze masu**	how to mix	**maze-kata**
insert	**ire-masu**	how to insert	**ire-kata**
extend/spread out	**hirogari-masu**	how to spread	**hirogari-kata**
use up	**tsukaikiri-masu**	how to use up	**tukaikiri-kata**

ENGLISH	MASU-FORM	METHOD (HOW TO)	VERB BASE + KATA
effect	kiki-masu	how to effect	kiki-kata
teach	oshie-masu	how to teach	oshie-kata
decrease	sage-masu	how to decrease	sage-kata
enter/include	hairi-masu	how to enter	hairi-kata
increase	age-masu	how to increase	age-kata
pay	harai-masu	how to pay	harai-kata
apply (eyedrops)	sashi-masu	how to apply	sashi-kata
inform/notify	shirase-masu	how to inform/notify	shirase-kata
empty/disappear/die	nakunari-masu	how to empty/disappear/die	nakunari-kata

2. The constructions NOUN + no hōhō and STEM VERB + hōhō

The noun **hōhō** means "method" and can also be used in sentences to say how to do something. There are two kinds of sentence structures, with no difference in meaning:

NOUN + **no hōhō**
Kusuri no chōgō no hōhō o oshiete kudasai.
Please tell me the method for preparing this medication

Kuruma no unten no hōhō o shitte masu ka.
Do you know how to drive a car?

STEM VERB + **hōhō**
Kusuri o chōgō suru hōhō o oshiete kudasai.
Please tell me the method for preparing this medication.

Kuruma o unten suru hōhō o shitte masu ka.
Do you know how to drive a car?

3. The suffix -inai ni

The noun suffix -**inai** is used with the particle **ni** and means "within" or "less than" with respect to time.

San-ji kan inai ni geri-dome o nonde kudasai.
Please take an antidiarrheal medicine within three hours.

Ichi-ji kan inai ni kensa o hajimemasu.
We will start the examination in an hour.

Sanjyu-ppun inai ni kusuri ga demasu.
The medicine will be ready in less than thirty minutes.

4. The construction **ichi-nichi ni** + NUMBER + **-kai** or **-do**

The expression **ichi-nichi ni** plus the compound suffixes -**kai** or -**do** means "how many times per day." **Kai** and **do** express frequency/time, and there is no difference in meaning between them. Both words are used interchangeably by the Japanese. In other contexts, **kai** expresses "how often", and **do** means "degree."

ichi-nichi ni i-kkai	**ichi-nichi ni ichi-do**	once a day
ichi-nichi ni ni-kai	**ichi-nichi ni ni-do**	twice a day
ichi-nichi ni san-kai	**ichi-nichi ni san-do**	three times a day
ichi-nichi ni yon-kai	**ichi-nichi ni yon-do**	four times a day
ichi-nichi ni go-kai	**ichi-nichi ni go-do**	five times a day

Ichi-nichi ni nan-kai kyōshin-zai ga nomemasu ka.
How many times a day am I supposed to take the cardio tonic?

Ichi-nichi ni san-kai nonde kudasai.
You should take it three times a day.

Kono kusuri wa ichi-nichi ni nan-jyō made nomemasu ka.
Up to how many tablets can I take a day? (*lit.*, Is this medicine possible to take how many tablets a day?)

Ichi-do ni san-jyō nonde kudasai.
You should take three tablets at a time.

5. The counters **i-kkai ni** and **ichi-do ni**

To express dosage, you use either of the counters **i-kkai ni** or **ichi-do ni** and a counter of medicine (**jyō**, **hai/pai**, **fukuro**, **teki**). **Jyō** is a counter for tablet medicine, **hai/pai** is for cups/spoons, **fukuro** is for packages, and **teki** is for drops.

Kono kōgan-zai wa i-kkai ni san-jyō nonde kudasai.
For this anticancer drug, you take three tablets at a time (*lit.*, This anticancer drug please take three tablets at a time).

Kono kusuri wa nan jō ichido ni nomeba ii desu ka.
How many tablets do I take at a time?

Kono kōsei-bushitsu wa i-kkai ni supūn ni-hai nonde kudasai.
You should take two spoonfuls of the antibiotic at a time.

6. The suffix -ika

The suffix -**ika** means "not more than, under" and is used to express a minimum age in the following examples. The suffix -**ika** is used with the verb suffix -**naide** for expressing prohibition.

> **Nijyū-issai ika wa osake o noma-naide kudasai.**
> Please don't drink if you are under the age of twenty-one.
>
> **Nana-sai ika wa (kono kusuri o) noma-naide kudasai.**
> Do not take (this medicine) if you are under age of seven.

Miman can replace -**ika** in this construction to convey "less than, below."

> **Go-sai miman wa (kono kusuri o) noma-naide kudasai.**
> Please do not take (this medicine) if you are less than 5 years old.
>
> **Go-sai miman no kodomo niwa kono kusuri o nomase-naide kudasai.**
> Please do not give this drug to children less than 5 years of age

7. The construction X ga Y ni kikimasu

To say that medicine X is effective against disease Y or works well against disease Y, use the construction MEDICINE **ga** DISEASE **ni kikimasu**. When the sentence is negative (in other words, the medicine isn't effective or doesn't work well), the subject marker **ga** changes to **wa**. To review the subject markers **ga** and **wa**, please see the grammar points in Lesson 2.

> **Kono kōsei-bushitsu ga kaze ni yoku kikimasu.**
> This antibiotic works well against the flu.
>
> **Kono kōgan-zai wa gan ni yoku kiki-masen deshita.**
> This anticancer drug wasn't effective against his/her cancer.

8. The verb kikimasu

The verb **kikimasu** also means "possible to accept/use; cover, be effective."

Hoken ga kikimasu ka.	Do you accept my insurance?
Hai, hoken ga kikimasu.	Yes, we do accept that insurance.
Iie, hoken wa kikimasen.	No, we don't accept that insurance.

> **Kono kō-hisutamin-zai wa kaze ni kikimasu ka.**
> Is this antihistamine effective for colds?

Hai, kiku to omoimasu.	Yes, I think it is effective (for colds).
Iie, kikanai to moimasu.	No, I don't think it is effective (for colds).

Useful Expressions (CD 15-3)

Listen to the CD and repeat the sentences.

1. **Kono kusuri no nomi-kata o setsumei shimasu.** I'll explain/tell you how to take these pills.
2. **Kono kusuri wa mai-shoku-go nonde kudasai.** Please take (this medicine) after eating.
3. **Kono kusuri wa shoku-go sanjyu-ppun inai ni nonde kudasai.** Please take this medicine within thirty minutes after every meal.
4. **Ichi-nichi ni ni-kai fukyō shite kudasai.** Please take this medication twice a day.
5. **Mai-shoku-go kono kusuri o nonde kudasai.** Please take this medicine after every meal.
6. **Zutsū ni(wa) asupirin o onomi kudasai.** (polite) Please take aspirin for your headache.
7. **Kono kōsei-bushitsu wa nakunaru made nonde kudasai.** Continue taking the antibiotic until you've used it up.
8. **Kaze ni yoku-kiku kusuri ga ikutsu ka arimasu.** We have several kinds of medication that are effective against a cold.
9. **Chintsū-zai wa itai toki dake nonde kudasai.** Please take this pain reliever only when you absolutely need it.
10. **Fukusayō no shinpai ga aru-kamo shitemasen.** I'm worried about the side effects.

Key Sentences (CD 15-4)

Listen to the CD and repeat the sentences.

1. **Kono kusuri no tsukai-kata o setsumei shimasu.** I'll explain how to take this medicine properly.
2. **Mai-shoku-go, san-jyu ppun inai ni, aspirin ni jyō o fukuyō shite kudasai.** Please take two aspirin within thirty minute after each meal.
3. **Kono kōsei bushitsu ga kaze ni yoku kikimasu.** This antibiotic works well against the flu.
4. **Kono kōsei-bushitsu wa ikkai ni san-jyō, rokuji-kan oki ni nonde kudasai.** Take two of the antibiotic tablets every six hours.
5. **Shinpai shinai-de [kudasai]. Hoken ga kikimasu yo.** Don't worry. Your insurance covers it.

Additional Words

nuru/nurimasu apply/spread
atatameru/atatamemasu warm
shiharai payment
todoku reach/arrive
oshirase information/notice
mai-shoku-go after every meal
shūshin-go after sleep
kūfuku-ji on an empty stomach
hokan keep/store
shōdoku-zai antiseptic
gendo maximun/limitation
menseki-gaku/jiko futan gendo-gaku deductible

hiyasu/hiyashimasu cooling
nakunaru/nakunarimasu become
    empty/use up/disappear/die
shiraseru/shirasemasu inform/notify
dake only
mai-shoku-zen before every meal
shūshin-mae before bed
shokkan between meals
chūi warning
yōdochinki iodine
jiko-futan kihon-ryōkin copayment

Language Notes

1. Directions for use (**shiyō-hōhō**): The following are possible replies to the question often asked of a pharmacist: **Kono kusuri no shiyō-hōhō wa nan desu ka.** "What are the instructions for taking this?" or "How do I take this (medicine/drug)?"

   1. **Ni-jyō o shoku-zen ni fukuyō shite kudasai.**
      Please take two capsules before meals.

   2. **Kono kusuri o shokkan ni ichi-jyō fukuyō shite kudasai.**
      Please take one pill between meals.

   3. **Kono kusuri o mai-shoku-go fukuyō shite kudasai.**
      Please take this medicine after every meal.

   4. **Kono kusuri wa kūfuku-ji ni fukuyō shite kudasai.**
      Please take this medicine on an empty stomach.

   5. **Kono kusuri wa kūfuku-ji ni fukuyō shinaide kudasai.**
      Please do not take this medicine on an empty stomach.

   6. **Kono kusui o ichi-nichi san-kai fukuyō shite kudasai.**
      Please take this medicine three times a day.

   7. **Kono kusuri wa shūshin-mae ni fukuyō shite kudasai.**
      Please take this medicine before going to bed.

   8. **Kono kusuri wa san-jyō o yo-jikan-oki ni fukuyō shite kudasai.**
      Please take two pills every four hours.

   9. **Kono kusuri wa mizu de fukuyō shite kudasai.**
      Please swallow this medicine with water.

10. **Kono kusuri wa owaru made nonde kudasai.**
    Please continue taking this medicine until the prescription runs out/you've used it up.

11. **Kono kusuri wa hitsuyō ni ōji-te nonde kudasai.**
    Please take this medicine as needed.

2. Dosage (**yōryō**): The following are possible answers to questions about dosage, such as **Kono kusuri no yōryō wa nan desu ka.** "What is the dosage on/for this medicine?" and **Kono kusuri wa nan-jō ichido ni nomeba ii desu ka.** "How many tablets/pills should I take at a time?"

> **Kono kōsei-bushitsu wa otona wa ikkai (ni) supūn ni hai, kodomo wa ippai nonde kudasai.**
> Please take two spoonfuls of this antibiotic for an adult at one time, and one for child.

> **Yōryō wa otona wa supūn ni-hai, kodomo wa i-pai, rokuji-kan okini nonde kudasai.**
> The dose is two spoonfuls for adults, or one spoonful for a child, every six hours.

> **Kono ichō-yaku wa otona wa ikkai (ni) san-jyō, nana-sai ijyō, jyū-go-sai miman wa ni-jō, nana-sai ika wa ichi-jyō nonde kudasai.**
> For this intestinal medicine, the dose is three tablets for adults, two tablets for children ages seven to fifteen, or one tablet for children under age seven.

> **Otona wa ikkai ni-jyō, kodomo wa ichi-jyō, nana-sai miman wa nomanaide kudasai.**
> The dose is two tablets for adults and one for children. Don't give this medicine to children under seven.

The following are counters of dosage for medicine.

Counters for drugs

NUMBERS	-KAI (FREQUENCY)	-JYŌ (TABLET/PILL)	-HAI/PAI (CUP/SPOON)	-FUKURO (PACKAGE)	-TEKI (DROPS)
1	i-kkai	ichi-jyō	i-ppai	hito-fukuro	i-tteki
2	ni-kai	ni-jyō	ni-hai	futa-fukuro	ni-teki
3	san-kai	san-jyō	san-pai	mi-fukuro	san-teki
4	yon-kai	yon-jyō	yon-pai	yo-fukuro	yon-teki
5	go-kai	go-jyō	go-hai	itsu-fukuro	go-teki
6	ro-kkai	roku-jyō	ro-ppai	ro-ppukuro	roku-teki

NUMBERS	-KAI (FREQUENCY)	-JYŌ (TABLET/PILL)	-HAI/PAI (CUP/SPOON)	-FUKURO (PACKAGE)	-TEKI (DROPS)
7	nana-kai	nana-jyō	nana-hai	nana-fukuro	nana-teki
8	ha-kkai	hachi-jyō	ha-ppai	ha-ppukuro	ha-tteki
9	kyū-kai	kyū-jyō	kyū-hai	kyū-fukuro	kyū-teki
10	jyu-kkai	jyū-jyō	jyu-ppai	jyu-ppukuro	jyu-tteki

NUMBERS	-DO (FREQUENCY)	-KAPUSERU (CAPSULES)
1	ichi-do	ichi-kapuseru
2	ni-do	ni-kapuseru
3	san-do	san-kapuseru
4	yon-do	yon-kapuseru
5	go-do	go-kapuseru
6	roku-do	roku-kapuseru
7	nana-do	nana-kapuseru
8	hachi-do	hachi-kapusru
9	kyū-do	kyū-kapuseru
10	jyū-do	jyū-kapuseru

OINTMENTS (APPLY)	
sukoshi nurimasu	(sparingly, a modest amount)
teki-ryō nurimasu	(moderately, a moderate amount)
yoku nurimasu	(good amount/apply well)
tappuri nurimasu	(amply, an ample amount)

Note: To make a question, add **nan** as a prefix, which makes: **nan-kai** (how many times?), **nan-jyō** (how many tablets?), **nan-pai** (how many cups/spoonfuls), **nan-fukuro** (how many packages?), and **nan-teki** (how many drops?).

3. Expressions of general warning

Moshi, itami ni taerarenai-yō deshita ra, kono chintsū-zai o fukuyō shite kudasai.
If you can't stand the pain, please take this pain reliever/painkiller.

Kono kusuri o nondara, ni-ji-kan wa unten shinai de kudasai.
Do not drive for two hours after taking this medicine.

Kono kusuri o nondara, arukōru wa noma-naide kudasai.
Do not drink alcohol when you're taking this medication.

Kodomo no te no todokanai tokoro-ni hokan shite kudasai.
Please keep this (medicine) out of the reach of children.

Kono kusuri wa suzushii tokoto-de hokan shite kudasai.
Keep/store this medicine in a cool place.

Kono kusuri o nonde ijyō o kanjitara suguni i-shi ni sōdan shire kudasai.
Consult your physician immediately if you notice any side effects from this medicine.

Kono nankō o nuru-mae ni, yoku te o aratte kudasai.
Wash your hands thoroughly before applying the ointment.

4. The common Japanese expression **kekkō desu** has two different meanings: 1) Yes, thank you; splendid; nice; wonderful; sufficient; fine; good enough; or 2) No, thank you. The meaning, and how you use the expression, depends on the context. However, the meaning can be inferred from the particle used. When used with the particle **de**, it is usually positive, and with a subject marker **wa** (**mō**), it is usually negative.

Kono kusuri de kekkō desu. This medicine is fine.
Kono kusuri wa (mō) kekkō desu. As for this medicine, no, thank you.

5. The verb **nomimasu** (drink) is used for "take (medicine)," whether the medication is swallowed in solid form or drunk as a liquid. The verb **fukuyō shimasu** has the same meaning but is a polite form.

Asupirin-o nomimasu. I will take the aspirin.
Asupirin-o fukuyō shimasu. I will take the aspirin. (polite)

Note that these verbs are not the ones that translate most meanings of the English verb *take*. Instead, for that purpose use **torimasu/toru**. Japanese never say *Kusuri o torimasu*. "I will take a medicine." However, they do say **Eiyō o torimasu**. "I will take nutrition," and **Kyūyō o torimasu**. "I will take a rest."

Language Roots

The prefix **kō-** (抗) means "against," like the English prefix *anti-*.

kō-sei bushitsu antibiotics
kō-gan-zai anticancer drug
kō-tai antibodies
kō-gi protest

The prefix **kyō-** (強) indicates strength or potency.

kyō-shin-zai	cardio tonic
kyō-sō-zai	restorative
kyō-ryoku	powerful

Culture Notes

The Japanese expression for "take (medicine)"

Japanese use a verb meaning "drink," **nomimasu**, when they speak of taking a medicine or medication. Before the advent of modern medicine in Japan, Japanese used medicinal plants to cure illness. A decoction would be made from plants and then drunk. Ever since, the verb "to drink" has been used for "take medicine" as well. The Japanese call medicine **kusuri**, a word that derives from **kusa iri**. **Kusa** is "medicinal plants," and **iri** (from **iru**) means "boiling" Literally, **kusuri** means "boiled medicinal plants" from ancient times.

The Japanese verb **nakunaru** and understanding death

Japanese express "die" as **nakunaru**. The literal meaning of **nakunaru** is "disappear, become empty, use up." Japanese understand death as the body disappearing, becoming emptiness, or all the energy in this body and life being exhausted or used up.

Health-related Japanese proverbs VI

Laughter is the best of all medicine.
Warai wa hyaku-yaku no chō.
笑いは百薬の長

Taking good care of your health is better than medicine.
Kusuri yori yōjyō.
薬より養生

Comprehension

Answer the following questions.

1. Which of the following does NOT belong with the others?
    a. **Kōfun-zai**   b. **Shiyō-hōhō**
    c. **Yōryō**   d. **Tenpu-bunsho**

2. Which of the following could be used to say "effect"?
   a. **Kusuri ga yoku kimasu.**   b. **Kusuri ga yoku kiemasu.**
   c. **Kusuri ga yoku kikimasu.**   d. **Kusuriga yoku kikemasu.**

3. Which of the following best completes the sentence below?
   Mai-shoku-go san-jyu ppun inai (   ) kono kusuri o fukuyō shite kudasai.
   Please take this medicine within thirty minute after every meal.
   a. **wa**   b. **ni**
   c. **de**   d. **o**

4. You are suggesting how much ointment to apply to the skin irritation. How do you say, "Apply a moderate amount" in Japanese?
   a. **Sukoshi nutte kudasai.**   b. **Tottemo nutte kudasai.**
   c. **Takusan nutte kudasai.**   d. **Tekiryō o nutte kudasai.**

Select the appropriate meaning from the list below.

---

5. **Kono kusui o ichi-nichi san-kai fukuyō shite kudasai.**   (   )
6. **Kono kusuri o mai-shokugo fukuyō shite kudasai.**   (   )
8. **Kono kusuri wa kū-fuku-ji ni fukuyō shinaide kudasai.**   (   )
8. **Kono kusuri o shoku-zen ni fukuyō shite kudasai.**   (   )
9. **Kono kusuri o shokkan ni fukuyō shite kudasai.**   (   )

a. Please take this medicine between meals.
b. Please take this medicine before meals.
c. Please do not take this medicine on an empty stomach.
d. Please take this medicine three times a day.
e. Please take this medicine after every meal.

Practice

Respond to the following in Japanese using the cues that have been provided.

---

1. Explain when to take this medicine:
   (Patient)   (Healthcare professional)
   1. **Kono kusuri wa itsu nomimasu ka.**   _____
                                              (before meals)

   2. **Kono kusuri wa itsu nomimasu ka.**   _____
                                              (between meals)

   3. **Kono kusuri wa itsu nomeba ii desu ka.** _____
                                              (after every meal)

4. **Kono kusuri wa itsu nomeba ii desu ka.** _____
   (on an empty stomach)
5. **Kono kusuri wa itsu nomeba ii desu ka.** _____
   (not on an empty stomach)

2. How much of the medicine should the patient take?
   (Patient)   (Healthcare professional)
   1. **Kono kusuri no yōryō wa nan desu ka.** _____
      (two spoonfuls)
   2. **Kono kusuri no yōryō wa nan desu ka.** _____
      (one tablespoon)
   3. **Kono kusuri wa nan-jyō ichido ni** _____
      nomeba ii desu ka.   (three tablets)
   4. **Kono kusuri wa nan-jyō ichido ni** _____
      nomeba ii desu ka.   (two capsules)

3. How do you give the following safety warnings to clients.
   (Warning)   (Healthcare professionals)
   1. Don't drive for two hours after taking this _____
      medicine.
   2. Don't drink alcohol when you take this _____
      medicine.
   3. Keep this medication out of the reach of _____
      your children.
   4. Please keep this medicine in a cool place. _____
   5. Tell your physician immediately if you _____
      notice any side effects.

4. Dialogue comprehension. Based on the dialogue, answer the following questions.
   1. **Kusuri wa itsu nomimasu ka.** _____
   2. **Kusuri wa ichi-nichi (ni) nan-kai nomimasu ka.** _____
   3. **Otona wa ikkai (ni) nan-jō kusuri o nomimasu ka.** _____
   4. **Nana-sai ika wa kusuri o nomemasu ka.** _____
   5. **Kusuri wa ikura desu ka.** _____
   6. **Hoken ga kikimasu ka.** _____

5. Free response questions.
   (Questions)   (Answers)
   1. **Kanpō-yaku o nomimasu ka.** _____
   2. **Chūi-jikō o setsumei shimasu ka.** _____

3. **Kōhatsu-iyaku-hin wa takai desu ka.** _____

4. **Jenerikku iyaku-hin wa yasui desu ka.** _____

5. **Seishin-antei-zai o nonde imasu ka.** _____

Exercises

1. Say the following words in Japanese.
   A. Anticancer drug _____
   B. Intestinal medicine _____
   C. Itchy lotion/medicine _____
   D. Antibiotic _____
   E. Contraceptive/pill _____

2. Say the following expressions in Japanese.
   A. I will explain how to use the disinfectant. _____
   B. Please take this antihypertensive drug within _____
      thirty minute after every meal.
   C. This anti-diarrhea medicine works well on diarrhea. _____
   D. Please take this sleeping pill as needed. _____
   E. Please take the pain reliever only when you need it. _____

3. In speaking to patients, how do you say the following in Japanese?
   A. Please don't drive for two hours after taking this _____
      medicine.
   B. Please don't drink alcohol when you take this _____
      medicine.
   C. Please keep this out of reach of your children. _____
   D. Please tell (us) immediately if you notice any strange _____
      side effects from this medicine.

4. Answer the following questions in Japanese.

   Q: **Kono kusuri wa nan-jō ichido ni nomeba ii desu ka.**
   A: _____
      (Please take three tablets for adults, two tablets for children, and do not
      give this medicine to a child under 5 years old.)

   Q: **Kono kusuri wa itsu nome-ba ii desu ka.**
   B: _____
      (Please take this medicine before going to bed.)

16 Infectious Diseases
(Densen-byō)

Basic Vocabulary (CD 16-1)

Listen to the CD and repeat the vocabulary.

1.	influenza/flu	**infuruenza**	インフルエンザ
2.	immunization	**yobō-sesshu**	予防接種
3.	inoculation/shot	**sesshu**	接種
4.	blister	**sui-hō**	水泡
5.	pus	**umi**	膿
6.	streptococcal infection	**yōren-kin kansen-shō**	溶連菌感染症
7.	Koplik spot	**kopurriku-han**	コプリック斑
8.	infectious hepatitis	**ryūkōsei kan-en**	流行性肝炎
9.	mumps	**otafuku kaze**	おたふく風邪
10.	leprosy/Hansen's disease	**rai-byō**	らい病
11.	yellow fever	**ō-netsu-byō**	黄熱病
12.	malaria	**mararia**	マラリア
13.	rabies	**kyōken-byō**	狂犬病
14.	measles	**hashika**	麻疹
15.	German measles	**fūshin/mikka-bashika**	風疹/三日麻疹
16.	smallpox	**tennen-tō**	天然痘
17.	vaccination	**shutō**	種痘
18.	chicken pox/varicella	**sui-tō/mizu-bōsō**	水痘/水疱瘡
19.	typhoid fever	**chō-chifusu**	腸チフス
20.	cholera	**korera**	コレラ
21.	pest	**pesuto/kokushi-byō**	黒死病
22.	scarlet fever/scarlatina	**shōkō-netsu**	猩紅熱
23.	DPT vaccine (also DTP)	**DPT fukugō-wakuchin**	DPT複合ワクチン
24.	diphtheria	**jifuteia**	ジフテリア
25.	whooping cough/pertussis	**hyaku-nichi-zeki**	百日咳
26.	tetanus	**hashōfū**	破傷風
27.	dysentery	**sekiri**	赤痢
28.	MMR vaccine	**sanshu-kongō-wakuchin**	三種混合ワクチン
29.	germs	**sai-kin/bai-kin/kin**	細菌/ばい菌/菌
30.	specimen	**kentai**	検体

Dialogue (CD 16-2)

Listen to the CD and repeat the dialogue.

At the Medical Specialist's Office

Mrs. Kato (patient's mom): **Sakuya kara, musuko no mune to senaka ni hosshin ga arawarete kimashita.**
My son broke out in eruptions on his chest and back last night.

Kesa wa suihō o kayu-gatte imasu.
This morning he was showing signs of blisters and complaining of itchiness.

Dr. Harris (male doctor): **Netsu o hakari mashita ka.**
Did you take his temperature?

Mrs. Kato: **Kesa wa san-jyū hachi-do hachi-bu (hyaku ni do) deshita.**
(His temperature) this morning was 38.8 degrees (102).

Dr. Harris: **Saikin, musuko-san no mawari de dareka mizu-bōsō no ko ga ima-sen deshita ka.**
Have any children around him had chicken pox recently?

Mrs. Kato: **Ni-san-shū-kan hodo mae ni, onaji gakkō de sū-nin, mizu-bōsō no ko ga demashita.**
A few students in the same school broke out in chicken pox about two or three weeks ago.

Dr. Harris: **Musuko-san wa mizu-bōsō ni chigai arimasen.**
I think there is no doubt he has chicken pox.

Musuko-san no chikaku ni iruhito ni kansen shite shimaimasu kara, gakkō o isshū-kan yasunde kudasai.
Your son is contagious, so please keep him home from school for a week.

Mrs. Kato: **Nani-ka yoi chiryō ga arimasu ka.**
Do you have any good treatments?

Dr. Harris: **Sō desu ne. Mizu-bōsō uirusu ni taishite nomi-gusuri, kayumi ni taishite kō-hisutamin-zai o shohō shimasu.**
Let's see. I will prescribe an oral medicine for the chickenpox virus and antihistamines for his itching.

Grammar

1. ### The construction PLACE **ni** SUBJECT **ga arawarete kimasu**

   The construction PLACE **ni** SUBJECT **ga arawarete kimasu** is used to say that someone or something has become visible or is manifesting.

   > **Otoko no hito ni byōki ga arawarete kimasu.**
   > The illness is showing on the man.

   > **Anata no kao ni fukide-mono ga arawarete kimasu.**
   > A pimple is breaking out on your face.

   > **Migi ude ni shisshin ga arawarete kimashita.**
   > The rash appeared on her right arm.

   > **Kao ni suihō ga awarete kimashita.**
   > The blister appeared on his face.

2. ### The **i**-adjective stem + **-garu**

   The **i**-adjective stem plus the suffix **-garu** means "to show signs of (a wish and desire)." To use this construction, first drop the **-i** ending from the adjective and replace it with **-garu** (or **-gatte imasu** in the present progressive tense). The suffix **-garu** requires a subject (the thing manifested by the signs, such as pain, itchiness, discomfort, etc.) and follows the object marker **o**.

   > **(Kanjya wa) Me ga itai(n) desu.**
   > The patient has eye pain.

   > **(Kanjya wa) Me o ita-garu.**
   > The patient shows signs of having pain in his eye.

   > **(Kanjya wa) Me o ita-gatte imasu.**
   > The patient is showing signs of having pain in his eye.

   > **(Kanjya wa) Mune ga kurushii desu.**
   > The patient has chest discomfort.

   > **(Kanjya wa) Mune o kurushi-garu.**
   > The patient shows signs of having discomfort in her chest.

   > **(Kanjya wa) Mune o kurushi-gatte imasu.**
   > The patient is showing signs of having discomfort in her chest.

The **i**-adjectives of feeling in the chart below commonly take **-garu**.

ENGLISH	ADJECTIVE DROP -I	REPLACE WITH -GARU (SHOW SIGNS OF)
painful/sore	**ita-i**	**ita-garu**
difficult/suffering/discomfort	**kurushi-i**	**kurushi-garu**
itchy	**kayu-i**	**kayu-garu**
difficult	**mazukashi-i**	**mazukashi-garu**
ticklish/extremely sensitive	**kusuguta-i**	**kusuguta-garu**
hot	**atsu-i**	**atsu-garu**
cold (weather/feeling/room)*	**samu-i**	**samu-garu**
cold (touch/body/drinks)*	**tsumeta-i**	**tsumeta-garu**
want/wish	**hoshi-i**	**hoshi-garu**
happy	**ureshi-i**	**ureshi-garu**
interesting	**omoshiro-i**	**omoshiro-garu**
wonderful	**subarashi-i**	**subarashi-garu**
lonely	**sabishi-i**	**sabishi-garu**
sad	**kanashi-i**	**kanashi-garu**
scary	**kowa-i**	**kowa-garu**
envious	**urayamashi-i**	**urayamashi-garu**

* Japanese has two different words for the meanings of the English word *cold*: **samui** and **tsumetai**. **Samui** is used for feeling cold with respect to weather and the human mind (the perception of cold). **Tsumetai** is used for cold to the touch (for example, ice) and human relationships.

3. The construction verb + -garu

There are also verbs that can attach to **-garu** to mean "show signs of (a wish/ want)." To form this construction, use the **masu** form first to identify the verb base, add the sufffix **-tai** (for "wish *or* want"), and finally drop the **-i** from the **tai**-form and replace it with **-garu**. To remember how to identify **tai**-form, see Lesson 12.

> **Kanjya wa mune o kaki-tai desu.**
> The patient wants to scratch his/her chest.

> **Kanjya wa mune o kaki-ta-garu.**
> The patient shows signs of wanting to scratch his/her chest.

> **Sensei wa kanjya o mi-tai desu.**
> The doctor wants to see the patient.

Sensei wa kanjya o mi-ta-garu.
The doctor shows signs of wanting to see the patient.

Kodomo ga gohan o tabeta-garu.
The children show signs of wanting to have a meal. (informal)

Kodomo ga gohan o tabeta-garimasu.
The children show signs of wanting to have a meal.

Kodomo ga onaka o ita-gatte imasu.
The children are showing signs of stomach pain.

Kodomo ga onaka o ita-gatte imashita.
The children were showing signs of stomach pain. (past tense)

The following verbs might also be used with **-garu**.

ENGLISH	VERB (-**MASU**)	VERB (-**TAI** FORM) WISH/WANT	-**GARU** (SHOW SIGNS OF WISH/WANT)
see/look/watch/examine	mi-masu	mi-tai	mi-ta-garu
eat	tabe-masu	tabe-tai	tabe-ta-garu
drink	nomi-masu	nomi-tai	nomita-garu
buy	kai-masu	kai-tai	kai-ta-garu
sleep	ne-masu	ne-tai	ne-ta-garu
rest/be absent	yasumi-masu	yasumi-tai	yasumi-ta-garu
sit down	suwari-masu	suwari-tai	suwari-ta-garu
stand up	tachi-masu	tachi-tai	tachi-ta-garu
speak	hanashi-masu	hanashi-tai	hanashi-ta-garu
do/play	shi-masu	shi-tai	shi-ta-garu
scratch	kaki-masu	kaki-tai	kaki-ta-garu
take off (clothes)	nugi-masu	nugi-tai	nugi-ta-garu
allow to do	sase-masu	sase-tai	sase-ta-garu
continue	tsuzuke-masu	tsuzuke-tai	tsuzuke-ta-garu
transmit/transfer	utsuri-masu	utsuri-tai	utsuri-ta-garu
anger/upset	okori-masu	okori-tai	okori-ta-garu
inform/teach	oshie-masu	oshie-tai	oshie-ta-garu
vomit	haki-masu	haki-tai	haki-ta-garu

4. The expression **no mawari-de**

The expression **no mawari-de** can be used to say that something is happening in a surrounding area, neighborhood, or locality. When preceded by a place or person, it means "around (the place/person)."

Byōin no mawari-de kyūkyū-sha ga sairen o narashite imasu.
The ambulance siren is wailing around the hospital.

Kaisha no mawari-de hashika ga ryūkō shite imasu.
Measles is spreading around/all over the company.

In the same construction, **no chikaku-ni/de** means "near."

Gakkō no chikaku-de hashika ga hirogatte imasu.
The measles are spreading near the school.

Machi no chikaku-ni yobō-sesshu-jyō ga arimasu.
Immunization services are available near the town.

5. The expression **ni chigai arimasen**

The expression **ni chigai arimasen** states a definite judgment about a diagnosis, as in "I think etc.," or "There is no doubt that etc." Often, healthcare professionals prefer something like **no yō desu** ("it looks like, seems to"). However, when the examination or test results are certain and it's necessary for the patient to understand clearly, healthcare professionals can choose to use **ni chigai arimasen**. Please see Lesson 11 for other expressions.

Kono shōjyō wa otafuku-kaze ni chigai arimasen.
I think there is no doubt that this symptom is the mumps (*lit.*, This symptom is mumps without doubt).

Kensa no kekka kara mararia ni chigai arimasen.
There is no doubt that the result of the test shows malaria.

Shōjyō kara, hyaku-nichi-zeki ni chigai arimasen.
There is no doubt that the symptom is whooping cough.

6. The **te** form + **shimau**

The **te**-form of the verb plus **shimau/shimaimasu** expresses the idea of the completion of an action, as in "have done."

Gakkō no mawari ni hashika ga hirogatte shimau.
The measles have spread around the school.

Byōin-nai-de ryūkō-sei kan-en ga kansen shite shimaimasu.
Hepatitis has infected the hospital. (*lit.*, Infectious hepatitis has spread in the hospital.)

7. The set phrase NOUN + **ni taishite**

A noun plus the preposition **ni taishite** is used to express a person's action or attitude with respect to someone or something (expressed by the noun).

> **Uirusu ni taishite kōsei-bushitsu o nonde kudasai.**
> Please take antibiotics for the virus.

> **Kangoshi-san wa dare ni taishite mo shinsetsu desu.**
> The nurse is kind to everybody.

NOUN plus **ni taishite** is also used to express an action or attitude in opposition to something.

> **Kono kodomo wa byōki ni taishite ganbatte imasu.**
> This child is doing his best against the illness.

> **Oisha wa kanjay no yōkyū ni taishite okotte imasu.**
> The doctor is getting angry about the patient's claim.

Ni taishi can replace **ni taishite** in formal speech.

> **Uirusu ni taishi(te) kōsei-bushitsu o nonde kudasai.**
> Please take antibiotics for the virus.

> **Infuruenza ni taishi, yobō-sesshu ga hitsuyō desu.**
> It's necessary to have immunization against flu.

The expression **ni taishite** can also be abbreviated to only **ni**.

> **Uirusu ni (taishite) kōsei bushitsu o nonde kudasai.**
> Please take antibiotics for the virus.

8. The adverbs **motto** and **takusan**

In Lesson 4, we studied the adverb **takusan** (many). The adverbs **motto** (more) and **takusan** are used to modify verbs in both positive ("even more") and negative ("any more") sentences. These two adverbs can be used together for emphasis.

Motto kensa ga hitsyō desu.	You need more tests.
Suibun o takusan totte kudasai.	You should drink more liquids.
Motto takusan yasun-de kudasai.	Please get even more rest.

> **Motto takusan no kusuri wa hitsuyō arimasen.**
> There's no need to take any more medicine.

Useful Expressions (CD 16-3)

Listen to the CD and repeat the sentences.

1. **Kodomo-san ni yobō-chūsha ga hitsuyō desu ka.** Does your child need immunization?
2. **Aka-chan ni karui netsu ga aruyō desu.** The baby seems to have a slight fever.
3. **Karui netsu ga detemo shinpai wa irimasen.** Don't worry if you have a slight fever.
4. **Hashika ni chigai arimasen.** I think there is no doubt it's measles.
5. **Sarani kuwashii kensa o shimasu node, yokaku o shite kudasai.** Please make an appointment for further tests.
6. **Sūjitsu nyūin saseta hō ga ii desu.** It might be best to bring him/her into the hospital for a few days.
7. **Seki ga ikka-getsu ijyō tsuzuite imasu ka.** Have you been coughing for more than a month?
8. **Chi o haitari ketsu-ben ga detari shimasu ka.** Have you ever coughed up blood or had bloody stool?
9. **Infuruenza no kensa o suru node, hana ni menbō o irete kentai o tori-masu ne.** We will take a nasal swab to check for the flu.
10. **Itaku arimasen node, rirakkusu shite kudasai. Sugu ni owarimasu.** It won't hurt at all, so just stay still and relax. It will be over in a few seconds.

Key Sentences (CD 16-4)

Listen to the CD and repeat the sentences.

1. **Kao ni mukumi ga arawarete kimashita.** Puffiness is appearing on/around the face.
2. **Kanjya wa mune o ita-gatte imasu.** The patient showing signs of having chest pain.
3. **Gakkō no mawari de infuruenza ga ryūkō shite imasu.** The influenza is infecting the area around the school.
4. **Kono shōjyō wa fūshin-ni chigai arimasen.** I think there is no doubt that this symptom is German measles.
5. **Gakkō de otafuku-kaze ni kansen shite shimai-mashita.** I have been in-fected by mumps at school.

Additional Words

arawareru/arawaremasu be visible/appear
saseru/sasemasu make/allow someone to do
utsuru/utsurimasu infect/transmit
taipu type
chikai nearby
uirusu virus
shin-gata new type

okoru/okorimasu angry
kansen infection
mawari surrounding
ryūkō-sei epidemic
menbō cotton swab
kyū-gata old type
machi town

Language Notes

1. There are two types of expressions for complaints: **itai** and **kurushii**. **Itai** should be used for pain, but **kurushii** can be used for a difficulty or discomfort, such as suffering with tightness.

2. When you read the temperature in Celsius, you can use the words "**ten . . . do**" or "**do . . . bu**" to say "point . . . degrees."

    38.6 = **Sanjyū hachi ten roku do desu.**
    39.8 = **Sanjyū-kyū do hachi bu desu.**

3. The time expression **kara** (since, from) can be used as follows:

kesa kara	since this morning
saku-ban kara	since last evening
saku-ya kara	since last night
saku-jitsu kara	since yesterday
sūjitsu mae kara	since a few days ago

Language Roots

The word **netsu** (熱) indicates fever and temperature.

ō-netsu-byō	yellow fever
shōkō-netsu	scarlet fever
kō-netsu	high fever/high temperature
hei-netsu	normal temperature
bi-netsu	slight fever

The word **shi** (死) indicates death and decease.

shi-bō	death
shi-nin	dead person

shi-tai	dead body
shizen-shi	natural death
fu-shizen-shi	unnatural death
byō-shi	death by disease
jiko-shi	death by accident
tō-shi	freezing to death
ga-shi	starving to death
totsuzen-shi	sudden death
soku-shi	instant death
anraku-shi	euthanasia

Culture Notes

The current Japanese vaccination requirements

Since April 2006, all Japanese are required to receive the MR vaccines (measles and German measles), between the ages of twelve and fifteen months for measles and thirty-six months for German measles. The government also requires a total of five immunizations for Japanese encephalitis (**nihon-noēn**). The vaccines for mumps and chickenpox are currently not mandatory in Japan. BCG (Bacille de Calmette et Guerin) must be administered within six months of birth. The polio vaccine is administered two times between three months and eighteen months. DPT (diphtheria, pertussis/whooping cough, and tetanus) is given three times from after three months to twelve months from birth. One additional DPT shot is required between twelve months and eighteen months of birth. (SOURCE: Ministry of Health, Labor, and Welfare of Japan)

New types of influenza (**shin-gata infuruenza**)

Recently, many new types of influenza have been spreading around of the world, with names like H1N1 and other strains of avian influenza, swine flu, bird flu, etc. Japanese call all these new influenzas **shin-gata** (new type) as compared to **kisetsu-fū** (seasonal) influenza.

Comprehension

Answer the following questions.

1. Which of the following does NOT belong with the others?
   a. **Hashika**
   b. **Haykunichi-zeki**
   c. **Fūshin**
   d. **Kisei-chū**

2. Which of the following could be used for say, "shows signs of being itchy?"
   a. **Daru-garu**
   b. **Kawarita-garu**
   c. **Mita-garu**
   d. **Kayu-garu**

3. Which of the following best completes the sentence below?
   Byōin-nai ni ryūkō-sei kan-en ga kansen (   ) imasu.
   (Infectious hepatitis has spread in the hospital.)
   a. **made**
   b. **kamo**
   c. **kara**
   d. **shite**

4. You are asking, "Was anyone infected with chicken pox around the children." How do you say "around the children?"
   a. **Kodomo no hidari de**
   b. **Kodomo no migi de**
   c. **Kodomo no mawari de**
   d. **Kodomo no shita de**

Select the appropriate meaning from the list below.

---

5. **Suibun o takusan totte kudasai.**   (   )
6. **Kanjya wa amari tabete imasen.**   (   )
7. **Motto takusan yasunde kudasai.**   (   )
8. **Kanjya wa kensa o zenzen ukemasen.**   (   )
9. **Motto kensa ga hitsyō desu.**   (   )

a. Please get even more rest.
b. The patient does not like having tests very much.
c. The patient is not eating much.
d. You should drink lots of liquids.
e. You need more tests.

Practice

Respond to the following in Japanese using the cues that have been provided.

---

1. Asking the cause of an illness:
   (Patient)   (Healthcare professional)
   1. **Nani ga genin desu ka.**   _____
                                            (streptococcal infection)
   2. **Don-na byōgen-kin desu ka.**   _____
                                            (virus)
   3. **Dōshite byōki ni narimashita ka.** _____
                                            (bacteria)

4. **Byōgenkin wa nan desu ka.** _____

(new type of virus)

5. **Infuruenza no taipu wa nan desu ka.** _____

(seasonal type)

2. Saying what kind of symptoms.
   (Patient)   (Healthcare professional)
   1. Eruption on the chest   _____
   2. Blister on the neck   _____
   3. Eczema on the upper back   _____
   4. Sore on the lip   _____
   5. High fever   _____

3. Giving the patient advice.
   (Patient)   (Healthcare professional)
   1. **Kensa ga hitsyō desu ka.**   _____

   (need more tests)

   2. **Suibun ga hitsuyō desu ka.** _____

   (need more liquid)

   3. **Kyūyō ga hitsuyō desu ka.** _____

   (need more rest)

   4. **Don-na kusuri o nome ba ii desu ka.** _____

   (take antibiotics)

   5. **Netsu ni nani ga hitsuyō desu ka.** _____

   (cool down)

4. Dialogue comprehension. Based on the dialogue, answer the following questions.
   1. **Dare ga kanjya desu ka.**   _____
   2. **Itsu kara hosshin ga demashita ka.** _____
   3. **Kesa wa don-na jyōtai desu ka.**   _____
   4. **Netsu wa nan-do desu ka.**   _____
   5. **Musuko-san no byōmei wa nan-desu ka.** _____

5. Free response questions.
   (Questions)   (Answers)
   1. **Shingata infuruenza no yobō-sesshu
      o ukemashita ka.**   _____
   2. **Ryūkōsei kan-en no kanjya ga imasu ka.** _____
   3. **Kodomo no toki ni otafuku-kaze ni
      kakarimashita ka.**   _____

4. **Sanshu-kongō wakuchin o ukemashita ka.** _____

5. **Hashōfū no chūsha o shimashita ka.** _____

Exercises

1. Say the following words in Japanese.
   A. Bacteria _____
   B. Measles _____
   C. Tetanus _____
   D. Immunization _____
   E. Streptococcus _____

2. Say the following sentences in Japanese.
   A. A tumor has appeared on the abdomen.

   _____

   B. The patients are showing signs of feeling itchy on their backs.

   _____

   C. Whooping cough is infecting the area around the school.

   _____

   D. I think there is no doubt that this symptom is infectious hepatitis.

   _____

   E. Please take this antibiotic for the flu.

   _____

3. In speaking to patients, how do you say the following in Japanese?
   A. Have you ever coughed up blood or had bloody stool?

   _____

   B. Don't worry if you have a slight fever.

   _____

   C. It won't hurt at all, so just stay still and relax.

   _____

   D. It might be best to bring him/her to the hospital immediately.

   _____

   E. We will take a nasal swab to check for the flu.

   _____

4. Answer the following questions in Japanese.

   Q: **Sensei, byōmei wa nan desu ka.**
   A: _____
   (I think there is no doubt it is measles.)

Q: **Sensei, kodomo ni netsu ga arumasu ka.**

B: _____

(The child looks like he/she has a slight fever.)

Q: **Sensei, mizu o nonde-mo ii desu ka.**

C: _____

(Yes, you should drink lots of liquids.)

Respiratory System
(Kokyūki-kei)

Basic Vocabulary (CD 17-1)

Listen to the CD and repeat the vocabulary.

1.	pulmonary function tests	**hai-kinō kensa**	肺機能検査
2.	respiratory illness	**kokyū-ki shikkan**	呼吸器疾患
3.	bronchoscopy	**kikanshi-kyō-kensa**	気管支鏡検査
4.	respiratory failure	**kokyū-fuzen**	呼吸不全
5.	asthma	**zensoku**	喘息
6.	bronchitis	**kikanshi-en**	気管支炎
7.	bronchial asthma	**kikanshi zensoku**	気管支喘息
8.	lung cancer/pulmonary cancer	**hai-gan**	肺癌
9.	pneumonia	**hai-en**	肺炎
10.	lung abscess	**hai-nōyō**	肺膿瘍
11.	tuberculosis	**kekkaku**	結核
12.	pulmonary tuberculosis/ lung TB	**hai kekkaku**	肺結核
13.	pleurodynia	**kyōmaku-tsū**	胸膜痛
14.	pleurisy	**kyōmaku-en**	胸膜炎
15.	peritonitis	**fukumaku-en**	腹膜炎
16.	pharyngitis/sore throat	**intō-en**	咽頭炎
17.	thyroiditis	**kōjyōsen-en**	甲状腺炎
18.	chills	**okan**	悪寒
19.	apnea	**mu-kokyu**	無呼吸
20.	oxygen deficiency	**sanso ketsubō-shō**	酸素欠乏症
21.	insomnia/sleeplessness	**fumin-shō**	不眠症
22.	dyspnea/shortness of breath	**kokyū kon-nan**	呼吸困難
23.	wheezing/stridor	**zenmei**	喘鳴
24.	expectorant	**kyotan-yaku**	去痰薬
25.	cough medicine	**seki-dome/ chingai-yaku**	咳止め/鎮咳薬
26.	bronchodilator	**kikanshi-kakuchō-zai**	気管支拡張剤
27.	pleural effusion	**kyō-sui**	胸水
28.	orthopnoea	**kiza-kokyū**	起座呼吸
29.	vocal cords	**seitai**	声帯
30.	cyanosis	**chianōze**	チアノーゼ

Dialogue (CD 17-2)

Listen to the CD and repeat the dialogue.

At the Medical Specialist's Office

Dr. Harris: **Kyō wa dō shimashita ka.**
How are you feeling today?

Mrs. Tanaka: **Futsu-ka mae kara, zei-zei to sekiga dete, tan ga tsuzuite, net-su-ppoi(n) desu.**
I have a hoarse cough, the phlegm keeps coming up, and I've been feeling feverish since two days ago.

Dr. Harris: **Dewa, chotto, chōshin-ki-de mune no oto o kiite mimashō.**
Well then, let me listen to your chest with the stethoscope.

Shatsu o agete, iki o ōkiku sutte, hai, tomete kudasai. Hai, (iki o dashite) ii desu yo.
Please lift up your shirt, take a deep breath, yes, hold it. Now (breathe out) . . . Okay, done.

Mrs. Tanaka: **Nandaka, zei-zei shite, mune ga itakute, chikara ga hairimasen.**
I feel like I'm sort of wheezing, my chest hurts, and I feel weak.

Iki o suru to rokkotsu no shita ga sasuyō ni itamimasu.
I also have terrible stabbing pains under my ribs when I breathe in.

Dr. Harris: **Tashikani, hai zentaini tan ga tsumatte, zenmei ga kikoemasu.**
Yes, you definitely have diffused congestive wheezing on the lungs.

Nodo mo akaku natte imasu.
Your throat also looks red and inflamed.

Osoraku, uirusu-sei no kikanshi-en dato omoimasu.
I think you most likely have viral bronchitis.

Mrs. Tanaka: **Eē, hontō desu ka.**
No, really?

Dr. Harris: **Nen-no-tame ni, kyōbu-rentogen o totte, hai-en ni natte inai ka tashikamete mimasu.**
I would like to take a chest X-ray to determine whether it has become pneumonia or not.

Soreni, ketsueki-kensa o shite, hakkekyū o shirabete, enshō o CRP de mimashō.

Also, I would like to do a blood test to examine your white cell count and check for inflammation using the CRP, the C-reactive protein test.

Mrs. Tanaka: **Zensoku o okoshite iru no dewa naika to shinpai desu.**
I'm worried about the risk of getting asthma.

Dr. Harris: **Toriaezu kensa o shimashō.**
Anyway, let's do some tests.

Kyō wa, kyotan-yaku to kikanshi-kakuchō-zai o shohō shimasu ne.
I'll prescribe an expectorant and bronchodilator for you.

Kono kusuri o nomeba yokunarimasu yo. Sū-jitsu-kan yōsu o mimashō.
I think, if you take these medications, you'll get well soon. I'll need follow your progress closely for several days.

Kokyūki-kei (Respiratory System)

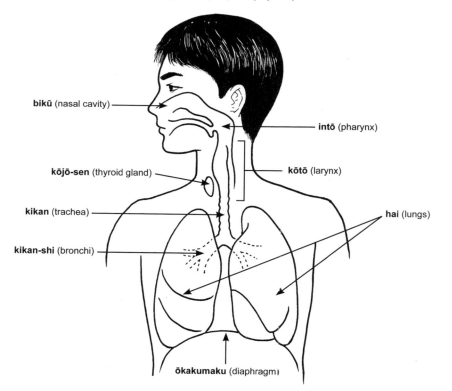

bikū (nasal cavity)

intō (pharynx)

kōjō-sen (thyroid gland)

kōtō (larynx)

kikan (trachea)

hai (lungs)

kikan-shi (bronchi)

ōkakumaku (diaphragm)

Grammar

1. The constructions STEM VERB + **-yō (ni)** and i-ADJECTIVE + **-yō (ni)**

In Lesson 9, we studied the suffix **-yō (na)** (looks like), and in Lesson 12 we studied the construction TIME plus **no yō(ni)** (almost every). The constructions STEM VERB plus **-yō (ni)** and i-ADJECTIVE plus **-yō (ni)** mean "is like; sounds like; or is similar to."

Saku-yō ni itai(n) desu.	It's like a tearing pain.
Sasu-yō ni itai(n) desu.	It's like a stabbing pain.

(Kodomo wa) kurushii yōni seki o shite imasu.
The child's coughing sounds like he/she is suffering.

2. The constructions NOUN + **no yō-ni** and na-ADJECTIVE + **na yō-na**

The constructions NOUN plus **no yō-ni** and na-ADJECTIVE plus **no yō-na** also mean "like" or "similar." **Ni** can substitute for **na** to make **no yō-na.**

Hai-en no shōjyō no yō ni seki ga dete imasu
You're coughing like you have pneumonia (*lit.*, Like symptom of pneumonia, you're coughing).

Sensei no yō ni natrita-katta desu.
I want to become like you, doctor.

Attū no yō na itami ga koshi ni arimasu.
I have a pain like (someone's) pressing on my back.

3. The expression **ni natte inai ka tashikamete mimasu**

The expression **ni natte inai ka tashikamete mimasu** means "I am trying to ascertain/see/be sure whether it has become X or not." The **te**-form used with **mimasu** means "try to (do something)."

Kakumaku-en ni natte inai ka tashikamete mimasu.
I am trying to ascertain whether it has become pleurisy or not.

Kekkaku ni natte inai ka shirabete mimasu.
I am trying to see whether it has become tuberculosis or not.

Kikanshi-zensoku ni natte inai ka kensa shite mimasu.
I am trying to determine whether it has become bronchial asthma or not.

4. The construction BODY PART + **zentai-ni**

The construction BODY PART plus **zentai-ni** means "the whole/entire (body part)." The adverb **zentai-ni** by itself means "generally," so be careful where you place it.

> **Hai zentai-ni enshō o okoshite imasu.**
> There is inflammation across the entire lungs.

> **Karada zentai-ni chikara ga hairimasen.**
> My whole body feels weak.

> **Senaka zentai-ni itami ga arimasu.**
> I have pain in my whole upper back.

> **Zentai-ni, chōshi ga ii desu ka.**
> Generally, is your condition good?

> **Zentai-ni hentō-sen wa yokunatte kite imasu.**
> Generally, your tonsils are getting better.

5. The construction i-ADJECTIVE + **ku-naru**

The **i**-adjective can express the meaning "become, turn" by dropping the suffix **-i** and replacing it with **-ku-naru** or **-ku-narimasu**. If you want to use two or more adjectives in this way in a single sentence, drop the **-masu** ending and end instead with **-ku-naru**.

ENGLISH	I-ADJECTIVE	BECOME (**KU-NARU**)
red	**aka-i**	**aka-ku-naru**
blue	**ao-i**	**ao-ku-naru**
painful/sore	**ita-i**	**ita-ku-naru**
tired	**daru-i**	**daru-ku-naru**

> **Enshō de hentōsen ga akaku-narimashita.**
> Your tonsils have become red with inflammation.

> **Mune ga kakketsu shite itaku-naru.**
> My chest has become sore from hemoptysis.

> **Fuminshō de karada ga daruku-natta.**
> I became tired because of insomnia/sleeplessness.

> **Hentōsen ga akaku-nari, nodo ga itai(n) desu.**
> My throat is becoming red, and it's getting sore.

> **Mune ga itaku-nari, kao ga aoku narimashita.**
> My chest is becoming painful, and my face is turning blue.

The verb **naru/narimasu** (become, turn) is conjugated with the noun or **na**-adjective followed by **ni** (**naru**).

Kikanshi-en ni narimasu. You're getting bronchitis (*lit.*, becoming bronchitis.)

Hai ga kirei ni narimashita. Your lungs have cleared up.

6. Changing the **i**-adjective to the **te**-form with the suffix **-kute**

Another way to string multiple adjectives together in a sentence is to change the **i**-adjective to the **te**-form. You do this by dropping the suffix **-i** and replacing it with the suffix **-kute**.

ENGLISH	I-ADJECTIVE	TE-FORM	KU-NARU (BECOME/TURN)
red	aka-i	aka-kute	akaku-naru
blue	ao-i	ao-kute	aoku-naku
black	kuro-i	kuro-kute	kuroku-naru
white	shiro-i	shiro-kute	shiroku-naru
yellow	kiiro-i	kiiro-kute	kiiroku-naru
brown	chairo-i	chairo-kute	chairoku-naru
painful/sore	ita-i	ita-kute	itaku-naru
tired	daru-i	daru-kute	daruku-naru

(Watakushi wa) Kyō wa karada ga darukute, atama ga itakute, chōshi ga warui(n) desu.
My body feels tired, I have a headache, and I feel generally bad (*lit.*, I am in a bad condition) today.

Hentōsen ga itakute, nodo ga akakute, netsu ga arimasu.
My tonsils hurt, my throat is red, and I have a fever.

The verb **te**-form and adjective **te**-form can be joined in a single sentence.

Kinō kara seki ga dete, atama ga itakute, chōshi wa yoku-nai desu.
Since yesterday, I have not been feeling well and have a cough and a headache. (*lit.*, Since yesterday, I have coughing and a headache and not been in a good condition.)

7. The **te**-form + **iru no dewa naika(to) shinpai desu**

The **te**-form plus **iru no dewa naika(to) shinpai desu** means "I am worried about the risk of."

Zensoku o okoshite iru no dewa nai ka(to) shinpai desu.
I am worried about the risk of getting asthma.

Hai-gan ni natte iru no dewa nai ka(to) shinpai desu.
I am worried about the risk of getting lung cancer.

Rentogen no kekka kara, kekkaku ni natte inaika shinpai desu ka.
From the X-ray results, I am worried about the risk of a tuberculosis infection.

8. The adverbs **tashika-ni** and **toriaezu**

When you use adverbs to modify verbs, Japanese sentences come alive and sound natural. The adverbs **tashika-ni** (surely, certainly, definitely) and **toriaezu** (first of all; for the time being; anyway) are handy for healthcare professionals. Note that Japanese allows adverbs to be positioned at the beginning of the sentence or before the verb.

Kono shōjyō wa tashikani kikanshi-en desu ne.
This symptom is certainly bronchitis.

Toriaezu, sekidome o nonde kudasai.
Please take cough medicine for the time being.

9. The conjunction -ba

The conjunction **-ba** indicates that the preceding phrase expresses a provisional or conditional statement, or an if-statement, as in "If X, then Y." The conjunction is contained in the -r/eba provisional verb ending. To form the verb, first find the stem. (See Lesson 13 for the stem verb chart.) For a **u**-verb, drop the -**u** at the end and replace it with **e-ba**. For a **ru**-verb, drop -**u** from the stem verb and replace it with **e-ba**. Or, drop -**masu** from the **masu** form and replace it with -**reba**.

U-verbs

ENGLISH	MASU FORM	VERB BASE	STEM VERB	PROVISIONAL VERB
drink	nomi-masu	nomi(masu)	nomu	nome-ba
read	yomi-masu	yomi(masu)	yomu	yome-ba
go	iki-masu	iki(masu)	iku	ike-ba
speak	hanashi-masu	hanashi(masu)	hanasu	hanase-ba
cool down	hiyashi-masu	hiyashi(masu)	hiyasu	hiyase-ba
reach/arrive	todoki-masu	todoki(masu)	todoku	todoke-ba
continue	tsuzuki-masu	tsuzuki(masu)	tsuzuku	tsuzuke-ba

Ru-verbs

ENGLISH	MASU FORM	VERB BASE	STEM VERB	PROVISIONAL VERB
sleep	ne-masu	ne(masu)	ne-ru	ne-reba
eat	tabe-masu	tabe(masu)	tabe-ru	tebe-reba
warm up	atatame-masu	atatame(masu)	atatame-ru	atatame-reba
be visible/appear	araware-masu	araware(masu)	araware-ru	awaware-reba
inform/notify	shirase-masu	shirase(masu)	shirase-ru	shirase-reba
shiver	furue-masu	furue(masu)	furue-ru	furue-reba
go out/appear	de-masu	de(masu)	de-ru	de-reba
allow/make do	sase-masu	sase(masu)	sase-ru	sase-reba
apply/paint	nuri-masu	nuri(masu)	nu-ru	nu-reba
anger	okori-masu	okori(masu)	oko-ru	oko-reba
infect/transmit	utsuri-masu	utsuri(masu)	utsu-ru	utsu-reba
mix	majiri-masu	majiri(masu)	maji-ru	maji-reba
empty/die/use up	nakunari-masu	nakunari(masu)	nakuna-ru	nakuna-reba
choke	tsumari-masu	tsumari(masu)	tsuma-ru	tsuma-reba
see/look/examine	mi-masu	mi(masu)	mi-ru	mi-reba
wake up	oki-masu	oki(masu)	oki-ru	oki-reba
do/play	shi-masu	shi(masu)	su-ru*	su-reba
come	ki-masu	ki(masu)	ku-ru*	ku-reba

* Irregular

Kono kusuri o nomeba, suguni yoku nari masu.
If you take this medicine, you will get well soon.

Kono kensa o sureba, byōki no genin ga wakarimasu.
If you have this test done, you will know the cause of the illness.

Byōin ni ikeba, sensei ga chiryō shite kuremasu.
If you go to the hospital, the doctor will cure you.

Useful Expressions (CD 17-3)

Listen to the CD and repeat the sentences.

1. **Kekkaku no shoki shōjyō desu ne.** You have/are showing the early stage symptoms of tuberculosis.
2. **Taion-kei o shita no shita ni irete kudasai.** Please put the thermometer under your tongue.
3. **Kuchi o akete "Aā" to itte kudasai.** Please open your mouth and say, "Ah."
4. **Ima wa ii kusuri ga arimasu kara, nyūin shinaide ii desu yo.** There is good medicine now, so there is no need for you to be hospitalized.
5. **Kensa no kekka, tan no naka ni takusan kin ga dete imasu. Nyūin ga hitsuyō desu.** There are many germs in your sputum. You should remain in the hospital.
6. **Seki de nemure-nai koto ga arimasu ka.** Does coughing disturb your sleeping?
7. **Hentōsen ga harete iru yō desu.** I think your tonsils are swollen.
8. **Chi no majitta tan ga demasu ka.** Are you coughing up bloody phlegm?
9. **Iki o sū to, mune ga itami masu ka.** Do you have chest pain when you breathe?
10. **Nani-ka, kafun ni arerugī ga arimasu ka.** Do you have an allergy to any pollens?

Key Sentences (CD 17-4)

Listen to the CD and repeat the sentences.

1. **Toriaezu, ketsueki-kensa o shite, nyō-kensa mo shite mimasu.** For the time being, I would like to try a blood test and a urine test, too.
2. **Ototoi-kara yoku seki ga dete, atama mo itakute, chōshi ga yoku-nai(n) desu.** Since the day before yesterday, I haven't been feeling well, and I often have a cough and a headache, too.
3. **Tashikani, kesa-kara sukoshi age-ppoi(n) desu.** Since this morning, I have definitely felt a little nauseous.
4. **Tashikani, kekkaku no shōjyō no yōni seki ga dete imasu ne.** You are certainly coughing like it's tuberculosis.
5. **Toriaezu, hai-en ni natte inai ka kensa shite mimasu.** Anyway, I am trying to determine definitely whether it has become pneumonia or not.

Additional Words

tsumaru/tsumarimasu choke	**furueru/furuemasu** shiver
majiru/majirimasu mix	**ao-ppoi** bluish color
henka change	**sanso-nōdo** oxygen concentration
nisanka-nōdo carbon dioxide	**yō-tsū** lower backache
senaka no itami upper back pain	**hatsu netsu** onset of fever
mune no itami chest pain	**bi-netsu** slight fever
hei-netsu ordinary temperature	**kō-netsu** high temperature
fukai uncomfortable	**hentōsen** tonsil
rokkotsu rib	**nisanka-tanso** carbon dioxide
kokkaku-kin skeletal muscle	**hansha han-nō** reflex reaction
gaiki open air	**kyū-in** aspiration
kaikan pleasant feeling	**jiki** period/time
zentai whole	

Language Notes

1. There are many onomatopoetic expressions for chest pain.

Mune ga zei-zei shimasu.	My chest is wheezing.
Mune ga doki-doki shimasu.	My heart is beating furiously.
Mune ga zukin-zukin shimasu.	My chest is throbbing.
Mune ga chiku-chiku shimasu.	I have a prickly pain in my chest.
Mune ga muka-muka shimasu.	I feel like vomiting.

2. There are different expressions for certain stages of illness: **sho-ki** (early stage), **chū-ki** (middle stage), and **ma-kki** (late stage). For instance, **ma-kki** is used for cancer, as in **makki gan** (late stage cancer) and symptoms, **makki shōjyō** (a late stage symptom).

   Zensoku no shoki shōjyō desu.
   This is (you have) an early stage symptom of asthma.

   Kore wa kikanshi-en no chū-ki shōjyō desu.
   This is the middle stage symptom for bronchitis.

   Kono shōjyō wa hai-gan no makki shōjyō kamo shiremasen.
   This symptom is probably the late stage of lung cancer.

3. There are many expressions for allergies.

kafun arerugī	allergic to pollens, pollen allergy
sakana arerugī	allergic to fish, fish allergy
kusuri arerugī	drug allergy

miruku arerugī	allergic to milk, milk allergy, lactose intolerance
hausu dasuto arerugī	allergic to household dust
hokori arerugī	allergic to dust, dust allery
tamago arerugī	allergic to eggs, egg allergy
asupirin arerugī	allergic to aspirin, aspirin allergy
penishirin arerugī	allergic to penicillin, penicillin allergy
pīnattsu arerugī	allergic to peanuts, peanut allergy

4. In Lesson 8, we studied how the **te**-form can be repeated more than once in a sentence. By using **te**-form, many verbs and **i**-adjectives can be strung together so that multiple actions can be described in a single sentence.

Shatsu o agete, iki o sutte, tomete, haite kudasai.
Please roll up your shirt, inhale, hold (your breath), and exhale.

Ketsueki-kensa o shite, Rentogen o totte, sorekara, nyō o shirabete mimasu.
I would like to try a blood test, get a chest X-ray, and then test your urine.

The following chart shows the stem verbs and **te**-forms for several new verbs. See Lesson 7 for instructions on how to change to the **te**-form.

ENGLISH	MASU FORM	STEM VERB	TE-FORM
go out	de-masu	de-ru	de-te
roll up/vomit/give	age-masu	age-ru	age-te
inhale/smoke	sui-masu	su-u	su-tte
pierce/apply	sashi-masu	sa-su	sashi-te
unfasten/take off	hazushi-masu	hazu-su	hazushi-te
attach	tsuke-masu	tsuke-ru	tsuke-te
swell	hare-masu	hare-ru	hare-te
stop	tome-masu	tome-ru	tome-te
feel	kanji-masu	kanji-ru	kanji-te
put in/insert	ire-masu	ire-ru	ire-te
shiver/shake	furue-masu	furue-ru	furue-te
become	nari-masu	na-ru	na-tte
take	tori-masu	to-ru	to-tte
research	shirabe-masu	shirabe-ru	shirabe-te
continue	tsuzuki-masu	tsuzu-ku	tsuzu-ite
exhale/vomit	haki-masu	ha-ku	ha-ite
move	ugoki-masu	ugo-ku	ugo-ite
tear	saki-masu	sa-ku	sa-ite

Language Roots

The suffix **-gan** (癌) indicates cancer of the internal organs.

hai-gan	lung cancer
intō-gan	pharynx cancer
shokudō-gan	esophageal cancer

The suffix **-en** (炎) indicates an inflammatory disease and corresponds to the suffix *-itis*.

kikanshi-en	bronchitis
arerugī-sei bi-en	allergic rhinitis
hai-en	pneumonitis

Culture Notes

The Japanese social security system

The social security system in Japan consists of social welfare, social insurance, livelihood assistance, health, public sanitation, and unemployment insurance. The national health insurance system was begun in 1961, and it covers almost all Japanese. Public nursing care insurance was started in 2000. People qualified under this insurance plan can receive such services as nursing and rehabilitation at home and daycare or subsidized short stays at care facilities.

Health-related Japanese proverbs VII

Seeing is believing.
Hyaku-bun wa ikken ni shikazu.
百聞は一見にしかず

Moderation is the best physician.
Hara hachi-bun-me.
腹八分目

Comprehension

Answer the following questions.

1. Which of the following does NOT belong with the others?
   a. **Bi-netsu** b. **Ne-ase**
   c. **Gan** d. **Hatsu-netsu**

2. Which of the following could NOT be used to mean "chest sound"?
   a. **Mune ga zei-zei shimasu.**   b. **Mune ga gata-gata shimasu.**
   c. **Mune ga doki-doki shimasu.** d. **Mune ga chiku-chiku shimasu.**

3. Which of the following best completes the sentence below?
   Kinō kara yoku seki ga (   ), netsu ga atte chōshi ga warui desu.
   Since yesterday, I have been feeling poorly (*lit.*, I been in poor condition) and
   I have had a frequent cough and fever, too.
   a. **dete**   b. **kite**
   c. **akete**   d. **mite**

4. You are speaking to a patient who is having an X-ray done. How do you say,
   "Take a deep breath"?
   a. **Ōkiku iki o sutte**   b. **Ōkiku iki o haite**
   c. **Ōkiku iki o tomete**   d. **Ōkiku iki o dashite**

Select an appropriate meaning from the list below.

---

5. **Toriaezu, ketsueki-kensa to Rentogen kensa o shite mimasu.**   (   )
6. **Tashikani zensoku no shōjyō no yōni seki ga dete imasu.**   (   )
7. **Kesa kara yoku seki ga dete, netsu-pokute chōshi ga yoku nai desu.** (   )
8. **Tashikani, kinō kara sukoshi netsu-poi(n) desu.**   (   )
9. **Hai-gan ni natte inai ka kensa shite mimasu.**   (   )

a. I am trying to see whether it has become lung cancer or not.
b. Since yesterday, I have definitely felt a little feverish.
c. You are certainly coughing like it's asthma.
d. Since this morning, I have not been feeling well and have had a frequent
   cough and am feverish.
e. For the time being, I would like to try a blood test and have an X-ray done.

Practice

Respond to the following in Japanese using the cues that have been provided.

---

1. Giving instructions and informing the patient of the symptoms.
   (Patient)   (Healthcare professional)
   1. I have a fever.   _____

                                      (Put the thermometer under your tongue.)
   2. I have a sore throat.   _____

                                      (Open your mouth and say, "Ah.")

3. I have lung TB.

_____

(You need to be hospitalized.)

4. I have a cough.

_____

(Your tonsils are swollen.)

2. Telling the patient what kind of illness she or he has.

(Patient)   (Healthcare professional)

1. **Kakketsu shite imasu.** _____ (lung TB)

2. **Furuete imasu.** _____ (pneumonia)

3. **Kōnetsu ga arimasu.** _____ (bronchitis)

4. **Hentōsen ga harete imasu.** _____ (asthma)

3. Telling the patient about the progress of an illness.

(Patient)   (Healthcare professional)

1. **Byōki no shinkō wa dō desu ka.** _____

(early state)

2. **Watakushi no gan wa dono jiki desu ka.** _____

(middle stage)

3. **Hai-kekkaku no shōjyō wa dō desu ka.** _____

(late state)

4. How do you say the following symptoms in Japanese?

(Questions)   (Healthcare professional)

1. Prickly pain _____

2. Wheezing _____

3. Throbbing _____

4. Beating furiously _____

5. Dialogue comprehension. Based on the dialogue, answer the following questions.

1. **Itsu kara chōshi ga warui(n) desu ka.** _____

2. **Tanaka-san wa don-na shōjyō desu ka.** _____

3. **Tanaka-san wa doko ga itai(n) desu ka.** _____

4. **Don-na itami desu ka.** _____

5. **Don-na kensa o shimasu ka.** _____

6. Free response questions.

(Questions)   (Answers)

1. **Fumin-shō desu ka.** _____

2. **Yōtsū ni natta koto ga arimasu ka.** _____

3. **Byōin ni zensoku no kanjya ga imasu ka.** _____

4. **Hentō-sen ga harete imasu ka.** _____

5. **Kekkaku ni kakatta koto ga arimasu ka.** _____

Exercises

1. Say the following words in Japanese.
   A. Lung cancer   _____
   B. Pleurisy   _____
   C. Tuberculosis   _____
   D. Pneumonia   _____
   E. Bronchitis   _____

2. Say the following sentences in Japanese.
   A. For the time being, I would like to try a blood test.

   _____

   B. Since yesterday, I have not been feeling well and I often have a backache.

   _____

   C. You are certainly coughing like it's pleurisy.

   _____

   D. Since this morning, I have definitely had chills.

   _____

   E. I am definitely trying to examine whether it has become lung cancer or not.

   _____

3. In speaking to patients, how do you say the following in Japanese?
   A. Please open your mouth and say, "Ah."

   _____

   B. Please put in the thermometer under your tongue.

   _____

   C. I need to follow you closely for several days.

   _____

   D. Please roll up your shirt, and then inhale, hold, and exhale.

   _____

   E. There is good medicine now, so there is no need for you to be hospitalized.

   _____

Circulatory/Cardiovascular System
(Junkan-ki/Shinzō-kekkan-kei)

Basic Vocabulary (CD 18-1)

Listen to the CD and repeat the vocabulary.

#	English	Romaji	Japanese
1.	blood vessel	kekkan	血管
2.	artery	dō-myaku	動脈
3.	vein	jyō-mayku	静脈
4.	arrhythmia/irregular pulse	fusei-myaku	不整脈
5.	valvular/disease of the heart	shinzō-benmaku-shō	心臓弁膜症
6.	heart attack	shinzō-hossa	心臓発作
7.	enlarged heart	shinzō-hidai	心臓肥大
8.	arteriosclerosis/hardening of arteries	dōmyaku kōka-shō	動脈硬化症
9.	clogged arteries	dōmyaku-kessen	動脈血栓
10.	coronary artery disease	kan-dōmyaku-shukkan	冠動脈疾患
11.	acute myocardial infarction	kyūsei shinkin-kōsoku	急性心筋梗塞
12.	thrombosis	kessen-shō	血栓症
13.	embolism	sokusen-shō	塞栓症
14.	angina	kyōshin-shō	狭心症
15.	cardiomyopahty	shinkin-shō	心筋症
16.	acute pericarditis	kyūsei-shinmaku-en	急性心膜炎
17.	leukemia	hakketsu-byō	白血病
18.	hyperglycemia	kō-kettō	高血糖
19.	cerebral anemia	nō-hinketsu	脳貧血
20.	cerebral infarction	nō-kōsoku	脳梗塞
21.	meningitis	nōmaku-en	脳膜炎
22.	stroke	nō-socchū	脳卒中
23.	heartbeat	shinzō no kodō	心臓の鼓動
24.	brain hemorrhage/apoplexy	nō-shukketsu	脳出血
25.	cerebral thrombosis	nō-kkesen	脳血栓
26.	encephalitis	nō-en	脳炎
27.	cardiac/heart failure	shin-fuzen	心不全

28.	hemophilia	**ketsuyū-byō**	<ruby>血<rt>けつ</rt></ruby><ruby>友<rt>ゆう</rt></ruby><ruby>病<rt>びょう</rt></ruby>
29.	liver cirrhosis	**kankōhen**	<ruby>肝<rt>かん</rt></ruby><ruby>硬<rt>こう</rt></ruby><ruby>変<rt>へん</rt></ruby>
30.	hepatitis	**kan-en**	<ruby>肝<rt>かん</rt></ruby><ruby>炎<rt>えん</rt></ruby>

Dialogue (CD 18-2)

Listen to the CD and repeat the dialogue.

At the Primary Care Physician's Office

Dr. Simon: **Tanaka-san, kyō wa dō shita no (desu ka).**
Are you concerned about anything today, Mrs. Tanaka?

Mrs. Tanaka: **Saikin undō o suru to, dōki ga shimasu.**
When I exercise, I feel palpitations.

Dr. Simon: **Don-na shōjyō ga tsuzuite iru no (desu ka).**
What kind of symptoms do you have all the time?

Mrs. Tanaka: **Nandaka, tokidoki mune ga shimetsuke-rareru yōna kanji ga sū-fun tsuzuite, fukai-kan ga arimashita.**
I sometimes feel a sort of squeezing pain in my chest for a few minutes, and then discomfort.

Demo, kesa kara sugoku kibun ga waruku-nari, kokyū ga shi-nikui(n) desu.
However, since this morning I have felt really sick, and breathing is difficult.

Dr. Simon: **Suguni, shinden-zu to toroponin tesuto o shimashō ne.**
I am going to do an ECG and tropnin test immediately.

Ima, kango-shi ga sanso-masuku to tenteki no yōi o shimasu ne.
The nurse will prepare an oxygen mask and intravenous drip now.

Mrs. Tanaka: **Sensei, shinden-zu kensa no kekka wa dō desu ka.**
Doctor, what is the result of the ECG test?

Dr. Simon: **Shinzō-hossa no yō desu yo. Kyūsei shinkin-kōsoku ni chigai arimasen.**
It looks like a heart attack. I think there is no doubt you are having an acute myocardial infarction.

Mrs. Tanaka: **Eē, hontō desu ka. Korekara dō sureba ii(n) desu ka.**
Really? What should I do now?

Dr. Simon: **Hayaku nyū-in shite, shinzō senmon-i ni kuwashiku shin-satsu to chiryō o shite morai mashō.**
You need to be hospitalized immediately, and then let's check you out in detail and arrange for treatment by a specialist.

Shinzō-kekkan-keis (Cardiovascular System)

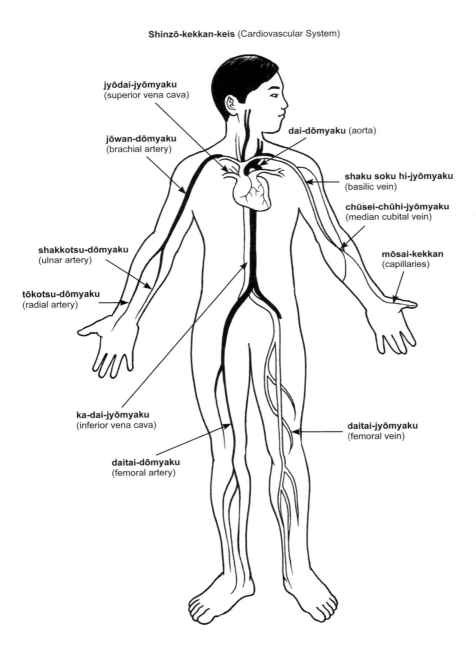

jyōdai-jyōmyaku
(superior vena cava)

jōwan-dōmyaku
(brachial artery)

dai-dōmyaku (aorta)

shaku soku hi-jyōmyaku
(basilic vein)

chūsei-chūhi-jyōmyaku
(median cubital vein)

shakkotsu-dōmyaku
(ulnar artery)

mōsai-kekkan
(capillaries)

tōkotsu-dōmyaku
(radial artery)

ka-dai-jyōmyaku
(inferior vena cava)

daitai-jyōmyaku
(femoral vein)

daitai-dōmyaku
(femoral artery)

Grammar

1. **The pattern** STEM VERB + SENTENCE-FINAL PARTICLE **no.**

    The stem verb plus the sentence-final particle **no** indicates a question. This is an abbreviation of **desu ka** and conveys a friendly feeling.

Kyō wa dō shita no (desu ka).	What is happening today?
Nani o shite iru no (desu ka).	What are you doing?
Dō shite iru no (desu ka).	How are you doing?

    The **i**-adjective and **na**-adjective can also use the sentence-final particle **no** for making a question.

Itai no (desu ka).	Do you have pain?
Kore wa kirei na no (desu ka).	Is this pretty?

    The question formed with the sentence-final particle **no** used to be considered a form for women or children but now is used by males, too.

2. **The pattern** STEM VERB + PARTICLE **to** for when- or if-clauses

    The stem verb and particle **to** can be used to form clauses beginning with "when" and "if." The particle **to** is a connective for two sentences. The first sentence should use the stem verb even if expressing past events and actions. The second sentence specifies tense and cannot be a request or command.

    Kanjya o miru to yōsu ga okashii (deshita).
    When I examined the patient, he looked like something was wrong (*lit.*, he was strange).

    Shisatsu o suru to tashika ni dōmyaku kōkashō deshita.
    When I examined her, she clearly had arteriosclerosis.

    Myaku o toru to shōjyō ga wakarimasu.
    If I take your pulse, I can/will be able to understand your symptom.

3. **The suffix -rare-ru or -rare-masu for the passive**

    The suffix -**rare-ru**/-**rare-masu** is the ending for the passive voice. In Japanese, the passive is used when someone or something is affected by an action or event or one cannot control an action or event oneself (which is a different understanding of the passive than in English). In the health fields, it often expresses the patient's point of view. In the following pairs of sentences, the second example illustrates this ending.

Kyō wa shinden-zu no kensa o shimashita.
I had an ECG test today.

Kyō wa shinden-zu no kensa o shuji-i kara sase-rare-mashita.
I was required to take an ECG test today by my primary care doctor.

Ima kensa no kekka o mise-mashita.
I showed the test result just now.

Ima kensa no kekka o mise-rare-mashita.
I was shown the test result just now.

Shinsatsu no toki ni, kanjya ni karorī-ryō o oshiemashita.
I taught the patient the proper amount of calories during consultation.

Watakushi wa karoii-ryō o oshie-rare-mashita.
I was taught the proper amount of calories by the doctor

Nani-ka mune o shimetsukemasu.
Something is squeezing/pressing my chest.

Mune ga shimetsuke-rareru yōna itami desu ka.
Do you have pain like squeezing (is happening) in your chest?

For verbs with stems ending in -**ru**, the passive ending is -**sase-raresu**, There are two rules for forming the passive in these verbs: 1) Drop the -**ru** suffix and replace it with -**sase-rareru**. 2) If the last syllable before -**masu** in the **masu** form is -**ri**, drop the -**ru** and replace it with -**ra**, then add -**sase-rareru**. The exceptions to this rule are the verbs for "do" (**shimasu**), "come" (**kimasu**), and "wake up" (**okimasu**).

Ru-verbs

ENGLISH	**MASU** FORM	VERB BASE	STEM VERB	-SASE-RARERU (PASSIVE)
sleep	**ne-masu**	**ne(masu)**	**ne-ru**	**ne-sase-rareru**
eat	**tabe-masu**	**tabe(masu)**	**tabe-ru**	**tebe-sase-rareru**
warm, warm up	**atatame-masu**	**atatame(masu)**	**atatame-ru**	**atatame-sase-rareru**
inform/notify	**shirase-masu**	**shirase(masu)**	**shirase-ru**	**shirase-sase-rareru**
shiver	**furue-masu**	**furue(masu)**	**furue-ru**	**furue-sase-rareru**
go out/ appear	**de-masu**	**de(masu)**	**de-ru**	**de-sase-rareru**

ENGLISH	**MASU** FORM	VERB BASE	STEM VERB	**-SASE-RARERU** (PASSIVE)
infect/ transmit	utsuri-masu	utsuri(masu)	utsu-ru	utsu-sase-rareru
see/look/ examine	mi-masu	mi(masu)	mi-ru	mi-sase-rareru
tighten	shime-masu	shime(masu)	shime-ru	shime-sase-rareru
open	ake-masu	ake(masu)	ake-ru	ake-sase-rareru
wear (clothes)	ki-masu	ki(masu)	ki-ru	ki-sase-rareru
feel	kanji-masu	kanji(masu)	kanji-ru	kanji-sase-rareru
become	nari- masu	nari(masu)	na-ru	na-ra-sase-rareru
apply/paint	nuri-masu	nuri(masu)	nu-ru	nu-ra-sase-rareru
mix	majiri-masu	majiri(masu)	maji-ru	maji-ra-sase-rareru
empty/die/ use up	nakunari-masu	nakunari(masu)	nakuna-ru	nakuna-ra-sase-rareru
choke	tsumari-masu	tsumari(masu)	tsuma-ru	tsuma-ra-sase-rareru
measure	hakari-masu	hakari(masu)	haka-ru	haka-ra-sase-rareru
begin/start	hajime-masu	hajime(masu)	hajime-ru	hajime-sase-rareru
stop/end	yame-masu	yame(masu)	yame-ru	yame-sase-rareru
wake up*	oki-masu	oki(masu)	oki-ru	oko-sase-rareru
do/play*	shi-masu	shi(masu)	su-ru	shi-sase-rareru
come*	ki-masu	ki(masu)	ku-ru	ko-sase-rareru

* Irregular

For **u**-verbs, if the stem verb ends with -**u**, change the -**u** to -**a**, then add -**se-rareru**. If the stem verb ends with **u** preceded by a vowel, drop the -**u** and add **wa**, then add -**se-rareru**.

U-verbs

ENGLISH	**MASU** FORM	VERB BASE	STEM VERB	-SE-RARERU (PASSIVE)
drink	nomi-masu	nomi(masu)	nomu	noma-se-rareru
read	yomi-masu	yomi(masu)	yomu	yoma-se-rareru
go	iki-masu	iki (masu)	iku	ika-se-rareru
listen	kiki-masu	kiki(masu)	kiku	kika-se-rareru
smell/sniff	kagi-masu	kagi(masu)	kagu	kaga-se-rareru
rub	momi-masu	momi(masu)	momu	moma-se-rareru
speak	hanashi-masu	hanashi(masu)	hanasu	hanasa-se-rareru
pull down	oroshi-masu	oroshi(masu)	orosu	orosa-se-rareru
cool, cool off	hiyashi-masu	hiyashi(masu)	hiyasu	hiyasa-se-rareru
send out/ prescribe	dashi-masu	dashi(masu)	dasu	dasa-se-rareru
reach/arrive	todoki-masu	todoki(masu)	todoku	todoka-se-rareru
throw up	hakidashi-masu	hakidashi(masu)	haki-dasu	hakidasa-se-rareru
try	tameshi-masu	tameshi(masu)	tamesu	tamesa-se-rareru
vomit	haki-masu	haki(masu)	ha-ku	haka-se-rareru
stretch	nobashi-masu	nobashi(masu)	nobasu	nobasa-se-rareru
wait	machi-masu	machi(masu)	matsu	mata-se-rareru
stand up	tachi-masu	tachi(masu)	tatsu	tata-se-rareru
buy	kai-masu	kai(masu)	ka-u	kawa-se-rareru
say	ii-masu	ii(masu)	i-u	iwa-se-rareru
follow/obey	shitagai-masu	shitagai(masu)	shitaga-u	shitagawa-se-rareru
inhale/ smoke	sui-masu	sui(masu)	su-u	suwa-se-rareru

4. The i-ADJECTIVE + **ku-narimasu** in conjoined sentences

In Lesson 17, we studied the construction i-ADJECTIVE plus **ku-naru** (meaning "become, turn"). When a sentence ending in **ku-naru** is connected to another sentence, **ku-naru** changes to **ku-nari**.

Mune ga itaku-nari, kibun ga waruku narimashita.
I had chest pain and began to feel (*lit.*, became feeling) bad.

Kao ga shiroku-nari, hinketsu o okoshimashita.
My face turned white, and I became sluggish/began to feel sluggish.

Tōbun ga takaku-nari, ketsuatsu ga agarimashita.
My blood sugar level became high, and my blood pressure rose.

5. The construction VERB BASE + -**yasui(n)** or -**nikui(n)**

Yasui means "easy to do," and **nikui** means "difficult to do." When attached to a verb base, the suffix -**nikui(n)** expresses the difficulty of an action. Similarly, the construction VERB BASE plus -**yasui** (easy) expresses the ease of an action. For example, **naori-yasui** (easy to recover/heal); **naori-nikui** (difficult to recover/heal); **nomi-yasui** (easy to swallow); **nomi-nikui** (difficult to swallow). If the subject is under focus, the subject particle **ga** is used.

Shinfuzen wa kensa shi-nikui(n) desu.
It's difficult to diagnose cardiac failure.

Byōin-shoku wa tabe-nikui(n) desu.
Hospital meals are difficult to eat.

Kono kona-gusuri wa choto nomi-nikui(n) desu.
This powdered medication is difficult to drink.

Kono shinden-zu wa yomi-nikui(n) desu.
This ECG is difficult to read.

Jyō-zai no kusuri wa nomi-yasui desu ka.
Is it easy to take a tablet?

Kensa ga shi-yasui desu.
The test is easy to perform.

Moji ga yomi-nikui desu.
The letter is difficult to read.

6. The pattern **te**-form + SUFFIX **morau**

The **te**-form plus the suffix **morau** expresses the notion of receiving some benefit from someone's action or getting someone to do something for your sake. The present/future tense is **te-moraimasu**, and past tense is **te-moraimashita.**

Watakushi wa sensei ni kusuri o dashite moraimasu.
I will have my doctor prescribe some medicine for me.

Kanjya wa kango-shi ni ketusatsu o hakatte moraimashita.
The patient had the nurse take his/her blood pressure.

Anata wa senmon-i ni shinsatsu to chiryō o shite moratte kudasai.
Please have a heart specialist examine and treat you.

The **te**-form plus the suffix **itadaku** is the polite form.

Watakushi wa sensei ni shinsatus o shite-itadakimasu.
I will have my doctor examine me. (polite)

7. The question **dō sureba ii(n) desu ka** means "What shall I do?"

In Lesson 17, we studied the provisional or if-statement suffix -**ba**. The idiom **dō sureba ii(n) desu ka** is used to ask what to do to resolve some question, matter, or problem in connection with a conditional statement using **no toki wa** (when) or **no baai wa** (in case/in case of).

Kusuri o nomu toki wa dō sureba ii(n) desu ka.
To take the medicine, what do I to do? (*lit.*, When I take the medicine, what shall I do?)

Shinzō ga doki-doki suru baai wa dō sureba i(n) desu ka.
In case of rapid heartbeat, what should I do?

Teiketsu-atsu no toki wa dō sureba ii(n) desu ka.
When/if I have low blood pressure, what should I do?

Dō sureba ii ka wakarimasen.
I am at loss as to what to do.

Dō sureba hinketsu ga yoku naru no deshō ka.
What should I do in order to treat anemia?

Dō sureba kyōshin-shō ga naoseru-noka oshiete kudasai.
Please tell me how I can get well from angina.

8. The construction INTERROGATIVE + -**daka**

The construction INTERROGATIVE plus -**daka** expresses the notion of "some" in connection with the meaning of the interrogative. For example, **nan-daka** means "somewhat, somehow, sort of"; **doko-daka** "somewhere"; **itsu-daka** "sometime ago"; **dō-daka** "somehow, wondering"; and **dare-daka** "someone, someone else."

Nan-daka kimochi ga warui(n) desu.
I feel sort of sick.

Itsu-daka, dōki ga shimasita.
Sometime ago, I had palpitations.

Dare-daka, shnzō no ishoku o shimashita.
Someone else did the heart transplant.

9. **Changing the i-adjective to an adverb: kuwashiku and sugoku**

Adverbs modify verbs, and when you use adverbs in Japanese sentences, the sentences become lively and more natural. To change i-adjectives to adverbs, drop the suffix -i, and replace it with -ku.

ENGLISH	I-ADJECTIVES	ADVERBS
detailed	**kuwashi-i**	**kuwashi-ku**
awful/difficult	**sugo-i**	**sugo-ku**
remarkable/notable	**ichijirushi-i**	**ichijirushi-ku**

(Anata no) fusei-myaku o kuwashi-ku shirabete mimashō.
Let's take a close look at your arrhythmia.

Hakketsu-byō wa sugoku muzukashi-i byōki desu.
Leukemia is a very difficult disease to treat.

Kankōhen no kanjya no yōtai wa ichijirushi-ku warui yō desu.
The patient with cirrhosis of the liver seems in remarkably bad condition.

Useful Expressions (CD 18-3)

Listen to the CD and repeat the sentences.

1. **Shinzō-hossa o okoshita koto ga arimasu ka.** Have you ever had a heart attack?
2. **Kokyū ga shi-nikui desu ka.** Do you have difficulty breathing?
3. **Sugoku iki-gire ga shimasu ka.** Do you have extreme shortness of breath?
4. **Dōki ga hageshiku-naru koto ga arimasu ka.** Does your heart start beating very rapidly?
5. **Osake wa donokuri nomi masu ka?** How much alcohol do you drink?
6. **Itami wa asupirin de hayaku herasu koto ga dekimasu.** The pain can be reduced quickly with aspirin.
7. **Tabako to osake wa karada ni yokunai node, yameta hō ga ii desu yo.** It's better for your health to give up smoking and drinking.
8. **Yoku memai ga shimasu ka.** Do you have frequent dizzy spells?
9. **Nō-socchu no yobō niwa seikatsu yōshiki no kaizen ga hitsuyō desu yo.** You need to change your lifestyle in order to reduce your risk of stroke.

10. **Enbun sesshu to karorī-ryō o herasu koto ga taisetsu desu.** It is important for you to reduce your salt and calorie intake.

Key Sentences (CD 18-4)

Listen to the CD and repeat the sentences.

1. **Kensa o suru to kankōhen deshita.** When I examined her, she had cirrhosis of the liver.
2. **Mune-yake-sase-rareru yōna kibun desu.** I have a feeling like heartburn.
3. **Ketsuyū-byō wa kensa shinikui(n) desu.** It's difficult to diagnose hemophilia.
4. **Kanjya wa sensei ni fusei-myaku o mite moraimashita.** The patient had the doctor check his irregular pulse.
5. **Nōhinketsu no toki wa dō sureba ii(n) desu ka.** If I have cerebral anemia, what should I do?

Additional Words

Toroponin Tesuto Troponin Test
fuyasu increase
hajimeru/hajimemasu begin/start
en-bun sodium
kō-shibō-shoku high-fat diet
fukai-kan discomfort
hageshii intense/violently
tetsu-bun iron
taisetsu important/valuable
shinzō-ishoku heart transplant
dō-myaku-ryū aneurysm
shinzō-zensoku cardiac asthma
kō-ketsuatsu hypertension/high blood pressure
tei-ketsuatsu hypotension/low blood pressure
kakuchō-gata shinkin-shō dilated cardiomyopathy
hidai-gata shinkin-shō hypertrophic cardiomyopathy
kōsoku-gata shinkin-shō restrictive cardiomyopathy
shinzō massāji cardiac massage/heart massage

herasu decrease
yameru/yamamasu end/stop/quit
ikigire shortness of breath
tō-bun sugar
kō-seni-shoku high-fiber diet
moji letters/characters
hayaku fast
sesshu intake
nai-shukketsu internal bleeding
jō-mayku-ryū varix
jyū-ketsu/ukketsu congestion

Language Notes

1. The suffix **-kan** indicates feeling and sense.

   fukai-kan   unpleasant feeling, discomfort
   sōkai-kan   refreshed feeling, exhilarating felling

datsuryoku-kan	weakness
fuan-(kan)	anxiety, anxious feeling, insecurity
anshin-kan	peace of mind, sense of security, safe feeling
kaku-yasu kan	like feeling cheap

Shinzō ni fukai-kan ga arimasu.
I feel discomfort in my heart.

Karada ni datsuryoku-kan ga arimasu ka.
Do you have a feeling of lassitude all over (your body)?

2. The following expressions are used in asking about heart pain.

Shinzō ga itai(n) desu ka.
Do you have heart pain?

Shinzō ga doki-doki shimasu ka.
Is your heart racing?

Shinzō ga chiku-chiku shimasu ka.
Do you have a prickly pain in your chest?

Shinzō ga shimetsuke-rarete imasu ka.
Do you have a squeezing pain in your chest?

Shinzō ga appaku sarete imasu ka.
Do you have a pressing pain in your chest?

Shinzō ga zuki-zuki shimasu ka.
Do you have a throbbing pain in your chest?

3. Japanese has no distinction between dizziness and vertigo and only one word for them, which is **memai**. However, **kaiten-sei no memai** can be used to specify vertigo, and **hi-kaiten-sei no memai** can specify dizziness. **Kaiten** means "turning"; **hi-kaiten** is "non-turning."

4. There are many other expressions regarding dizziness:

Memai ga shite, ki o ushinai mashita.
I feel dizzy and faint.

Myaku ga hayaku nari, memai ga shimashita.
I had a rapid heartbeat and (feel) dizziness.

Memai ga shite, muka-muka to modoshi sō desu.
I feel dizzy and nauseous.

Kurikaeshi memai ga shite, miminari ga shite, nanchō ga airmashita.
I had recurrent attacks of dizziness, tinnitus, and decreased hearing.

5. Japanese has many expressions for vomiting (**ōto/modosu**) and nausea (**ha-kike**).

gero o haku	throw up
hedo o haku	vomit
tabeta mono o ōto suru	vomit the food ingested (refined expression)
tabeta mono o hakidasu	spit out the food eaten
tabeta mono o modosu	spit up /return the food eaten
tabeta mono ga komiageru	nauseous from the food
tabeta mono ni hakike o moyōsu	feel nausea from the food I ate

Language Roots

Shin (心) indicates the heart and corresponds to the prefix *cardio-*.

shin-zō-byō	heart diseases
shin-fuzen	cardiac failure
shin-zō hossa	heart attack
shin-zō kekkan-shō	cardiovascular disease

Shō (症) indicates illness and corresponds to the suffix *-sis*.

kafun-shō	pollen allergy
en-shō	inflammation
jyū-shō	serious illness/wound/injury
kei-shō	minor injury
shō-jyō	symptom
kessen-shō	thrombosis

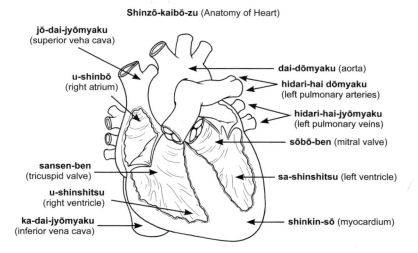

Shinzō-kaibō-zu (Anatomy of Heart)

jō-dai-jyōmyaku (superior veha cava)

u-shinbō (right atrium)

sansen-ben (tricuspid valve)

u-shinshitsu (right ventricle)

ka-dai-jyōmyaku (inferior vena cava)

dai-dōmyaku (aorta)

hidari-hai dōmyaku (left pulmonary arteries)

hidari-hai-jyōmyaku (left pulmonary veins)

sōbō-ben (mitral valve)

sa-shinshitsu (left ventricle)

shinkin-sō (myocardium)

Culture Notes

Location of heart and mind in Japanese culture

Japanese makes no distinction between heart and mind and uses the word **koko-ro** for both. Traditionally, Japanese believe that both the heart and the mind are located in the chest in the human body. In contrast, Western culture recognizes that the heart is located in the chest, while the mind is associated with the brain. Japanese also uses the word **kokoro** for "spirit." In Japanese culture, the organ called **kokoro** that unites the heart, mind, and spirit in the chest is the most important part of the body.

Health-related Japanese proverbs VIII

Learn much and play much.
Yoku asobi, yoku manabe.
よく学びよく遊べ

In the coffin, all men are equal.
Meido no michi wa ō mo nashi.
冥土の道は王もなし

Comprehension

Answer the following questions.

1. Which of the following does NOT belong with the others?
   a. **Hinketsu**   b. **Dōki**
   c. **Haketsu-byō**   d. **Fusei-myaku**

2. Which of the following could NOT be used to say "vomiting?"
   a. **Hedo o haku**   b. **Tabemono o modosu**
   c. **Gero o haku**   d. **Kutsu o haku**

3. Which of the following best completes the sentence below?
   Watakushi wa sensei (   ) shinsatsu o shte itadaki tai desu.
   I would like my doctor to examine me.
   a. **o**   b. **ni**
   c. **to**   d. **wa**

4. You are asking a patient what kind of chest pain he or she has. How do you say "prickly pain?"
   a. **muka-muka**   b. **chiku-chiku**
   c. **doki-doki**   d. **jin-jin**

Select an appropriate meaning from the list below.

5. **Kessen-shō wa kensa shinikui(n) desu.** ( )
6. **Shinzō-hossa sase rareru yōna kibun desu.** ( )
7. **Shinzō-benmaku-shō no toki wa dō sureba ii(n) desu ka.** ( )
8. **Kensa o suru to kyūsei shinkin-kōsoku deshita.** ( )
9. **Kanjya wa sensei ni kō-ketsuatsu o mite morai-mashita.** ( )

a. When I examined him, he had an acute myocardial infarction.
b. I have a feeling like a heart attack
c. It's difficult to diagnose thrombosis.
d. The patient had the doctor check her high blood pressure.
e. If I have valve disease, what should I do?

Practice

Respond to the following in Japanese using the cues that have been provided.

1. Recognizing and characterizing a patient's state.
   (Patient)   (Healthcare professional)
   1. Discomfort   _____
   2. Refreshed feeling   _____
   3. Languid feeling   _____
   4. Anxiousness   _____
   5. A safe feeling   _____

2. Asking the patient about earlier symptoms.
   (Patient's condition)   (Healthcare professional)
   1. **Shinzō ga itai(n) desu.**   _____
   2. **Ikigire ga shimasu.**   _____
   3. **Kokyū ga shi-nikui desu.**   _____
   4. **Memai ga shimasu.**   _____
   5. **Shinzō ga doki-doki shimasu.** _____
   6. **Shinzō ga shimetsuke-rarete imasu.** _____
   7. **Shinzō ga chiku-chiku shimasu.** _____

3. Giving the patient some suggestions.
   (Patient's situation)   (Healthcare professional)
   1. **Enbun ga takusan desu.**   _____
   2. **Amai-mono o takusan tabemasu.** _____
   3. **Osake o takusan nomimasu.**   _____

4. **Undō o shimasen.**　　　　　　　　　　_____

5. **(O)niku o takusan tabemasu.**　　　_____

4. Dialogue comprehension. Based on the dialogue, answer the following questions.

1. **Tanaka-san no shōjyō wa nan desu ka.**

_____

2. **Kesa kara Tanaka-san wa doko ga itai(n) desu ka.**

_____

3. **Shimon-sensei wa don-na kensa o shimashita ka.**

_____

4. **Tanaka-san no byōmei wa nan desu ka.**

_____

5. **Tanaka-san wa nani ga hitsuyō desu ka.**

_____

5. Free response questions.

(Questions)　　　　　　　　　　　　　　　(Answers)

1. **Chikagoro, dōki ga shimasu ka.**　　_____

2. **Hinketsu-gimi desu ka.**　　　　　　_____

3. **Ketsu-atsu wa dō desu ka.**　　　　_____

4. **Saikin, shinzō ga itaku narimasu ka.**　_____

5. **Saikin, sinzō no kensa o saserare-mashita ka.**　_____

Exercises

1. Say the following words in Japanese.

A. Cirrhosis of the liver　　　　　　_____

B. Arrhythmia/irregular pulse　　　_____

C. Stroke　　　　　　　　　　　　_____

D. Cardiac failure　　　　　　　　_____

E. Angina　　　　　　　　　　　　_____

2. Say the following sentences in Japanese.

A. It's difficult to cure leukemia.　　_____

B. The patient had the doctor check her for internal bleeding.　_____

C. When I examined him, he had pulmonary tuberculosis.　_____

D. If I think I have a thrombosis, what should I do?　_____

E. I have a feeling like anemia.　　_____

3. How do you ask patients the following questions in Japanese?
    A. Do you have frequent spells of dizziness?   _____
    B. Are you having a heart attack?   _____
    C. Do you have a squeezing pain in your chest?   _____
    D. Does your heart start beating very rapidly?   _____
    E. How much alcohol do you drink?   _____

4. Answer the following questions in Japanese.
    Q: **Sumimasen, dō sureba hinketsu ga yoku naru deshō ka.**
    A: _____
    (Please eat foods high in iron.)

    Q: **Kono shinden-zu wa yomi-nikui(n) desu.**
    B: _____
    (No, it's easy to read.)

    Q: **Nō-socchū no yobō wa dō sureba ii(n) desu ka.**
    C: _____
    (You need to change your lifestyle in order to reduce your risk of stroke.)

Digestive/Gastrointestinal System
(Shōkaki-ka/Ichō-ka-kei)

Basic Vocabulary (CD 19-1)

Listen to the CD and repeat the vocabulary.

1.	piles/hemorrhoids	ji	痔
2.	ultrasound test	chō-onpa-kensa	超音波検査
3.	stomach acid	i-san	胃酸
4.	digestive enzymes	shōka-kōso	消化酵素
5.	gastroptosis	i-kasui	胃下垂
6.	gastritis	i-en	胃炎
7.	nonulcer dyspepsia	shinkeisi-i-en	神経性胃炎
8.	gastrospasm/stomach cramps	i- keiren	胃痙攣
9.	gastritis ulcer/stomach ulcer	i-kaiyō	胃潰瘍
10.	hyperacidity	i-san-kata-shō	胃酸過多症
11.	stomach cancer	i-gan	胃癌
12.	gastroesophageal reflux disease	i-shokudō-gyakuryū-shō	胃食道逆流症
13.	duodenitis	jyūnishichō-en	十二指腸炎
14.	duodenitis ulcer	jyūnishichō-kaiyō	十二指腸潰瘍
15.	enteritis	chō-en	腸炎
16.	intestinal catarrh	chō-kataru	腸カタル
17.	intestinal TB	chō-kekkaku	腸結核
18.	volvulus	chō-nenten	腸捻転
19.	appendicitis	chūsui-en	虫垂炎
20.	colitis	daichō-en	大腸炎
21.	cirrhosis of the liver	kankō-hen	肝硬変
22.	gallstones	tan-seki	胆石
23.	cholelithiasis	tan-seki-shō	胆石症
24.	cholesystitis	tannō-en	胆嚢炎
25.	laparoscopic surgery	fuku-kōkyō-shujyutsu	腹腔鏡手術
26.	anal fistula	jirō	痔瘻
27.	bowel movement disorder	ben-tsū shōgai	便通障害
28.	food poisoning	shoku-chūdoku	食中毒
29.	mucous membrane	nen-maku	粘膜
30.	parasite	kiseichū	寄生虫

Shōkaki-ka/Ichō-ka Kei (Digestive/Gastrointestinal System)

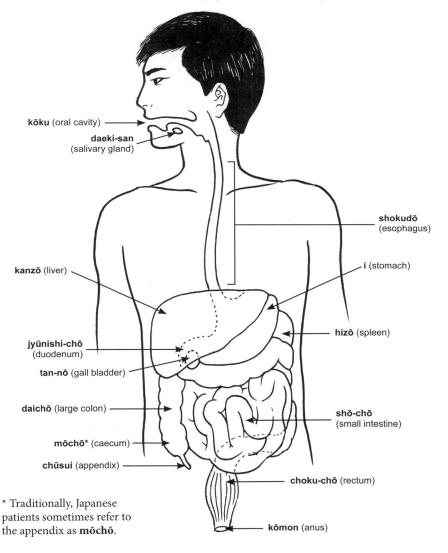

kōku (oral cavity)

daeki-san
(salivary gland)

shokudō
(esophagus)

kanzō (liver)

i (stomach)

hizō (spleen)

jyūnishi-chō
(duodenum)

tan-nō (gall bladder)

daichō (large colon)

shō-chō
(small intestine)

mōchō* (caecum)

chūsui (appendix)

choku-chō (rectum)

* Traditionally, Japanese
patients sometimes refer to
the appendix as **mōchō**.

kōmon (anus)

Dialogue (CD 19-2)

Listen to the CD and repeat the dialogue.

At the Primary Care Physician's Office

Dr. Diab (female doctor): **Satō-san, kyō wa dō shimashita ka.**
Do you have any complaints, Mr. Satō?

Mr. Satō: **Kinō kara onaka ga itakute itakute.**
I have had a stomachache since yesterday.

Shoku-yoku ga nakute, ugoku to (onaka ga) itai(n) desu.
I don't have an appetite, and it (my stomach) hurts when I move.

Dr Diab: **Kesa no guai wa ikaga deshita ka.**
How were you feeling this morning?

Kinō yori yoku-natte imasu ka. Soretomo, waruku-natte imasu ka.
Is it getting better or worse?

Mr. Satō: **Chotto, hakkiri shimasen.**
Well, I'm not sure.

Aruitari, seki o suru to (onaka ni) hibiite itai(n) desu.
It (my stomach) hurts whenever I walk or cough.

Dr. Diab: **Soredewa, onaka o shinsatsu shimasu.**
Then I would like to check your stomach.

Uwagi o nuide, beddo no ue ni aomuke ni natte kudasai.
Could you take off your shirt, and please lie down on this bed with your face up?

Koko o osu-to itami ga arimasu ka.
Does it hurt when I push here?

Mr. Satō: **Hai, sukoshi itai(n) desu.**
Yes, it hurts a little.

Dr. Diab: **Dewa, ashi o magete, onaka no chikara o nuite, yukkuri shinkokyū o shite (kudasai).**
Well then, could you bend your knees, relax your stomach, and breathe in and out slowly and deeply.

Dewa, onaka kara kyū ni te o hanasu to itami ga aru-ka oshiete kudasai.
Could you tell me if it hurts when I release my hand quickly from your stomach?

Soko wa dō desu ka. Koko wa dō desu ka.
Is there pain there? Is there pain here?

Mr. Satō: **Itai, itai. Te o hanasu to, soko wa itaku-nakute, koko ga sugoku itami-masu.**
Ouch. It hurts. It's not painful there but very painful here when you release your hand.

Koko o osae-rareru to, onaka zentai ga itakute itakute, haki-sō ni narimasu.
If you push here, my whole abdomen hurts. I feel like I'm going to vomit.

Dr. Diab: **Dōmo, kore wa ikasui dewa nakute, kyūsei chūsui-en no yō desu.**
It looks like you don't have gastroptosis but acute appendicitis.

Suguni, kensa ga hitsuyō desu ne.
You need some tests immediately.

Saiketsu, ken-nyō, fukubu ekō to fukubu CT nado no kensa o shimasu.
We'll test your blood, and do a urinalysis, ultrasound, and a CT scan of your stomach.

Kensa wa sorehodo tsurakuwa arimasen. Sugu ni owarimasu yo.
These tests aren't too painful. They can be done quickly.

Grammar

1. Sentences ending with -te

Sentences ending with **-te** are used to express requests, instructions, and commands. Note that the verb **kudasai** that would normally appear at the end of the sentence has been dropped.

Kochira ni kite (kudasai).	Come here.
Kono kusuri o nonde (kudasai).	Take this medicine.
Hiza o magete (kudasai).	Bend your knees.

The following are more **te**-forms. For a reminder about how to make the **te**-form, see Lesson 12.

ENGLISH	MASU FORM	STEM FORM	TE-FORM
numb	shibire-masu	shibire-ru	shibire-te
bend	mage-masu	mage-ru	mage-te
hold	osae-masu	osae-ru	osae-te
shiver	furue-masu	furue-ru	furue-te
be visible/appear	araware-masu	araware-ru	araware-te
begin/start	hajime-masu	hajime-ru	hajime-te
end/stop/quit	yame-masu	yame-ru	yame-te
feel	kanji-masu	kanji-ru	kanji-te

ENGLISH	MASU FORM	STEM FORM	TE-FORM
build up/collect/save	tamari-masu	tama-ru	tama-tte
infect/transfer	utsuri-masu	utsu-ru	utsu-tte
anger/be angry	okori-masu	oko-ru	oko-tte
work well/be effective	kiki-masu	ki-ku	ki-ite
move	ugoki-masu	ugo-ku	ugo-ite
walk	aruki-masu	aru-ku	aru-ite
release/pull out	nuki-masu	nu-ku	nu-ite
shake/vibrate	hibiki-masu	hibi-ku	hibi-ite
walk	aruki-masu	aru-ku	aru-ite
undress	nugi-masu	nu-gu	nu-ide
bite	kami-masu	ka-mu	ka-nde

2. The expression **no guai wa ikaga desu ka**

The expression **no guai wa ikaga desu ka** is a polite way to ask about the patient's medical condition.

I no guai wa ikaga desu ka. How is your stomach? (polite)
I no guai wa dō desu ka. How is your stomach?

Ji no guai wa ikaga desu ka. How is your hemorrhoid? (polite)
Ji no guai wa dō desu ka. How is your hemorrhoid?

I-san-kata-shō no guai wa ikaga desu ka.
How is your hyperacidity? (polite)

I-san-kata-shō no guai wa dō desu ka.
How is your hyperacidity?

3. The particle **yori** as a comparative marker

The particle **yori** is used to indicate a subject or object that is being compared with another subject or object.

Mae no kensa kekka yori, kyō no kensa kekka no hō ga yokunatte imasu.
This test result shows improvement over the last one (*lit.*, Today's test result becomes better than the previous test result).

Sutēki yori (o)sakana no hō ga suki desu ka.
Do you like steak more than fish?

Ikaiyō wa i-en yori itai(n) desu.
A gastric ulcer is more painful than gastritis.

Sono kensa wa omotta yori itakuwa arimasen deshia.
The test was not as painful as I thought.

4. The expression **ka oshiete kudasai**

The expression **ka oshiete kudasai** means "Could you tell me if/whether?" and can be used with nouns, adjectives, and stem verbs.

Onaka no itami wa tannō-en ka oshiete kudasai.
Could you tell me if my stomach pain is cholesystitis?

Kono kusuri wa nigai ka amai ka oshiete kudasai.
Could you tell me whether this medicine is bitter or sweet?

Tanseki-shō ga aru ka oshiete kudasai.
Could you tell me whether I have cholelithiasis or not?

5. The negative **te**-form of i-adjectives is **ku(wa)-nakute** (not X but Y).

In Lesson 17, we studied how to change i-adjectives to the **te**-form by dropping the -i ending and replacing it with **-kute**. In Lesson 8, we saw that the **te**-form can be used to link two or more statements in one sentence, as in the following examples:

Onaka ga ita-kute kurushii desu.
I have stomach pain and am suffering.

I ga ita-kute, mune ga kurushi-kute, karada ga darui(n) desu.
I have stomach pain, chest pain, and my body feels tired.

To make the negative **te**-form of i-adjectives, drop the -i and replace it with **-ku(wa)-nakute**. This negative form can be translated as "not X but Y."

Onaka wa ita-ku-nakute, kayui(n) desu.
My stomach doesn't hurt, but it does itch.

Atama wa kayu-ku-nakute, itai(n) desu.
My head doesn't itch, but it hurts.

I wa kurushi-ku-nakute, itai(n) desu.
My stomach isn't upset but painful.

The following chart shows a list of i-adjectives, the **te**-form with **-kute**, and the negative **te**-form of the adjectives.

ENGLISH	ADJECTIVE/ DROP -I	REPLACE WITH -KUTE	NEGATIVE TE-FORM (-NAKUTE)
good	yo-i/ii	yo-kute	yo-ku-nakute
bad	waru-i	waru-kute	waru-ku-nakute
painful/sore	ita-i	ita-kute	ita-ku-nakute
suffering	kurushi-i	kurushi-kute	kurushi-ku-nakute
itchy	kayu-i	kayu-kute	kayu-ku-nakute
tired/listless	daru-i	daru-kute	daru-ku-nakute
ticklish	kusuguta-i	kusuguta-kute	kusuguta-ku-nakute
hot	atsu-i	atsu-kute	atsu-ku-nakute
cold (weather/ feeling)	samu-i	samu-kute	samu-ku-nakute
cold (touch/ body temp)	tsumeta-i	tsumeta-kute	tsumeta-ku-nakute
happy	ureshi-i	ureshi-kute	ureshi-ku-nakute
interesting	omoshiro-i	omoshiro-kute	omoshiro-ku-nakute
wonderful	subarashi-i	subarashi-kute	subarashi-ku-nakute
lonely	sabishi-i	sabishi-kute	sabishi-ku-nakute
sad	kanashi-i	kanashi-kute	kanashi-ku-nakute
scary	kowa-i	kowa-kute	kowa-ku-nakute
envious	urayamashi-i	urayamashi-kute	urayamashi-ku-nakute

6. The construction VERB BASE + sō ni narimasu

The construction VERB BASE plus **sō ni narimasu** means "I feel like I am going to (do something); I feel like doing (something)."

> **Haki sō ni narimasu.**
> I feel like I'm going to vomit.

> **I-san-kata-shō wa kowai desu ga, osake o nomi sō ni narimasu.**
> I feel like drinking alcohol even if I am afraid of hyperacidity.

> **Jirō wa kowai desu ga, karai-mono o tabe sō ni narimasu.**
> I feel like eating hot foods even though I have an anal fistula.

> **Osake o nomi sō ni narimasu ka.**
> Do you feel like you're going to drink alcohol?

7. **The negative te-form of nouns ends in dewa naku(te).**

To make the negative **te**-form of nouns, add **dewa nakute**. This negative form links nouns in statements of the form "not X but Y." In negative sentences, the **-te** in the ending can be dropped for more concise expression.

> **Byōmei wa i-en dewa naku(te), chō-en desu yo.**
> The name of your illness is not gastritis but enteritis.

> **Shōjyō wa i-kaiyō dewa naku(te), i-san-kata-shō no yō desu.**
> Your symptoms don't look like gastritis but hyperacidity.

> **Chō-en no genin wa kiseichū dewa naku(te) pirori-kin deshita.**
> The cause of the enteritis was not a parasite but Helicobacter pylori.

8. **The polite form of the negative i-adjective is kuwa arimasen.**

In Lesson 5, we studied the negative form of the i-adjective, **-kunai (desu)**. The i-adjective also has a polite negative form using the suffix **-kuwa arima-sen**. To make this, drop the **-i** and replace it with the **-kuwa arimasen** ending. For the past tense, add **deshita** after **kuwa arimasen**.

> **Chūsha wa itakuwa arimasen.**
> The injection is not painful.

> **Mōchō no shujyutsu wa kowakuwa arimasen deshita.**
> My appendectomy wasn't scary. (*lit.*, The operation on my appendicitis wasn't scary.)

> **Gakkō no shoku-chūdoku wa omokuwa arimasen deshita.**
> The food poisoning at school wasn't serious.

9. **The construction i-ADJECTIVE + kuwa nai(n)-desu ka**

The construction **i** ADJECTIVE plus **kuwa nai(n)-desu ka** is used for asking questions beginning "Don't you have . . . ?" To form this construction, drop the **-i** and replace it with **-kuwa nai(n)desu ka**.

> **Ji-rō wa itakuwa nai(n)-desu ka.**
> Don't you have anal fistula pain?

> **Mōchō wa kowakuwa nai(n)-desu ka.**
> Aren't you scared of appendicitis?

> **Shōka-furyō de onaka ga omokuwa nai(n)-desu ka.**
> Don't you have the heaviness of indigestion in your stomach?

10. The suffixes -nado and -ya

The suffix -**nado** means "et cetera; and the like; and so forth; and so on." -**nado** can be used with stem verbs and adjectives as well nouns. The suffix -**ya** can be used only with nouns.

> **Sensei ya, kango-shi nado ga shujyutsu o okonaimasu.**
> A doctor, nurse, et cetera are performing operations.

> **Kono byōin wa i-gan, i-kaiyō, jyūnishichō-kaiyō nado no shujyutsu o shimasu.**
> This hospital performs operations on stomach cancer, stomach ulcers, duodenitis ulcers, etc.

> **Shōka-ki no byōki wa i-kasui, i-en, i-san-kata-shō nado o fukumimasu.**
> Digestive diseases include gastroptosis, gastritis, hyperacidity, and so forth.

> **Tai-in-go wa osake o nomu-nado shinai-de kudasai.**
> After being discharged from the hospital, please do not drink alcohol and the like.

> **Chūsui-en no shujyutsu no ato wa itai nado no shōjyō ga arimasu.**
> After the appendectomy, you may have (the symptom of) pain and so forth.

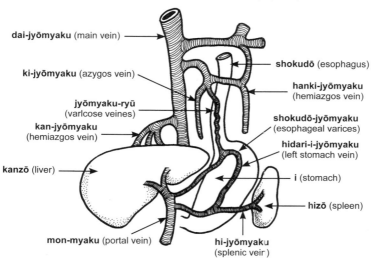

Tan-kan-kei (Liver, Gall Bladder, Biliary System)

- **dai-jyōmyaku** (main vein)
- **ki-jyōmyaku** (azygos vein)
- **jyōmyaku-ryū** (varicose veines)
- **kan-jyōmyaku** (hemiazgos vein)
- **kanzō** (liver)
- **mon-myaku** (portal vein)
- **hi-jyōmyaku** (splenic veir)
- **shokudō** (esophagus)
- **hanki-jyōmyaku** (hemiazgos vein)
- **shokudō-jyōmyaku** (esophageal varices)
- **hidari-i-jyōmyaku** (left stomach vein)
- **i** (stomach)
- **hizō** (spleen)

Useful Expressions (CD 19-3)

Listen to the CD and repeat the sentences.

1. **Sū-jitsu wa zesshoku o shite, zettai(ni) ansei ni shite kudasai.** You should fast completely for a few days, and you should get absolute rest.

2. **Tanseki-shō kamo shiremasen.** You may have cholelithiasis.
3. **I ga motarete imasu.** My stomach feels heavy.
4. **I ni appaku-kan ga arimasu ka.** Do you have a pressing feeling in your stomach?
5. **Shōka-furyō dato omoimasu.** I think you have indigestion.
6. **Kono fuku-tsū ni(wa) tae-rare-masen.** I can't stand this stomachache.
7. **Onaka ni gasu ga tamatte imasu.** You have gas in your abdomen.
8. **Onaga ga ippai ni naru to i ga itami masu ka.** Does your stomach hurt after a meal?/Is your stomach painful after a meal?
9. **Aruku to masu-masu itaku-nari masu.** The pain is much worse when I walk.
10. **Itami ga i no bubun kara kafukubu e uttsuta yō desu.** The pain feels like it moved from the stomach area to the abdomen.

Key Sentences (CD 19-4)

Listen to the CD and repeat the sentences.

1. **Kafukubu ga itakute kurushii desu ka.** Do you have abdominal pain and distress?
2. **I ga itakuwa naidesu ka.** Don't you have stomach pain?
3. **Onaka no guai wa ikaga desu ka.** How is your stomach feeling?
4. **Mae no kensa kekka yori, kyō no kensa kakka no hō ga yokunatte imasu.** This test result shows improvement over the last one.
5. **Kono kusuri wa yoku kiku ka oshiete kudasai.** Could you tell me if this medicine is effective?

Additional Words

fukumu/fukumimasu include	**nen-maku** mucous membrane
pirori-kin Helicobacter pylori	**hakkiri** clearly
nan-ben loose bowels	**shin-kokyū** deep breath
hana no nen-maku nose membranes	**(o)sakana** fish
stēiki steak	**niku** meat
chō-onpa kensa-tanshi ultrasound probe	**bubun** part/section

Language Notes

1. The first questions a doctor or nurse may ask are: How are you today? Do you have any complaints? Are you concerned about anything? Japanese has several ways of posing a question that contains all of these meanings, namely **Dō shimashita ka, Dō sare mashita ka**, and **Dō nasare mashita ka** in order of politeness. The level of politeness one should use depends on the person,

social status, context, and situation. The Japanese sense of politeness is very different from that in English-speaking countries, so it may help to understand better what situation calls for a polite form as opposed to how a doctor or nurse or any healthcare professional would or should normally speak to a patient.

Dō shita. (informal, for an emergency or quick expression)
Dō shimashita ka. (standard, for all people and situations)
Dō sare mashita ka. (polite expression of respect for elders)
Dō nasare mashita ka. (super polite expression for a person not known to the speaker or a person of high social status)

2. The question BODY PART/CONDITION **no guai wa ikaga desu ka** is a very polite way to ask a patient how he or she is doing.

Onaka no guai wa ikaga desu ka.	How is your stomach?
Tanseki-shō no guai wa ikaga desu ka.	How is your cholelithiasis?

3. In response to a general question about health, patients may reply with one of the following general expressions using **yoi/yoku** (well) or **warui** (ill).

Tottemo yoku narimashita.	I am feeling very well/quite fine.
Yoku narimashita.	I am fine.
Sukoshi yoku narimashita.	I feel pretty good/okay.
Mā-mā desu.	So-so; nothing special
Mada, sukoshi yokunai desu.	I am not quite well yet.
Mada, yokunai desu.	I am not well yet.
Mada, wari(n) desu.	I am still ill.
Sugoku, warui(n) desu.	I am very ill.
Hontō-ni, warui(n) desu.	I feel terrible./ I feel really bad.

4. Japanese use **i**-adjectives to express their feelings. To emphasize the feeling, the adjective is usually repeated twice in the **te**-form.

Onakaga itakute itakute.	My stomach is very painful.
Mume ga kurushi-kute, kurushi-kute.	My chest hurts a lot.
Atamaga kayu-kute, kayu-kute.	My head is very itchy.

5. In Lesson 11, we studied the ten **i**-adjectives relating to taste. The following chart shows the twelve tastes in Japanese and provides a complete list of Japanese taste expressions.

ENGLISH	I-ADJEC-TIVE	TE-FORM	-KU-NARU (BECOME/ TURN TO)	NEGATIVE (NOT)	PAST TENSE
good taste	oishi-i	oishi-kute	oishi-ku-naru	oishi-ku-nai	oishi-katta
bad taste	mazu-i	mazu-kute	mazu-ku-naru	mazu-ku-nai	mazu-katta
sweet	ama-i	ama-kute	ama-ku-naru	ama-ku-nai	ama-katta
salty	shoppa-i	shoppa-kute	shoppa-ku-naru	shoppa-ku-nai	shoppa-katta
hot/spicy	kara-i	kara-kute	kara-ku-naru	kara-ku-nai	kara-katta
bitter	niga-i	niga-kute	niga-ku-naru	niga-ku-nai	niga-katta
sour	suppa-i	suppa-kute	suppa-ku-naru	suppa-ku-nai	suppa-katta
tasty	uma-i	uma-kute	uma-ku-naru	uma-ku-nai	uma-katta
sweet and sour	ama-zupa-i	ama-zupa-kute	ama-zupaku-naru	ama-zupa-ku-nai	ama-zupa-katta
sweet and spicy	ama-kara-i	ama-kara-kute	ama-karaku-naru	ama-kara-ku-nai	ama-kara-katta
astringent	shibu-i	shibu-kute	shibu-ku-naru	shibu-ku-nai	shibu-katta
harsh	egu-i	egu-kute	egu-ku-naru	egu-ku-nai	egu-katta

6. The following statements are often used to express symptoms of the stomach.

I ni geki-tsū ga shimasu.	I have a sharp pain in my stomach.
I ni don-tsū ga shimasu.	I have a dull ache in my stomach.
I ni kiri-kiri suru itami ga airmasu.	I have a piercing pain in my stomach.
I ni sashi-komu yō na itami ga arimasu.	I have a pinlike pain in my stomach.
I ga motare masu.	I have a heavy, pressing feeling in my stomach.
I ga omoi desu.	I have a heavy feeling in my stomach/ My stomach feels heavy.
I ni chiku-chiku suru itami ga arimasu.	I have a prickly pain in my stomach.
I ni ana ga akisō na itami desu.	I feel pain like I have a hole in my stomach.

I ni appaku-kan ga airmasu.　　I have a pressing pain in my stomach.
I ni zuki-zuki suru itami ga　　I have a throbbing pain in my stomach.
arimasu.

To make questions of these statements, place the question marker **ka** at the end. Since there is no subject pronoun in the Japanese, there is no need to change the subject from "I" to "you" or a third-person pronoun.

I ni geki-tsū ga arimasu ka.
Do you have pain in your stomach?

I ni don-tsū ga arimasu ka.
Do you have a dull ache in your stomach?

I ni kiri-kiri suru itami ga arimasu ka.
Do you have a piercing pain in your stomach?

7.　The following forms can be used to express symptoms of gastrointestinal distress.

PATIENT'S STATEMENT:

| SYMPTOM **ga arimasu** (with some evidence) | I have a SYMPTOM. |
| **Netsu**　**ga arimasu** | I have a fever. |

| SYMPTOM **ga shimasu** (feeling) | I feel SYMPTOM. |
| **Memai**　**ga shimasu.** | I feel dizzy. |

SYMPTOM **ga demasu** (excrescences)	I have obvious/manifest SYMPTOM.
Chi　**ga demasu.**	I have bleeding/some bleeding.
Tan　**ga demasu.**	I have phlegm.
Kobu　**ga demasu.**	I have a bump.

HEALTHCARE PROFESSIONAL'S STATEMENT:

| SYMPTOM **ga mi-raremasu.** | I can see the SYMPTOM. |
| **Jirō**　**ga mi-rare masu.** | I can see your anal fistula. |

Symptoms expressed with **arimasu** words: SYMPTOM **ga arimasu.**

itami	pain
mukumi	edema
biran/tadare	irritation/abscess
fuku-bu no itami	upper abdominal pain
shukketsu	hemorrhage/bleeding

Symptoms expressed with **shimasu**: SYMPTOM **ga shimasu**.

BODY PART-**tsū**	PAIN IN BODY PART
onaka ga haru kanji	tightness/tight feeling in stomach
shoku-go ni mukatsuku kanji	nausea after eating
shokuyoku-fushin	no appetite
mune-yake	heartburn
haki-ke	nausea
hinketsu	anemia

Symptoms expressed with **demasu**: SYMPTOM **ga demasu**.

makkuroi ben	tarry stool
geppu	gas
onara/he	flatulence/fart/intestinal gases
isan	stomach acid

Language Roots

The prefix **i-** (胃) indicates the stomach and corresponds to the prefix *gastro-*.

i-gusuri	stomach medicine
i-kaiyō	gastritis ulcer
i-en	gastritis
i-kasui	gastroptosis

The suffix **-kei** (系) means "group, lineage, system."

i-chō-ki kei	gastrointestinal system
shōka-ki-kei	digestive system
seitai-kei	ecosystem

Culture Notes

Sounds in Japanese etiquette

There are two words for passing gas in Japanese. One is **he**, and the other is **onara**. **He** is standard Japanese for fart, but many people prefer not to use it and say **onara** instead. **Onara** is literary or bookish and literally means "make noise" or "make a sound." It derives from **o-narashi**, a word generally used by females. In Japanese culture, it is extremely rude to pass gas in public. Japanese are shy about making bodily noises such as burps, sneezes, snores, sniffles, and hiccups. The only exception to this discomfort with public noise making is noodle eating, where slurping is even welcomed.

Health-related Japanese proverbs IX

Short temper is the loser.
Tan-ki wa son-ki.
短気は損気

Much meat, much malady.
Ōgui wa ta-byō no moto.
大食は多病のもと

Comprehension

Answer the following questions.

1. Which of the following does NOT belong with the others?
   a. **I-kaiyō**   b. **I-san-kata-shō**
   c. **I-keiren**   d. **I-en**

2. Which of the following could NOT be used to say "stomachache?"
   a. **Zuki-zuki**   b. **Chiku-chiku**
   c. **Doki-doki**   d. **Kiri-kiri**

3. Which of the following best completes the sentence below?
   Sono kensa wa omotta (   ) itakuwa arimasen deshia.
   (The examination was not as painful as I thought.)
   a. **nari**   b. **demo**
   c. **kara**   d. **yori**

4. You are asking a patient "Are you concerned about anything?" Which of the
   following may NOT be used to ask this question?
   a. **Dō nasare mashita ka.**   b. **Dō saremashita ka.**
   c. **Dō shimashita ka.**   d. **Dō yarase mashita ka.**

Select an appropriate meaning from the list below.

5. **Tanseki no guai wa ikaga desu ka.**   (   )
6. **I ga ita-kuwa nai(n)desu ka.**   (   )
7. **Kafukubu ga itakute kurushii desu ka.**   (   )
8. **Kono kensa-kekka wa yoku wakaru ka oshiete kudasai.**   (   )
9. **Mae no kusuri yori, ima no kusuri no hō ga yokunatte imasu.** (   )

a. Do you have abdominal pain and distress?
b. Don't you have stomach pain?
c. How is your gallstone condition?
d. It's improving much more with this medicine than with the previous one.
e. Could you tell me whether this test result is easy to understand or not?

Practice

Respond to the following in Japanese using the cues that have been provided.

1. Asking about a patient's physical conditions in a polite way.
   (Healthcare professional)   (Patient)
   1. _____ (stomach cramps) **Yoku narimashita.**
   2. _____ (stomach ulcer)   **Mada itai(n) desu.**
   3. _____ (gallstones)   **Mā-mā-desu.**
   4. _____ (appendicitis)   **Sukoshi yoku narimashita.**
   5. _____ (piles)   **Kayuku-narimashita.**

2. Confirming pains using the question marker **ka**.
   (Patient)   (Healthcare professional)
   1. **I ga motare masu.**   _____
   2. **I ni appaku-kan ga arimasu.**   _____
   3. **I ni zuki-zuki suru itami ga arimasu.** _____
   4. **I ni chiku-chiku suru itami ga arimasu.** _____
   5. **I ni sashi-komu yō na itami ga arimasu.** _____

3. How do you say the following kinds of pain?
   (Questions)   (Healthcare professional)
   1. **Don-na itami desu ka.**   _____ (sharp pain)
   2. **Don-na shōjyō ga arimasu ka.**   _____ (heavy, pressing feeling)
   3. **Onaka ni don-na itami ga arimasu ka.** _____ (piercing pain)
   4. **I no guai wa dō desu ka.**   _____ (heavy feeling)
   5. **Onaka wa dō desu ka.**   _____ (dull pain)

4. Dialogue comprehension. Based on the dialogue, answer the following questions.
   1. **Satō-san wa doko ga itai(n) desu ka.**   _____
   2. **Itsu kara itai(n) desu ka.**   _____
   3. **Satō-san no kesa no guai wa dō desu ka.**   _____
   4. **Onaka o osu to itai(n) desu ka, hanasu to itai desu ka.** _____
   5. **Satō-san no byōmei wa nan desu ka.**   _____

5. Free response questions.

(Questions)   (Answers)

1. **Kyō no i no guai wa dō desu ka.** _____

2. **Ji ni natta koto ga arimasu ka.** _____

3. **Dokoka onaka ga itai(n) desu ka.** _____

4. **Ben wa dō desu ka.** _____

5. **Shoku-chūdoku ni narimashita ka.** _____

Exercises

1. Say the following words in Japanese.
   A. Parasaites   _____
   B. Gastritis   _____
   C. Gastritis ulcer   _____
   D. Appendicitis   _____
   E. Duodenitis ulcer   _____

2. Say the following in Japanese.
   A. Don't you have stomach pain?   _____
   B. How is your stomach condition?   _____
   C. Do you have abdominal pain and distress?   _____
   D. It's getting better in this test result than the previous one. _____
   E. Could you tell me if this medicine works well?   _____

3. How do you ask patients the following questions in Japanese?
   A. Don't you have a stomachache?   _____
   B. Do you have a pressing feeling in your stomach?   _____
   C. Do you have gas in your abdomen?   _____
   D. Does your stomach have pain/hurt after a meal?   _____
   E. Is this pain much worse when you walk?   _____

4. Answer the following questions in Japanese.

   Q: **Sensei, konogoro sukoshi I ga itamimasu.**
   A: _____ (When do you have pain?)

   Q: **Onaka ga suku to itamimasu.**
   B: _____ (Do you drink alcohol or smoke tobacco?)

   Q: **Hai, mainichi osake o nonde, yoku tabako o suimasu.**
   C: _____ (You should cut down on alcohol and tobacco for a while.)

LESSON 20 Kidney and Urogenital System
(Jinzō, Hinyō, Sei-ki kei)

Basic Vocabulary (CD 20-1)

Listen to the CD and repeat the vocabulary.

1.	renal function tests	jin-kinō-kensa	腎機能検査
2.	cystoscopy	bōkō-kyō-kensa	膀胱鏡検査
3.	enlarged prostate	zenritsusen-hidai	前立腺肥大
4.	nephritis/kidney inflammation	jin-en	腎炎
5.	pyelitis	jin-u-en	腎盂炎
6.	chronic nephritis	mansei-jin-en	慢性腎炎
7.	nephrosis	nefurōze	ネフローゼ
8.	kidney stone/nephrolith	jinzō kesseki	腎臓結石
9.	hydronephrosis	suijin-shō	水腎症
10.	bladder cancer	bōkō-gan	膀胱癌
11.	bladder inflammation/cystitis	bōkō-en	膀胱炎
12.	bladder stone	bōkō kesseki	膀胱結石
13.	uremia	nyō-doku-shō	尿毒症
14.	urethritis	nyō-dō-en	尿道炎
15.	urinary tract stones	nyō-ro kesseki	尿路結石
16.	urinary problem	hai-nyō-shōgai	排尿障害
17.	sexually transmitted disease	sei-byō/sei-kōi-kansen-shō	性病 / 性行為感染症
18.	gonorrhea	rin-byō	淋病
19.	syphilis	bai-doku	梅毒
20.	impotence	bokki fuzen/funō	勃起不全/不能
21.	frequent urination	hin-nyō	頻尿
22.	bed wetting/enuresis	onesho/ya-nyō-shō	お寝小/夜尿症
23.	urinary sediment test	nyō-chin-sa-kensa	尿沈渣検査
24.	dialysis	jinkō-tōseki	人工透析
25.	AIDS test	eizu kensa	エイズ検査
26.	urine sample	sai-nyō	採尿
27.	urination	hai-nyō	排尿
28.	middle of urination	chūkan-nyō	中間尿
29.	blockage	heisoku	閉塞
30.	urinary incontinence	nyō-shikkin	尿失禁

Dialogue (CD 20-2)

Listen to the CD and repeat the dialogue.

At the Medical Specialist's Office

Dr. Harris: **Suzuki-san, kyō wa dō shimashita ka.**
Mrs. Suzuki, how are you feeling today?

Mrs. Suzuki: **Saikin, nando mo otearia ni ikitaku-nari, kinō kara nyō ni sukoshi chi ga majiru-yō ni narimashita.**
I've been having to go to the bathroom a lot recently, and since yesterday there has been a little blood mixed in my urine.

Dr. Harris: **Hai-nyō no toki (ni), itami ga airmasu ka.**
Do you have pain when you urinate?

Mrs. Suzuki: **Hai-nyō ga owaru toki (ni) itami o tomonaimasu.**
I feel some pain toward the end (of urination).

Dr. Harris: **Dewa mazu, fukubu ekō-kensa o ukete kudasai.**
First of all, you should have an abdominal sonogram.

Sorekara, suttafu ni sai-nyō o jyunbi sasemasu-node, chūkan-nyō o totte kudasai.
Then I'll have the staff take a sample of your urine for testing. Please use urine from the middle of the stream.

Chūkan-nyō wa nyō ga dehajitete kara, sukoshi tatta nyō no koto desu.
The middle of stream means you should allow the urine to flow for a few seconds before you take the sample.

Mrs. Suzuki: **Hai, wakarimashita.**
I understand.

Dr. Harris: **Suzuki-san, kensa no kekka ga demashita yo.**
Mrs. Suzuki, we have the exam result.

Kyūsei bōkō-en no yō desu.
It seems to be an acute bladder inflammation.

Mrs. Suzuki: **Harisu-Sensei, naoru-noni donokuri (jikan ga) kakari masu ka.**
Doctor Harris, how long do you think it will take to cure?

Dr. Harris: **Osoraku kusuri o nonde mikka teido de yoku-narimasu.**
You will probably be well within about three days with medication.

Hai-nyō wa gaman-sezu(ni), suibun o narubeku takusan toru yōni (shite kudasai.)

Don't hesitate to urinate, and you should drink as much liquid as possible.

Jinzō, Hinyō, Sei-ki Kei (Kidney and Urogenital System)

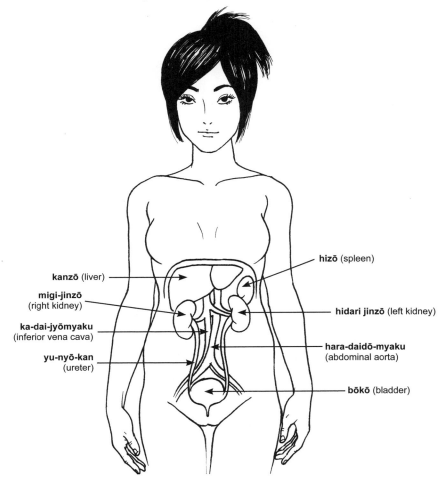

kanzō (liver)

migi-jinzō (right kidney)

ka-dai-jyōmyaku (inferior vena cava)

yu-nyō-kan (ureter)

hizō (spleen)

hidari jinzō (left kidney)

hara-daidō-myaku (abdominal aorta)

bōkō (bladder)

Grammar

1. The construction VERB BASE + **taku-naru/narimasu**

The construction VERB BASE plus **taku naru/narimasu** expresses the wish to begin an action that hasn't started yet.

Ban-gohan o tabe-taku narimashita ka.

Do you want to start having supper?

Nyō o shi-taku narimashita.
I want to begin urinating.

Onaka ga itai node, kusuri o nomi-taku narimashita.
I had a stomachache, so I wish to start medication.

Yasumi-taku narimashita.
I want to begin to rest.

2. STEM VERB + **toki(ni)**

The word **toki** means "time." When used with stem verbs, however, it means "when" or "at that time." The particle **ni** after **toki** is optional, but using the particle **ni** emphasizes the time phrase.

Masui ga kireru toki (ni) itami o tomonaimasu.
When the anesthetic wears off, you may have pain.

Byōki ga naoru toki (ni) kayumi o tomonaimasu.
When healing from illness, you may have itching.

Kesa okita toki (ni) kibun ga tottemo warukatta deshita.
At the time I awoke this morning, I felt very ill.

3. VERB BASE + **-seru/-saseru**

Seru/saseru is an auxiliary verb meaning "make, have, order." Adding **-seru/-saseru** to the verb base expresses the idea of an order or command in the sense of "make/have/order someone to do something." The subject ordering or commanding is marked by the particle **wa** or **ga**. The person who receives the order or command is marked by the particle **o** or **ni**. The negative form of **-seru** is **-senai**, and the negative form of **-saseru** is **-sasenai**.

Sensei wa kango-shi ni jyunbi o saseru yō desu.
The doctor seemed to have ordered a nurse to prepare it.

Sensei wa kanjya ni kusuri o nomaseru.
The doctor requests a patient to take her/his medicine.

Sensei wa kanjya ni kensa o saseru.
The doctor orders a patient to have a test.

Sensei wa kanjya o beddo ni suwaraseru.
The doctor made the patient sit on the bed.

Kanjya wa Eizu kensa o sasenai.
The patient is not allowed an AIDS test.

U-verbs and **ru**-verbs connect with the auxiliary verb differently. For **u**-verbs, change the last letter of the stem verb from -**u** to -**a**, and then add -**seru**. The negative form is -**senai**.

U-verbs

ENGLISH	**MASU** FORM	VERB BASE	STEM VERB	MAKE/ORDER -SERU
drink	nomi-masu	nomi(masu)	nomu	noma-seru
read	yomi-masu	yomi(masu)	yomu	yoma-seru
go	iki-masu	iki(masu)	iku	ika-seru
speak	hanashi-masu	hanashi(masu)	hanasu	hanasa-seru
return	kaeri-masu	kaeri(masu)	kaeru	kaera-seru
listen	kiki-masu	kiki(masu)	kiku	kika-seru
pull down	oroshi-masu	oroshi(masu)	orosu	orosa-seru
cool	hiyashi-masu	hiyashi(masu)	hiyasu	hiyasa-seru
paint/put/ spread	nuri-masu	nuri(masu)	nuru	nura-seru
cut	kiri-masu	kiri(masu)	kiru	kira-seru
sit down	suwari-masu	kuwari(masu)	suwaru	suwara-seru
roll up	makuri-masu	makuri(masu)	makuru	makura-seru
smell/sniff	kagi-masu	kagi(masu)	kagu	kaga-seru
become	nari-masu	nari(masu)	naru	nara-seru
wait	machi-masu	machi(masu)	matsu	mata-seru

For **ru**-verbs, drop the -**ru** and replace it with -**saseru/-sase-masu**. When the **masu** form ends with -**ri**, drop the stem verb suffix -**ru** and replace it with -**ra**, then add -**saseru**. **Okimasu, shimasu**, and **kimasu** are irregular.

Ru-verbs

ENGLISH	**MASU** FORM	VERB BASE	STEM VERB	MAKE/ORDER -SASERU
sleep	ne-masu	ne(masu)	ne-ru	ne-saseru
eat	tabe-masu	tabe(masu)	tabe-ru	tebe-saseru
warm, warm up	atatame-masu	atatame(masu)	atatame-ru	atatame-saseru
manifest/appear	araware-masu	araware(masu)	araware-ru	araware-saseru

ENGLISH	MASU FORM	VERB BASE	STEM VERB	MAKE/ORDER -SASERU
inform/notify	shirase-masu	shirase(masu)	shirasere-ru	shirase-saseru
shiver	furue-masu	furue(masu)	furue-ru	furue-saseru
go out/appear	de-masu	de(masu)	de-ru	de-saseru
allow/make to do	sase-masu	sase(masu)	sase-ru	sase-saseru
see/look/examine	mi-masu	mi(masu)	mi-ru	mi-saseru
tighten	shime-masu	shime(masu)	shime-ru	shime-saseru
leak	more-masu	more(masu)	more-ru	more-saseru
open	ake-masu	ake(masu)	ake-ru	ake-saseru
wear (clothes)	ki-masu	ki(masu)	ki-ru	ki-saseru
feel	kanji-masu	kanji(masu)	kanji-ru	kanji-saseru
become	nari- masu	nari(masu)	na-ru	na-ra-saseru
apply/paint	nuri-masu	nuri(masu)	nu-ru	nu-ra-saseru
mix	majiri-masu	majiri(masu)	maji-ru	maji-ra-saseru
empty/die/use up	nakunari-masu	nakunari(masu)	nakuna-ru	nakuna-ra-saseru
anger/be angry	okori-masu	okori(masu)	oko-ru	oko-ra-saseru
infect/transmit	utsuri-masu	utsuri(masu)	utsu-ru	utsu-ra-saseru
choke	tsumari-masu	tsumari(masu)	tsuma-ru	tsuma-ra-saseru
measure	hakari-masu	hakari(masu)	haka-ru	haka-ra-saseru
wake up*	oki-masu	oki(masu)	oki-ru	oko-saseru
do/play*	shi-masu	shi(masu)	su-ru	saseru
come*	ki-masu	ki(masu)	ku-ru	ko-saseru

* Irregular

4. The construction SUBJECT **wa** NOUN **no koto**

The expression **no koto** literally means "in fact; matter of fact; that is." **Koto** is a nominalizer that caps or concludes and identifies a noun phrase whose subject is indicated by the subject marker **wa**. Generally speaking, the construction SUBJECT **wa** NOUN **no koto desu** can be used by healthcare professionals to explain a symptom or rephrase a medical term.

Jin-en wa jinzō-en no koto desu.
Nephritis is in fact a kidney inflammation.

Oshikko wa nyō no koto desu.
Pee is in fact urine.

Chūkan nyō wa tochū no nyō no koto desu.
The middle of urination is in fact the urine between the beginning and the end.

5. STEM VERB **+ noni** (to/for/from)

When used with the stem verb, the conjunction **noni** indicates the purpose of or reason for doing something or the process of doing it and translates as "to, for, from." **Noni** with the past tense also means "as though, although, in spite of."

Seibyō no kensa o suru noni jikan ga kakarimasu.
It will take time to test for a sexually transmitted disease

Jinkō-tōseki o suru noni jikan to okane ga kakarimasu
It will take time and cost a lot for dialysis.

Kanjya wa kondōmu o tsukatta noni, seibyō ni natte shimatta.
Although the patient used a condom, he was infected with a sexually transmitted disease (*lit.*, The patient used a condom, but he/she was infected with a sexually transmitted disease).

Kinō nyō-kensa o shita noni, nyō-doku-shō wa wakarana-katta desu.
We could not diagnose uremia in spite of the urine test yesterday.

6. An interrogative followed by the suffix **-kurai**

An interrogative followed by the suffix **-kurai/-gurai** is used to ask about approximate quantity, length, or extent. **-kurai** and **-gurai** frequently replace each other without any difference in meaning.

dono-kurai/dono-gurai	how long/what extent
dore-kurai/dore-gurai	how much

Shinsatsu ni dono-kurai kakarimasu ka.
How long will it take for the physical?/About how long will the physical take?

Kensano kekka ga wakaru noni, dono-kurai kakarimasu ka.
How long will the test result take?

Dono-kurai bōkō-gan ga shinkō shite imasu ka.
How far/to what extent has the bladder cancer progressed?

Itsu-gurai ni byōki ga naorimasu ka.
How long will be needed to cure my illness?

Byōki ga naoru noni, san-ka-getsu-kan gurai kakari masu.
Approximately three months will be needed to cure your illness.

7. TIME + **teido de**

The noun **teido** means "degree, amount." The construction TIME plus **teido de** conveys the approximate time or duration and can be translated as "about." Thus, TIME plus **teido de** is synonymous with **gurai de** (about). The difference between the two is that **teido de** is more formal than **gurai de**, which makes it more suitable for professionals to use with patients.

Itsuka teido de/gurai de naorimasu.
It will be cured in about five days.

Nyōdoku-shō wa ni-shū-kan teido de yoku-narimasu.
Uremia will get/gets better in about two weeks.

Bōkō-kesseki wa ni-ka-getsu teido de naorimasu yo.
I am telling you that your bladder stones will be completely gone in about two months.

8. **Sezu(ni)** and its synonym **shinai-de**

Sezu(ni) is the negative form of **suru**, and like its synonym **shinai-de** it means "without (something)."

Shujyutsu o suru/shimasu.
You will have an operation.

Shujyutsu o sezu(ni), kusuri de chiryō o shimasu.
We will not do the operation, but treat you with medication. (*lit.*, Without the operation, but treat you with medication.)

Hai-nyō o shite kudasai.
Please urinate.

Hai-nyō (o) sezu(ni), sai-nyō wa dekimasen.
Without urination, we can't have a urine sample.

Nyō kensa o shimasu.
I'm having a urine test.

Nyō kensa o shinai-de, sei-byō wa wakarimasen.
Without a urine test, we won't understand what venereal disease you have.

9. The adverb **narubeku**

The adverb **narubeku** literally means "as much as possible; whenever practical" and can also be translated as "if possible" or "if you can." **Narubeku** is thus very useful in offering encouragement and suggestions to patients or making requests.

> **Narubeku mizu o takusan nonde kudasai.**
> Please drink water as much as possible, if you can.

> **Narubeku arukōru wa noma-naide kudasai.**
> Please do not drink alcohol, if possible.

> **Narubeku shigeki no aru tabemono wa hikaete kudasai.**
> Please restrain yourself from overeating stimulating foods as much as possible.

Useful Expressions (CD 20-3)

Listen to the CD and repeat the sentences.

1. **Kusuri o nonde, sekkusu ga shitaku narimashita ka.** After taking the medication, do you have sexual desire?
2. **Bōkō no atari ga itami masu ka.** Do you have pain around your bladder?
3. **Nyō ni umi no yōna mono ga demasu ka.** Does something like pus come out when you urinate?
4. **Jinkō-tōseki o ukete imasu ka.** Have you tried dialysis?
5. **Sensei wa kanjya ni Eizu kensa o ukesaseru hitsuyō ga arimasu.** It's necessary to have the patient take an AIDS test.
6. **Seibyō ni kakatte iru kamo shiremasen.** You may have contracted a venereal disease.
7. **Seikō suru toki [ni] itami ga arimasu ka.** Do you have pain during intercourse?
8. **Hai-ben no toki [ni] itami ga arimasu ka.** Do you have pain when you have bowel movements?
9. **Ni-shū-kan teido de te-ashi no mukumi ga nakurai-masu.** The swelling in your hand and legs will be cured in about two weeks.
10. **Izen(ni) nyō kara tanpaku-shitsu ga demashita ka.** Have you had albumin in your urine before?

Key Sentences (CD 20-4)

Listen to the CD and repeat the sentences.

1. **Ichi-nichi ni nankai oteari ni ikitaku-narimasu ka.** How often do you want to urinate in a day?

2. **Kensa o surru toki(ni), sukoshi itai kamo shiremasen.** When you have the test, you might feel a little pain.

3. **Sensei wa kanjya o beddo ni yokoni narasase-mashita.** The doctor had the patient lie down on the bed.

4. **Jin-en wa jinzō-en no kodo desu.** Nephritis is in fact kidney inflammation.

5. **Nyōdō-en wa itsuka teido de yoku narimasu.** Urethritis will heal in about five days.

Jyosei Hinyō Sei-ki Kei (Female Urogenital Systems)

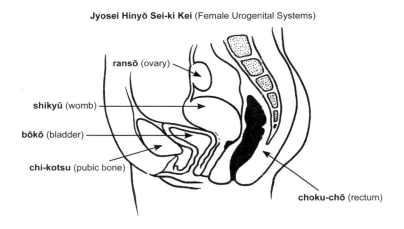

ransō (ovary)

shikyū (womb)

bōkō (bladder)

chi-kotsu (pubic bone)

choku-chō (rectum)

Dansei Hinyō Sei-ki Kei (Male Urogenital Systems)

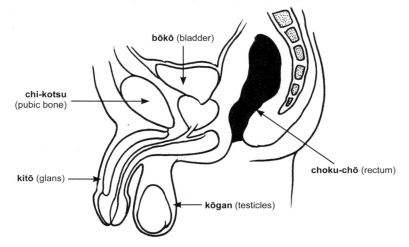

bōkō (bladder)

chi-kotsu (pubic bone)

choku-chō (rectum)

kitō (glans)

kōgan (testicles)

Additional Words

kireru/kiremasu can cut/apart
moreru/moremasu spill out
dehajimeru/dehajimemasu begin/start
  to go out
sei-yoku sexual desire
hōkei phimosis
hō-on keep warm
nyō-kan urinary duct; ureter
izen(ni) before
sei-kō fukan-shō sexual frigidity
tanpaku-shitsu protein
hito person

hikaeru/hakemasu restrain oneself
  from excessive
gaman restraint/patience
rōhai-butsu waste
sei-kō sexual intercourse
sōrō premature ejaculation
suibun-hokyū hydration
masui anesthesia
ekō-kensa sonogram
choku-chō-shin rectal examination
hai-ben bowel movement
ningen human

Language Notes

1. There are a number of expressions for pain and problems with urination. The following can be used with **ga arimasu** or **ga arimasu ka**.

    Shimiru yōna itami ga arimasu.   I have a penetrating pain.
    Shimiru yōna itami ga arimasu ka.   Do you have a penetrating pain?

shimiru yōna itami	penetrating pain
yakeru yō na itami	burning pain
karui itami	mild pain
tsuyoi itami	severe pain
geki-tsū	very severe pain
sasaru itami	piercing pain
shitsukoi itami	persistent pain
nibui itami	dull pain
hai-nyō kon-nan	urination problems
hin-nyō	pollakiuria; frequent urination
zan-nyō kan	feeling that one's bladder hasn't been completely emptied

2. The following common nouns can be used with **o suru/shimasu** (to do) or **o sezu(ni)/shinai de** (not to do).

    Shujyutsu o suru/shimasu.   I will do the operation.
    Shujyutsu o sezu(ni)/shinai de okimashō.   Let's not do the operation.

shujyutsu	operation	**kensa**	examination
chiryō/shochi	medical treatment	**kyūkei**	ordinary rest

shokuji	meal	**ryōri**	cooking
kaimono	shopping	**shigoto**	work
spōtsu	sport	**benkyō**	study
ryokō	travel	**sōji**	clean a room/clean up/
kenketsu	blood donation		sweep
sentaku	wash/washing	**nyūyoku**	bathe/bathing
jogingu	jog/jogging	**sanpo**	(a) walk, stroll
nyō sanpuru	urine sample		

3. The following are words for common sexually transmitted diseases (**sei-byō/ sei-kōi-kansen-shō**) and can be plugged into the statement: **STD ni kansen shite imasu** "You are infected with an STD."

kuramijia	chlamydia	**rin-byō**	gonorrhea
bai-doku	syphilis	**Eizu**	AIDS
B-gata kan-en	hepatitis B	**C-gata kan-en**	hepatitis C

senkei-konjirōma	genital warts; condyloma
seiki-kanshida-shō	genital candidiasis
chitsu-Torikomonasu-shō	Trichomonas virginals

Language Roots

Jin (腎) refers to the kidneys and corresponds to the prefix *nephr-*.

jin-en	nephritis/kidney inflammation
jin-zō kesseki	nephrolith/kidney stone
jin-fuzen	renal failure

Kyū (急) means "urgent, sudden, fast."

kyū-sei	acute
kin-kyū	urgent/emergency
kyū-kyū-sha	ambulance
ō-kyū-shochi	first aid
kyū-shi	sudden death

Culture Notes

Japanese words for "urine" and "stool"

Japanese use **oshikko** for "urine" in ordinary conversation. **Nyō** is used in formal or public speech and in healthcare settings. All Japanese study biology and human anatomy in school, and in these classes urine is called **shō-ben** (small excreta). Japanese use **unchi** for "stool" in ordinary conversation. **Dai-ben** (big excreta) is used in formal or public speech and in healthcare settings. There is also a term, **otsūji**, which is a very polite female word. **Unko** and **kuso** (shit) are rude male expressions that connote modest educational and social backgrounds.

Human desires and passions in Japanese

There are several expressions for human desires (**yokubō**) in Japanese. The usual construction might be NOUN **ga arimasu/arimasen** (there is/is not) or NOUN **ga ōi/sukunai desu** (have much/little).

sei-yoku	sexual desire	**shoku-yoku**	appetite
suimin-yoku	drowsiness	**meiyo-yoku**	fame
kin-yoku	greed	**kekkon-yoku**	marriage desire

The following are terms for human behaviors in Japanese. A common construction or sentence pattern for them might be "PERSON **ni** PASSION WORD **o suru** (to do)/**ga aru** (to be)/or **o iu** (to say)."

shitto	jealousy	**netami**	envy
iyagarase	harassment	**waru-guchi**	verbal abuse
tsuge-guchi	tattling	**age-guchi**	malicious gossip; backbiting
sei-teki iyagarase	sexual harassment		
ijime	teasing, bullying	**kage-guchi**	gossip

Sensei ni shitto o suru/shimasu.	I am jealous of the doctor.
Kanjya ga kango-shi ni iyagarase o suru/shimasu.	The patient is harassing the nurse.
Ningen ni netami ga aru/arimasu.	There is envy in human beings.
Ijime wa byōin de wa nai (desu).	Teasing is not allowed in the hospital.
Hito ni waru-guchi o iu/iimasu.	(She is) verbally abusing that person.
Hito no kage-guchi o iu/iimasu.	(He is) gossiping with that person.

Comprehension

Answer the following questions.

1. Which of the following does NOT belong with the others?
   a. **Bai-doku**   b. **Sei-byō**
   c. **Rin-byō**   d. **Hōkei**

2. Which of the following could NOT be used to say "stool"?
   a. **Unchi**   b. **Daiben**
   c. **Oshikko**   d. **Otsūji**

3. Which of the following best completes the sentence below?
   Chūkan nyō wa tochū no nyō (   ) koto desu.
   (The midstream of urination is in fact the urine between beginning and end.)
   a. **de**   b. **no**
   c. **ni**   d. **o**

4. You are asking a patient, "How do you feel when urinating?"
   Which of the following does NOT relate to urine conditions?
   a. **Zan-nyō kan**   b. **Attsū**
   c. **Hai-nyō kon-nan**   d. **Hin-nyō**

Select an appropriate meaning from list below.

---

5. **Jin-en wa jinzō-en no kodo desu.**   (   )
6. **Jinzō-kesseki wa san-ka-getsu teido de yoku narimasu.**   (   )
7. **Ichi-nichi ni nankai oteari ni itaku narimasu ka.**   (   )
8. **Kensa o suru toki ni sukoshi itai kamo shiremasen.**   (   )
9. **Sensei wa kanjya o beddo ni yokoni narasase-mashita.**   (   )

a. How often do you want to urinate in a day?
b. When you have the test, you might feel a little pain.
c. The doctor had the patient lie down on the bed.
d. Nephritis is in fact kidney inflammation.
e. The kidney stones will be cured/gone in about three months.

Practice

Respond to the following in Japanese using the cues that have been provided.

---

1. Asking the patient a question.
   (Patient)   (Healthcare professional)
   1. **Oshikko ga demasu.**   _____
                                          (Do you want to begin urination?)
   2. **Oshikko o shitai(n) desu.**   _____
                                          (Don't hesitate to urinate.)
   3. **Nyōdō-en wa itsu naorimasu ka.** _____
                                          (It will be cured in about a week.)
   4. **Osake o nomitai(n) desu.**   _____
                                          (Whenever possible, please don't drink alcohol.)

5. **Seiki ga itai(n) desu.**

_____

(Do you have pain when you have sexual intercourse?)

2. Explaining the meaning.
   (Patient)   (Healthcare professional)
   1. **Jin-en wa nan no koto desu ka.**

   _____
   (kidney inflammation)

   2. **Chūkan nyō wa nan no koto desu ka.**

   _____
   (midstream of urination)

   3. **Oshikko wa nan no koto desu ka.**

   _____
   (urine)

   4. **Funō wa nan no koto desu ka.**

   _____
   (impotence)

   5. **Bai-doku wa nan no koto desu ka.**

   _____
   (venereal disease)

3. How do you say the following pains?
   (Questions)   (Healthcare professional)
   1. **Hainyō no toki wa don-na itami desu ka.**

   _____
   (burning pain)

   2. **Don-na shōjyō ga arimasu ka.**

   _____
   (mild pain)

   3. **Bōkō ni don-na itami ga arimasu ka.**

   _____
   (dull pain)

   4. **Hai-nyō wa don-na guai desu ka.**

   _____
   (frequent urination)

   5. **Nyō-ga demasu ka.**

   _____
   (urination problems)

4. Dialogue comprehension. Based on the dialogue, answer the following questions.
   1. **Suzuki-san no shōjyō wa dō desu ka.**   _____
   2. **Harisu-sensei wa don-na kensa o mazu shimashita ka.** _____
   3. **Suzuki-san wa itsu itami ga arimasu ka.**   _____
   4. **Kensa no kekka, byōmei wa nan deshita ka.**   _____
   5. **Itsu yoku naru to Harisu sensei wa itte imasu ka.** _____

5. Free response questions.
    (Questions)   (Answers)
    1. **Hai-nyō no toki itami ga arimasu ka.**   _____
    2. **Sei-yoku wa arimasu ka.**   _____
    3. **Eizu-kensa o shimashita ka.**   _____
    4. **Hai-ben ni mondai ga arimasu ka.**   _____
    5. **Sei-byō ni natta koto ga arimasu ka.**   _____

Exercises

1. Say the following words in Japanese.
    A. Uremia   _____
    B. Nephritis   _____
    C. Pyelitis   _____
    D. Urinary tract stones   _____
    E. Urethritis   _____

2. Say the following expressions in Japanese.
    A. How often do you want to urinate in a day?   _____
    B. Please drink water as much as possible, if you can. _____
    C. Pee is in fact urine.   _____
    D. The doctor had the patient sit on the bed.   _____
    E. Urethritis will be cured in about three weeks.   _____

3. How do you ask your patients the following questions in Japanese?
    A. Without drawing blood, we can't have a blood test, can we?

    _____

    B. When you awoke this morning, did you felt intense pain in your bladder?

    _____

    C. Was the cystoscopy exam painful?

    _____

    D. How long will it take to get the result from the AIDS test?

    _____

    E. Do you want to start having your meal?

    _____

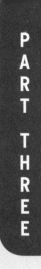

PART THREE

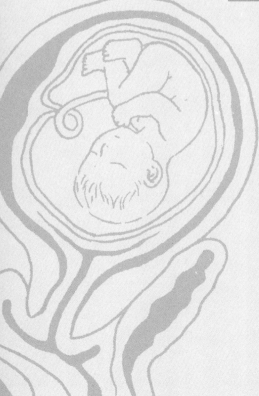

Internal Medicine
(Nai-ka)

Basic Vocabulary (CD 21-1)

Listen to the CD and repeat the vocabulary.

1.	subjective symptom	**jikaku shōjyō**	自覚症状
2.	constitution	**taishitsu**	体質
3.	aging process	**karei**	加齢
4.	heredity	**iden**	遺伝
5.	environment	**kankyō**	環境
6.	thyroid gland	**kōjyō-sen**	甲状腺
7.	lymph gland	**rinpa-sen**	リンパ線
8.	endocrine gland	**nai-bunpitsu-sen**	内分泌腺
9.	poisoning/addiction	**chū-doku**	中毒
10.	carbon monoxide poisoning	**issanka chū-doku**	一酸化中毒
11.	alcoholism	**arukōru chū-doku**	アルコール中毒
12.	acidosis	**sanketsu-shō**	酸欠病
13.	gout	**tsūfū**	痛風
14.	vitamin deficiency	**bitamin ketsubō-shō**	ビタミン欠乏症
15.	beriberi	**kakke**	脚気
16.	summer heat fatigue	**natsu-bate**	夏バテ
17.	pernicious anemia	**akusei hinketsu**	悪性貧血
18.	chronic pain	**mansei-tsū**	慢性痛
19.	motion sickness	**norimono-yoi**	乗り物酔い
20.	lump	**shikori**	しこり
21.	rheumatism	**ryūmachi**	リュウマチ
22.	heaviness of the head	**zujyū-kan**	頭重感
23.	carotid artery	**kei-dōmyaku**	頚動脈
24.	pulsation	**hakudō**	拍動
25.	vascular bruit	**kekkan-zatsuon**	血管雑音
26.	sign	**chōkō**	兆候
27.	organ transplantation	**zōki ishoku**	臓器移植
28.	homeostasis	**karada no baransu**	体のバランス/ホメオスタシス
29.	lifestyle	**seikatsu yōshiki**	生活様式
30.	improvement/betterment	**kaizen**	改善

Dialogue (CD 21-2)

Listen to the CD and repeat the dialogue.

At the Medical Specialist's Office

Dr. Mayo (female doctor): **Suzuki-san, kyō wa dō nasare-mashita ka.**
Mr. Suzuki, are you concerned about anything today?

Mr. Suzuki: **Saikin taichō ga warukute genki ga denai node, shinsatsu o onegai shimasu.**
I have bad a physical condition and haven't felt well recently, so I'd like to have a checkup.

Dr. Mayo: **Saikin, nani-ka jikaku-shōjyō wa gozaimasu ka.**
Have you noticed any (subjective) symptoms recently?

Tatoeba, zutsū, katakori, memai, hakike, mimi-nari, zujyū-kan, furatsuku nado no shōjyō ga arimasu ka.
For example, have you had any symptoms like headaches, stiff neck, dizziness, nausea, tinnitus, heaviness of the head, or a floating sensation?

Mr. Suzuki: **Tokidoki, memai to mimi-nari ga suru toki ga arimasu. Sonohoka wa nanimo (shōjyō wa) arimasen.**
Sometime, I have dizziness and tinnitus. Other than that I don't have any symptoms.

Dr. Mayo: **Monshin-hyō ni yoruto, tabako o sutte, sutoresu ga tamatte iruyō desu ne.**
According to your medical questionnaire, it looks like you like smoking cigarettes and have built-up stress, don't you?

Mazu, ketsu-atsu o hakarimashō.
First of all, let's take your blood pressure.

Uwagi o nuide itadake masu ka.
Could you take off your shirt?

Mr. Suzuki: **Hai.**
Yes.

Dr. Mayo: **Ketsuatsu wa ue wa 175 de, shita wa 105 desu. Shinpaku-sū wa 52 de hei-myaku desu.**
Your blood pressure is 175 over 105, and your pulse is a regular 52 beats per minute.

Dewa, mune to kubi ni chōshinki o atete-mimasu.
I will place a stethoscope on your chest and neck.

Migi-keidōmyaku no hakudō no toki (ni), zatsu-on ga shimasu.
On your right carotid artery I can hear a bruit.

Kekkan-zatsu-on wa dōmyaku-kōka no chōkō desu.
Vascular bruit is usually a sign of atherosclerosis.

Soredewa, ketsueki kensa o shimashō ka.
Then shall we take a sample of your blood?

Mr. Suzuki: **Hai, onegai-shimasu.**
Yes, please.

Grammar

1. ### The **na**-adjective **genki**

The **na**-adjective **genki** means "healthy and energetic." When modifying a noun, it takes on the suffix -**na**. Na-adjectives use the same conjugation with nouns as without, while **i**-adjectives drop the -**i** and replace it with -**kunai**.

(Watakushi wa) Genki desu.	I am fine/healthy/energetic.
(O)genki desu ka.	How are you? Are you doing well?
Kanjya wa genki desu.	The patient is fine/healthy/energetic.
Genki-na kanjya desu ne.	You are a healthy patient, aren't you?
Genki desu.	You are fine.
(Anata wa) Genki da.	You're fine. (informal)
(Anata wa) Genki dewa arimasen.	You are not healthy. (negative form)
(Anata wa) Genki deshita.	I was healthy. (past tense)
Genki dewa arimasen-deshita.	She was not healthy (past negative form)
Genki ni narimasu.	You will become healthy.

2. ### The conjunction **node**

The conjunction **node** expresses a reason or cause and translates as "so, since, because." The conjunction **kara** also expresses a reason (because, so), as was explained in Lesson 7, and Japanese uses both interchangeably for expressing this meaning. However, there is a difference in usage. **Node** is used when the subject information is acceptable or evident to the listener, while **kara** involves an assumption by the speaker and/or an emphasis on the reason. The stem verb and **i**-adjective use **node** by itself. The noun and **na**-adjective use **na-node**.

Mimi-nari no jikaku-shōjyō ga aru-node, tōnyō-byō kamo shiremasen.
As you have (self-)identified the symptom of tinnitus, you may have diabetes.

Zujyū-kan nanode, kō-ketsuatsu no yō desu ne.
You have heaviness of the head, so it looks like you may high blood pressure.

Himan-shō gimi nanode/dakara, seikatsu-shūkan o kaete kudasai.
Please change your lifestyle, because you are obese.

Kekkan-zatsu-on no chōkō ga aru-kara, suguni shinden-zu kensa o ukete kudasai.
You have signs of a vascular bruit, so please have a cardiogram test immediately.

3. The **na**-adjective + **de**

In Lesson 17, we studied how the construction i-ADJECTIVE plus **kute** conjoins two sentences. **Na**-adjectives also link statements in this way and require **de** to do so.

Genki-de hatarakimasu.	I will be healthy and work.
Genki-de imasu.	I am healthy and staying so. (present progressive tense)
Genki-de ite kudasai.	Please stay healthy.

Byōin wa shizukade, kirei desu.
The hospital is quiet and clean.

Anzende, eiyō no aru tabe-mono ga taisetsu desu
It is important that you eat safe and nutritious foods.

4. The **na**-adjective + **da-kara**

The dictionary form of the verb and **i**-adjective use **-kara** to express a reason. The noun and **na**-adjective use **da-kara** to express a reason, which can be translated as "so, because, since." The expression **da-kara** strongly indicates a speaker's opinion, reason, or motivation.

Genki-da-kara, jikaku-shōjyō ga arimasen.
Since I'm healthy, I have no (subjective) symptoms.

Tūfū da-kara, hiza ga tottemo itai(n) desu ka.
You have gout, so do you have knee pain?

Bitamin ketsubō-shō da-kara, kakke ni narimasu yo.
You may come to have beriberi, because you have a vitamin deficiency.

The following are **na**-adjectives:

ENGLISH	NA-ADJECTIVE	MODIFYING NOUN	DE/TO (COMBINE)	DA-KARA (REASON)
healthy/ energetic	genki	genki-na	genki-de	genki-da-kara
ill	byōki	byōki-na	byōki-de	byōki-da-kara
beautiful/ clean	kirei	kirei-na	kirei-de	kirei-da-kaka
quiet	shizuka	shizuka-na	shizuka-de	shizuka-da-kara
disgusting	kirai	kirai-na	kirai-de	kirai-da-kara
likable/ favorite	suki	suki-na	suki-de	suki-da-kara
lively	nigiyaka	nigiyaka-na	nigiyaka-de	nigiyaka-da-kara
not busy/idle	hima	hima-na	hima-de	hima-da-kara
handsome	hansamu	hansamu-na	hansamu-de	hansamu-da-kara
hateful	dai kirai	dai kirai-na	dai kirai-de	dai kirai-da-kara
loveable	dai suki	dai suki-na	dai suki-de	dai suki-da-kara
skillful/good at	jyōzu	jyōzu-na	jyōzu-de	jyōzu-da-kara
unskillful/ poor at	heta	heta-na	heta-de	heta-da-kara
useless/vain/ hopeless	dame	dame-na	dame-de	dame-da-kara
simple/easy	kantan	kantan-na	kantan-de	kantan-da-kara
comfort/ease	raku	raku-na	raku-de	raku-da-kara
very/difficult	taihen	taihen-na	taihen-de	taihen-da-kara
kind/helpful	shinsetsu	shinsetsu-na	shinsetsu-de	shinsetsu-da-kara
polite	teinei	teinei-na	teinei-de	teinei-da-kara
famous	yūmei	yūmei-na	yūmei-de	yūmei-da-kara
convenient	benri	benri-na	benri-de	benri-da-kara
inconvenient	fuben	fuben-na	fuben-de	fuben-da-kara
important	daiji	daiji-na	daiji-de	daiji-da-kara
safe	anzen	anzen-na	anzen-de	anzen-da-kara
rude	shitsurei	shitsurei-na	shitsurei-de	shitsurei-da-kara
wonderful/ lovely	suteki	suteki-na	suteki-de	suteki-da-kara

ENGLISH	NA-ADJECTIVE	MODIFYING NOUN	DE/TO (COMBINE)	DA-KARA (REASON)
necessary	**hitsuyō**	**hitsuyō-na**	**hitsuyō-de**	**hitsuyō-da-kara**
various	**iroiro**	**iroiro-na**	**iroiro-to**	**iroiro-da-kara**
nervous/annoying	**iraira**	**iraira-na**	**iraira-to**	**iraira-da-kara**
anxious	**dokidoki**	**dokidoki-na**	**doki-doki-to**	**dokidoki-da-kara**
odious	**fuyukai**	**fuyukai-na**	**fuyukai-de**	**fuyukai-da-kara**

5. The construction NOUN + **ni yoruto**

The construction NOUN plus **ni yoruto** means "according to."

> **Monshin-hyō ni yoruto dokomo warui-tokoro wa mattaku arimasen.**
> According to the questionnaire, there is nothing wrong with you.

> **Kensa kekka ni yoruto, ryūmachi no yō desu.**
> According to the test results, it looks like you have rheumatism.

> **Kono shōjyō ni yoruto, issanka-chūdoku deshō.**
> According to this symptom, you probably have carbon monoxide poisoning.

6. Adverbs with negative forms: **nani-mo, doko-mo, mettani, kesshite, sappari, sukoshi-mo,** and **chitto-mo**

The adverb **nanimo** usually occurs in negative sentences and means "(nothing) at all." It is used for things. **Nani-mo** is one of a group of adverbs that occur with negative predicates. The following are some examples.

nani-mo	nothing at all (things)	**doko-mo**	nothing at all (place/location/body parts)
zenzen	not at all (informal)	**mettani**	rarely/seldom
kesshite	never/by no means	**sappari**	not at all (informal)
sukoshi-mo	not at all	**chitto-mo**	not a bit (informal)
amari	not much	**a(n)mari**	not much (informal)

> **Karada wa doko-mo waruku (wa) arimasen.**
> Your body has nothing at all wrong with it

> **Kensa no kekka wa nani-mo waruku (wa) arimasen**
> The test result shows nothing at all wrong.

> **Karada wa sukoshi-mo waruku (wa) arimasen.**
> Your body has not a thing wrong with it. (*lit.,* Your body has not at all wrong with it.)

7. Itadake masu ka is a more polite kudasai.

Kudasai is the standard Japanese expression for requesting a favor and usually is translated as "please." However, Japanese also has an even more respectful way to say please with **itadake masu ka**, which is the best way of asking a favor or making a request.

Fuku o nuide kudasai.	Please take off your clothes.
Fuku o nuide itadake masu ka.	(polite)

Kuchi o akete kudasai.	Please open your month.
Kuchi o akete itadake masu ka.	(polite)

8. Gozaimasu ka is a more polite arimasu ka.

Gozaimasu is the super polite expression for **arimasu** (I have/there is) in Japanese. However, this form is more polite than most healthcare professionals would ordinarily be with patients.

Saikin, nani-ka jikaku-shōjyō ga gozaimasu ka. (super polite)
Saikin, nani-ka jikaku-shōjyō ga arimasu ka. (standard for healthcare professionals)
Saikin, nani-ka jikaku-shōjyō ga aru. (informal/friendly)
Have you had any self-identified symptoms recently?

9. Directionals and body parts: migi, hidari, ue, shita, naka, soto, man-naka

In Lesson 5, we began to study directionals. The following are Japanese expressions for directionals used with body parts: **migi** (right); **hidari** (left); **shita** (below/under); **naka** (inside); **soto** (outside); and **man-naka** (center).

Migi-hai ni zatsu-on ga kikoe masu.   Your right lung has a bruit.
Hidari-kata ga itai(n) desu ka.   Do you have pain in your left shoulder?

Himan no hito wa naishikyō-kensa de chō no naka o mirare-mashia.
Endoscopy was used to look inside the intestines of the obese person. (*lit.*, The person who has obesity was looked inside of intestines by endoscopy examination.)

BODY PART	LEFT SIDE (**HIDARI GAWA**)	RIGHT SIDE (**MIGI-GAWA**)
me (eye)	hidari me	migi me
mimi (ear)	hidari mimi	migi mimi
hoho (cheek)	hidari hoho	migi hoho

BODY PART	LEFT SIDE (**HIDARI GAWA**)	RIGHT SIDE (**MIGI-GAWA**)
kata (shoulder)	**hidari kata**	**migi kata**
hai (lung)	**hidari hai**	**migi hai**
ude (arm)	**hidari ude**	**migi ude**
hiji (elbow)	**hidari hiji**	**migi hiji**
te (hand)	**hidari te**	**migi te**
ashi (leg/foot)	**hidari ashi**	**migi ashi**
hiza (knee)	**hidari hiza**	**migi hiza**

10. The construction NOUN + **no chōkō ga arimasu**

The construction NOUN plus **no chōkō ga arimasu** means "show the signs of a disease, manifest a symptom." **Chōkō** conveys the sense of a very serious sign that raises doubts about someone's health. The expression **no kizashi** similarly translates as "sign, omen, or symptom." **Kizashi** is informal and is used in the sense of showing signs of/forecasting a positive result with respect to non-health-related phenomena, such as weather, the economy, and international relations.

Kono kanjya-san wa akusei-hinketsu no chōkō ga arimasu.
This patient shows signs of pernicious anemia.

Sono hito wa zenritsusen-hidai no chōkō ga gozaimasu. (polite)
That person is showing sign of prostate hypertrophy.

Ryūmachi no chōkō wa arimasen.
You do not have signs of rheumatism. (negative)

Kanjya wa kaifuku no kizashi ga arimasu.
The patient shows signs of recovery.

Useful Expressions (CD 21-3)

Listen to the CD and repeat the sentences.

1. **Tan ni chi ga majitte iru noni ki ga tsuki mashita ka.** Did you notice blood in your sputum?
2. **Mune ga doki-doki shite, ikigire mo shimasu ka.** Do you have an elevated heart rate and shortness of breath?
3. **Seki no hossa ya zensoku no hossa ga arimashita ka.** Have you had a coughing fit or asthma attack, et cetera?
4. **Seki ga derushi, netsu mo aruyō desu ne.** You have a cough and a high temperature.

5. **Nodo ga itakute, mono ga nomi-komi nikui yō dusu ne.** It looks like you have a sore throat that is making swallowing difficult, is that right?

6. **Kushami ya hanamizu ga hidoku(te), atama mo itamimasu.** I'm sneezing, and I have a runny nose and a headache.

7. **Kafukubu no itamini no ato(ni), chi no majitta geri ga arimashita.** I had lower abdominal pain followed by bloody diarrhea.

8. **Enbun to karori o herashite kudasai.** Please cut down on your salt and calorie intake.

9. **Ichi-nichi ni ichi-jikan teido, undō o shite kudasai.** Please exercise about an hour a day.

10. **Chūi-jikō o mamotte, san-ka-getsu-goni mata kite kudasai.** Please follow the guidelines and come back to see me again in three months.

Key Sentences (CD 21-4)

Listen to the CD and repeat the sentences.

1. **Monshin-hyō ni yoruto dokomo warui-tokoro wa mattaku arimasen.** According to the questionnaire, there is nothing at all wrong with you.

2. **Karada wa sukoshimo waruku (wa) arimasen.** Your body has nothing at all wrong with it.

3. **Beddo ni yokoni natte itadake masen ka.** Would you mind lying down on the bed?

4. **Hidari-hai ni zatsu-on ga kikoe masu.** Your left lung has a noise.

5. **Genki-na kango-shi-san desu ne.** You are an energetic nurse./You are a nurse with lots of energy.

Additional Words

kigatsuku/kitagaukimasu notice/re-alize

tamaru/tamarimasu accumulate

hiki-okosu/hiki-okoshimasu cause/induce

tan-jyū bile

yawarageru relieve/ease/soften

fusegimasu prevent

shinkō progressive

maebure sign/indication

dōmyaku-kōka atherosclerosis

furatsuki floating sensation

tokui taishitsu idiosyncrasy

kōzan-byō mountain sickness

kuru-byō rickets

kajyō-sesshu over intake

sesshu-busoku insufficient intake

taichō-furyō bad physical condition

hei-myaku normal pulse

kaiketsu-byō scurvy

chōshin-ki stethoscope

zatsu-on noise/bruit

uwa-gi coat/garment

pantsu underpants/briefs

Language Notes

1. The following expressions are for different kinds of headaches:

hidoi zutsū	severe headache
karui zutsū	light/mild headache
zuki-zuki suru zutsū	throbbing headache
hen-zutsū	migraine
wareru yōna itami no zutsū	splitting headache
gan-gan suru itami no zutsū	intense/pounding headache
zujyū-kan	heaviness of the head

2. The following are directionals for general use:

mae	front	**ushiro**	back
ue	up/on/above	**shita**	below/under
tonari	next	**yoko**	side
soba	near	**chikaku**	nearby
atari	around/in the vicinity		

3. When Japanese say that something is at about a 45-degree angle, they place **naname** before the directional. **Naname** means "45-degree angle" in any direction.

Naname	about a 45-degree angle
Naname ue	about 45 degrees up
Naname mae	about 45 degrees in front
Naname migi ue	about 45 degree up on the right side

Language Roots

The suffix **-kan** (感) indicates feeling and sense.

fukai-kan	unpleasant feeling, displeasure, discomfort
datsuryoku-kan	languor, feeling of exhaustion, lassitude
fuan-kan	anxiety, insecurity, unease
anshin-kan	peace of mind, sense of security, ease
shinmitsu-kan	feeling of closeness, intimate feeling

Dō (動) can be either a prefix or a suffix and indicates motion and movement.

dō-myaku kōka	arteriosclerosis	**kei-dō-myaku**	carotid artery
haku-dō	pulsation, pulse	**dō-ki**	heart beat
shin-dō	vibration	**un-dō**	exercise

Culture Notes

Japanese food and the risk of high blood pressure in modern society

The Japanese diet was developed in ancient times for workers engaged in hard, physical labor such as samurai and farmers, and in such staples as **miso** (soybean paste), **shōyu** (soy sauce), and **tsukemono** (pickles) it includes a lot of salt. In modern times, with much less demand for exercise in the work or social environments, many Japanese take in too much sodium, more than in Western diets. For this reason, there is a high probability among Japanese people of illnesses or conditions related to excessive dietary sodium, including high blood pressure, atherosclerosis, stroke, and acute myocardial infarction.

Health-related Japanese proverbs X

The mouth is the gate of evil.
Kuchi wa wazawai no mon.
口は禍（わざわい）の門

Sleep is better than medicine.
Sui-min wa ryō-yaku ni masaru.
睡眠は良薬にまさる

Comprehension

Answer the following questions.

1. Which of the following does NOT belong with the others?
    a. **Kaiketsu-byō**   b. **Kakke**
    c. **Torime**   d. **Norimono-yoi**

2. Which of the following could be used to say "a headache"?
    a. **Hen-zutsū**   b. **Shinkin-kan**
    c. **Zuki-zuki suru itami** d. **Fura-fura suru itami**

3. Which of the following best completes the sentence below?
    Tokidoki, memai to miminari ga suru (   ) ga arimasu.
    (Sometime, I feel dizzy and have tinnitus.)
    a. **made**   b. **toki**
    c. **ato**   d. **gogo**

4. You are asking a patient, "What kind of lifestyle do you have?" In order to prevent lifestyle-related disease, which of the following do you NOT need to be careful of?

    a. **Party**   b. **Sutoresu**

    c. **Enbun**   d. **Kitsuen**

Select the appropriate meaning from the list below.

---

5. **Monshin-hyō ni yoruto dokomo warui-tokoro wa mattaku arimasen.** ( )
6. **Karada wa sukoshimo waruku (wa) arimasen.** ( )
7. **Beddo ni yokoni natte itadake masen ka.** ( )
8. **Hidari-hai ni zatsu-on ga kikoemasu.** ( )
9. **Genki-na kango-shi-san desu ne.** ( )

a. According to the questionnaire, there is nothing at all wrong it.
b. You are an energetic nurse, aren't you?
c. Would you mind lying down on the bed?
d. Your body has nothing at all wrong it.
e. Your right lung has a noise.

Practice

Respond to the following in Japanese using the cues that have been provided.

---

1. Giving the opinion that nothing is wrong.

    (Patient)   (Healthcare professional)

    1. **Mimi-nari ga shimasu.**   _____

                                   (nothing is wrong at all)

    2. **Memai ga shimasu.**   _____

                                   (not a thing wrong)

    3. **Norimono-yoi ga shinpai desu.**   _____

                                   (don't worry too much)

    4. **Issanka chūdoku ni kakarimasu ka.**   _____

                                   (rarely happens)

    5. **[Watakushi wa] Kaiketsu-byō desu ka.**   _____

                                   (never happens)

2. Telling the patient what the symptoms show.

    (Patient's condition)   (Healthcare professional)

    1. Vitamin deficiency   _____

    2. Beriberi   _____

3. Rheumatism   _____

4. Alcoholism   _____

5. Obesity   _____

3. Understanding various types of headache. Express the following in Japanese.

(Patient's situation)   (Healthcare professional)

1. Severe headache

2. Mild headache

3. Migraine

4. Heaviness of the head

5. Throbbing headache

6. Pounding headache

7. Splitting headache

4. Dialogue comprehension. Based on the dialogue, answer the following questions.

1. **Suzuki-san no jikaku-shōjyō wa nan desu ka.**

2. **Suzuki-san no ketsu-atsu wa takai desu ka, hikui desu ka.**

3. **Suzuki-san no ketsu-atsu wa ikutsu desu ka.**

4. **Suzuki-san no mune kara don-na oto ga kikoemasu ka.**

5. **Suzuki-san no shōjyō wa nan desu ka.**

5. Free response questions.

(Questions)   (Healthcare professional)

1. **Saikin, nani-ka byōki no chōkō ga arimasu ka.**

2. **Sukoshi, himan-shō desu ka.**

3. **Nanika byōki no jikaku-shōjyō ga arimasu ka.**

4. **Tokidoki, miminari ga shimasu ka.**

5. **Kenkō-shindan de naishikyō-kensa o shimashita ka.**

Exercises

1. Say the following words in Japanese.
    A. Thyroid gland   _____
    B. Poisoning   _____
    C. Constitution   _____
    D. Heredity   _____
    E. Organ transplantation   _____

2. Say the following expressions in Japanese.
    A. Please stay healthy.   _____
    B. Do you have pain in your left lung?   _____
    C. The test results show nothing wrong.   _____
    D. According to the test result, it looks like gout.   _____
    E. Please open your month.   _____

3. How do you ask your patients the following questions in Japanese?
    A. Did you notice blood in your urine?   _____
    B. Do you have a fast heart rate and shortness of breath?   _____
    C. Would you mind lying down on the bed?   _____
    D. You look like you have a high temperature, don't you?   _____
    E. Do you exercise about an hour a day?   _____

4. Answer the following questions in Japanese.

    Q: **Kesa kara memai ga shite, atama ga itai(n) desu ga.**
    A: _____
    (Have you had any (subjective) symptoms like a heaviness of the head?)

    Q: **Sono-yōna shōjyō wa, mattaku nanimo arimasen.**
    B: _____
    (According to the questionnaire, you experienced a stroke.)

    Q: **Saikin, shigoto ga taihen de, sutoresu ga takusan arimasu.**
    C: _____
    (Please be careful about your lifestyle.)

Orthopedic Surgery
(Seikei-ge-ka)

Basic Vocabulary (CD 22-1)

Listen to the CD and repeat the vocabulary.

1.	spine/backbone	**se-bone**	背骨 (せぼね)
2.	cervical spine	**kei-tsui**	頚椎 (けいつい)
3.	thoracic spine	**kyō-tsui**	胸椎 (きょうつい)
4.	lumbar spine	**yō-tsui**	腰椎 (ようつい)
5.	breastbone	**kyō-kotsu**	胸骨 (きょうこつ)
6.	collarbone	**sa-kotsu**	鎖骨 (さこつ)
7.	spinal cord	**sekizui**	脊髄 (せきずい)
8.	rib	**rokkotsu**	肋骨 (ろっこつ)
9.	thigh bone	**daitai-kotsu**	大腿骨 (だいたいこつ)
10.	cartilage	**nan-kotsu**	軟骨 (なんこつ)
11.	pelvis	**kotsu-ban**	骨盤 (こつばん)
12.	pulled/torn muscle	**niku-banare**	肉離れ (にくばな)
13.	latissimus dorsi muscle	**(kō) hai-kin**	（広）背筋 (こう はいきん)
14.	Achilles tendon	**akiresu-ken**	アキレス腱 (けん)
15.	slipped disc	**tsui-kanban herunia**	椎間板ヘルニア (ついかんばん)
16.	strained back	**gikkuri-goshi**	ぎっくり腰 (ごし)
17.	sciatica	**zakotsu-shinkei-tsū**	坐骨神経痛 (ざこつしんけいつう)
18.	internal bleeding	**nai-shukketsu**	内出血 (ないしゅっけつ)
19.	abrasion	**surikizu**	擦り傷 (すりきず)
20.	contusion	**daboku(shō)**	打撲(症) (だぼくしょう)
21.	bump	**kobu**	瘤 (こぶ)
22.	sprains	**nenza**	捻挫 (ねんざ)
23.	broken bone/fracture	**kossetsu**	骨折 (こっせつ)
24.	ligament	**jintai**	靭帯 (じんたい)
25.	crack	**hibi**	罅 (ひび)
26.	tendonitis	**kenshō-en**	腱鞘炎 (けんしょうえん)
27.	arthritis	**kansetsu-en**	関節炎 (かんせつえん)
28.	dislocation	**dakkyū**	脱臼 (だっきゅう)
29.	cast	**gibusu**	ギブス
30.	crutches	**matsuba-zue**	松葉杖 (まつばづえ)

Kokkaku-kei-zu (Skeletal System)

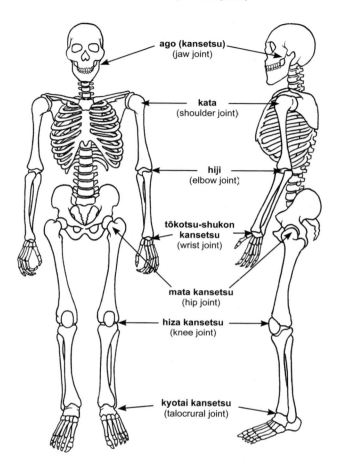

ago (kansetsu)
(jaw joint)

kata
(shoulder joint)

hiji
(elbow joint)

tōkotsu-shukon
kansetsu
(wrist joint)

mata kansetsu
(hip joint)

hiza kansetsu
(knee joint)

kyotai kansetsu
(talocrural joint)

Dialogue (CD 22-2)

Listen to the CD and repeat the dialogue.

At the Orthopedic Surgeon's Office

Dr. Gibson (male doctor):   **Kyō wa dō shimashita ka.**
                              Do you have any complaints today?

Mrs. Kato: **Nimotsu o mochiage yō to shita totan (ni), koshi o itamemashita.**
I hurt my back as (*lit.*, just as soon as) I tried to lift up my luggage.

Dr. Gibson: **Dewa, (kosi no) shinsatsu o shite mimashō.**
Well, let's take a look at your back.

Mazu, uwagi o nuide, kochira no beddo no ue ni utsubuse ni natte kudasai.
First of all, please take off your shirt, and could you lie face down on this bed?

Mrs. Kato: **Koshi o sukoshi ugokasu dake de(mo) gekitsū ga hashirimasu.**
Even if I move my back a little, I have a sharp pain running through it.

Koshi o mageru koto ga zenzen dekimasen.
I can't bend my back at all.

Dr. Gibson: **Sōdesu ka, wakarimashia. Sore wa taihen desu ne. Dewa, koshi o mimashō.**
Is that so? I understand. I am sorry to hear that. Then let's examine your back.

Tokorode, ashi ga shibire tari, tsumasaki-e-no hōsantsū ga ari-masen ka.
By the way, (tell me), don't you have numbness in your leg or a radiating pain toward the tip of your toe?

Mrs. Kato: **Tokuni, itami ya shibire wa nai-to omoimasu.**
I think I don't have any particular pains or numbness.

Dr. Gibson: **(Koshi o osu to) itamu-nowa kono atari desu ka.**
(When I press on your back,) Is the place you feel pain around here?

Dewa, kondo wa aomuke ni natte kudasai.
Well then, could you turn over and lie on your back?

Ashi o mochi-ageru kensa o shimasu. Koko wa dōdesu ka. Itai desu ka.
I am going to raise your legs up to examine them. How about here? Does this hurt?

Mrs. Kato: **Itai, itai. Migi-ashi o ageru toki, koshi no atari ni itami ga hashiri-masu.**
Ouch, ouch. I have a sharp pain shooting up my back when I raise my right leg.

Dr. Gibson: **Mita tokoro, tsuikanban herunia dewa naika to omoimasu.**
In my estimation, it's likely you have a slipped disc.

Yōtsui no MRI o totte moraimasu node, shinryō hōshasen-gishi no shiji ni shitagatte kudasai.
I would like to get an MRI of your lumbar spine, so please follow the medical radiographer's instructions.

Grammar

1. The expression **yōto shita totan (ni)**

The construction VERB BASE plus **yōto shita totan (ni)** indicates the moment of completion of an action. It is usually translated as "just as, at the moment, the moment, as soon as, as." The particle **ni** is optional.

> **Oki-yō to shita totan ni hidari-kata no kansetsu o itamemashita.**
> As soon as I got up, I hurt my left shoulder joint.

> **Kan o ake-yō to shita totan ni, hitosashi-yubi o kirimashita.**
> The moment I opened the can, I cut my index finger.

> **Fuku ni airon o ake-yō to shita totan (ni), migi-te o yakedo shimashita.**
> Just as I started ironing my clothes, I burned my right hand with the iron.

Other adverbs of time are **shunkan (ni)** (the instant, the exact moment), **totan (ni)** (just now, as soon as), and **toki (ni)** (when). The particle **ni** is optional. The meaning of **shunkan (ni)** is precise and punctual, while **totan (ni)** is a little less so, and **toki (ni)** denotes time in a more general way.

> **Subetta shunkan (ni) koronde ashi o orimashitra.**
> The instant I slipped and fell down, I broke my leg.

> **Doa o aketa totan (ni), naka-yubi o hasamimashita.**
> Just as I opened the door, I jammed my middle finger.

> **Sanpo o shita toki (ni), inu ni migi-ashi o kamaremashita.**
> When I was out taking a walk, I was bitten on the right leg by a dog.

2. STEM VERB + **dake de(mo)**

The phrase **dake de(mo)** expresses the notion of "even just doing" or "doing just enough for something to happen." It can also express the moment of an action taking place. The particle **mo** is optional.

> **Koko ni suwaru dake de(mo), koshi ga itai(n) desu.**
> I have back pain just sitting here. (*lit.*, Even just sitting, I have back pain.)

> **Koko ni butsukkata dake de, hiza ni hibi ga hairimashita.**
> I cracked my knee just hitting it here.

> **Ude o nobasu dake de(mo), kenshō-en ni narimasu.**
> You can get tendonitis even just stretching your arms.

> **Koronda dake de, dakkyū shimasu yo.**
> You can dislocate it even just by falling down.

3. The expression **dewa naika to omoimasu** and other expressions of possibility or probability

In Lessons 9 and 14, we studied some diagnostic expressions. The expression **dewa naika to omoimasu** includes an element of doubt but conveys the near certainty of a diagnosis based on familiarity with a symptom or illness. Culturally, the Japanese do not make a clear distinction between possibility and probability or likelihood. The following are other common diagnostic expressions.

Kossetsu mitai desu.	You look like you have broken bone.
Daboku no yō desu.	It seems that you have a bruise.
Nenza kamo shiremasen.	You might have a sprain.
Kenshō-en dewa naika to omoimasu.	I think you probably have tendonitis.
Dakkyū ni chigai arimasen.	This should be a dislocation. (offered as a clear, definite diagnosis)

4. The construction PAST TENSE VERB + **tokoro**

The dependent noun **tokoro** is used to express when someone has done something intentionally and takes a past tense verb.

Mita tokoro, kizu ga kanō shite iru yō desu.
In my estimation (*lit.*, When I looked/estimated), the wound has festered.

Kensa shita tokoro, sono kobu wa daboku kara dekita yō desu.
When I examined it, that bump was caused by a bruise.

Tabeta tokoro, byōin no shokuji wa oishikatta desu.
When I ate it, the hospital food was delicious.

5. The suffix **-morau** and the **te**-form

In Lesson 18, we studied the **te**-form plus the suffix -**morau**. The suffix -**morau** expresses to the notion of receiving some benefit from someone's action.

Kanjya wa sensei ni migi-ashi o kensa shite moraimashita.
The patient had his/her right leg examined by doctor.

Shinryō hōsha-sen-gishi ni MRI o totte moratte kudasai.
Please ask to have a MRI done by a medical radiographer.

Morau/moraimasu is one of several sets of giving and receiving verbs. Its usage is limited in one important way, in that it is used only when the status of the receiver is lower than that of the person who is giving.

Kanjya-san wa sensei kara shohōsen o dashite moraimashia.
The patient has received a prescription from the doctor.

Kanjya-san wa sensei ni gibusu to tsukete moraimasu.
The patient was put in a cast by the doctor.

As these examples show, **morau/moraimasu** takes both **ni** (by) and **kara** (from). The particle **ni** is for persons, and **kara** is both for persons and things other than persons. The particle **ni** contains the idea of direct contact with a person, while the particle **kara** conveys the idea of any source including a person, institution, or abstract concept. For example:

Byōin kara seikyū-sho o moraimashita.
I have received an invoice from the hospital.

Uketsuke kara an-nai o moraimasu.
I will receive information from the receptionist.

Sensei kara rihabiri-hōhō o oshiete moraimasu.
I will learn physical therapy from the doctor.

By way of comparison with the first example above, the following sentence is not acceptable in Japanese: *Byō-in ni tegami o moraimashita. As a rule, it's safe always to use the particle **kara** for **moraimasu**. The polite expression of **moraimasu** is **itadaku/itakakimasu**.

Sensei kara shoken o itadakimashita.
I received the doctor's remarks (*lit.*, I received remarks from the doctor).

Byōin kara matsuba-zue o itadaku to omoimasu.
I think that I will receive a pair of crutches from hospital.

6. The verbs ageru/agemasu and kureru/kuremasu

Other sets of verbs that mean "give" are **ageru/agemasu** and **kureru/kure-masu**. The verb **ageru/agemasu** requires the giver's point of view when describing an event, and the giver (subject) is an active agent.

Sensei wa matsuba-zue o kanjya ni ageta.
The doctor gives a crutch to the patient.

Uketsuke wa yoyaku-bangō o kanjya ni agemashita.
The receptionist gave a reservation number to the patient.

The polite form of **ageru/agemasu** is **sashi-ageru/sashi-agemasu**.

Sensei wa matsuba-zue o kanjya ni sashi-ageru.
The doctor gives a crutch to the patient.

Uketsuke wa yoyaku-bangō o kanjya ni sashi-agemashita.
The receptionist gave a reservation number to the patient.

The informal form of **ageru/agemasu** is **yaru**. However, **yaru** is very rude, and healthcare professionals should avoid using it.

Sensei wa matsuba-zue o kanjya ni yaru.
The doctor gives a crutch to the patient.

Uketsuke wa yoyaku-bangō o kanjya ni yaru.
The receptionist gave a reservation number to the patient.

The informal verb **yaru/yarimasu** also has the meaning conveyed by **suru/shimasu** (do/play), and so is its informal form.

(Sensei wa) kensa o shimasu.   The doctor will do the examination.
(Sensei wa) kensa o yaru.   The doctor will do the examination. (impolite)

However, **ageru/agemasu** can't be used if the receiver is the first-person subject (I, we) or within the group of family members or friends, in other words, a group that contains the first-person subject. In such cases, the verb **kureru/kuremasu** (give) is used instead.

Sensei wa matsuba-zue o watakushi ni kureta.
The doctor gave me a crutch.

Uketsuke wa yoayku-bangō o haha ni kuremashita.
The receptionist gave my mother a reservation number.

The polite form of **kureru/kuremasu** is **kudasaru/kudasai-masu**.

Sensei wa matsuba-zue o watakushi ni kudasaru.
The doctor will give me a crutch.

Uketsuke wa yoayku-bangō o haha ni kudasai-mashita.
The receptionist gave my mother a reservation number.

Kokkaku-kei Sokumen-zu (Skeletal System From Side)

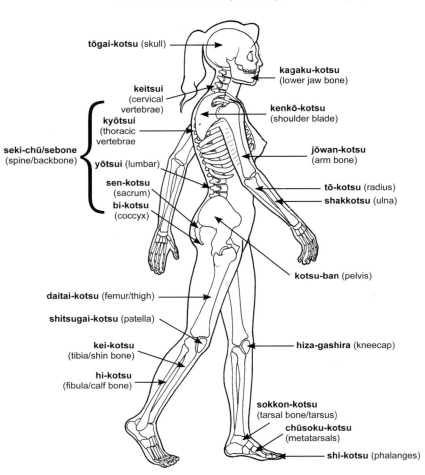

tōgai-kotsu (skull)

kagaku-kotsu
(lower jaw bone)

keitsui
(cervical
vertebrae)

kenkō-kotsu
(shoulder blade)

kyōtsui
(thoracic
vertebrae

seki-chū/sebone
(spine/backbone)

jōwan-kotsu
(arm bone)

yōtsui (lumbar)

sen-kotsu
(sacrum)

tō-kotsu (radius)

shakkotsu (ulna)

bi-kotsu
(coccyx)

kotsu-ban (pelvis)

daitai-kotsu (femur/thigh)

shitsugai-kotsu (patella)

kei-kotsu
(tibia/shin bone)

hiza-gashira (kneecap)

hi-kotsu
(fibula/calf bone)

sokkon-kotsu
(tarsal bone/tarsus)

chūsoku-kotsu
(metatarsals)

shi-kotsu (phalanges)

Useful Expressions (CD 22-3)

Listen to the CD and repeat the sentences.

1. **Koronde hidari-te-kubi o itame mashita.** Upon falling down, I hurt my left wrist.
2. **Garasu no hahen de hidari-te o kirimashita.** I cut my right hand on a piece of glass.
3. **Doa ni ko-yubi o hasami mashita.** I pinched my little finger in the door.
4. **Kono oya-yubi ni toge ga sasatte toremasen.** I can't get this splinter out of my thumb.
5. **Kaidan kara ochite, senaka o tsuyoku uchimashita.** I fell down the stairs and hit my back very hard.

6. **Daboku no ato ga arimasu.** You have a bruise mark.
7. **Kaidan o fumi hazushite, migi-ashi-kubi o nenza shita yō desu.** I missed a step on the stairs and sprained my right ankle.
8. **Hidari ude o kossetsu shite imasu yo.** You have broken/fractured your left arm.
9. **Koshi ga nobase masu ka.** Can you straighten out your back?
10. **Migi-te ga shibirete imasu ka.** Do you have numbness in your right hand?

Key Sentences (CD 22-4)

Listen to the CD and repeat the sentences.

1. **Dakkyū dewa nai-ka to omoimasu.** I think you probably have a dislocation.
2. **Mita tokoro, rokkotsu ni hibi ga haitte iru yō desu.** In my estimation, you have a cracked rib.
3. **Ryōri o shiyō to shita totan (ni), naka-yubi o yakedo shimashita.** As (at the moment) I was cooking, I burned my middle finger.
4. **Kanjya-san wa sensei kara kusuri no shohōsen o moraimashita.** The patient received a prescription for drugs from the doctor.
5. **Koko o sawaru dakede, kansetsu ga itai(n) desu ka.** Do you have joint pain when I just touch here?

Additional Words

mageru/magemasu bent	**ugokasu/ugokashimasu** move
osu/oshimasu push	**mochiageru/mochiagemasu** lift up
suberu/suberimasu slip	**sakeru/sakemasu** splinter
nū/nuimasu stitch	**nobasu/nobashimasu** stretch
ataru/atarimasu hit	**korobu/korobimasu** fall down
katameru/katamemasu bind/harden	**taoreru/taoremasu** collapse/fall down/smite
hako box	
kiru/resshō tear off	**enshō/akaku-naru** inflamed
ato mark	**kizuato** scar
garasu glass	**hahen** fragment/broken piece
sekkō plaster/gypsum	**hari** needle/counter for stitch
shiji instruction/order	**toge** thorn
taezu constantly	**nayamu** suffering
zenkai complete recovery	**fukkin** abdominal muscles
jiko accident	**kōtsū-jiko** car accident
gojyū-kata frozen shoulder	**kenin ryōhō** traction therapy
kotsu-sosō-shō osteoporosis	**gaihan-boshi** hallux valgus/bunion

rihabiri physical therapy
shinkei-tsū neuralgia
shinryō hōsha-sen-gishi medical
  radiographer
kansetsu-kō joint cavity
tsuki-yubi sprained finger

seitai chiropractic
yugami distortion
airon iron
rinshō kensa-gishi clinical
  laboratory technician

Language Notes

1. The literal meaning of the verb **hashiru/hashirimasu** is "run." However, Japanese also use **hashiru/hashirimasu** to express pain or thunderbolts.

Itami ga karada o hashirimashita.	I had a pain shooting through my body.
Shinkei ni gekitsū ga hashirimasu.	I have a severe pain shooting down my nerves.
Senaka ni itami ga hashirimasu ka.	Do you have a pain shooting down your back?

2. **Gekitsū o kanjiru** and **gekitsū o oboeru** both convey the same meaning of "feeling severe/sharp pain." There are two ways to express pain:

   Daboku ni-yoru gekitsū o kanjimashita.
   I felt a severe pain from (*lit.*, caused by) the bruise.

   Totsuzen, nenza ni-yoru gekitsū o oboemashita.
   I felt a sudden sharp pain caused by the sprain (*lit.*, cause by being sprained).

3. Radiating pain is called **hōsan-tsū** in Japanese. Literally, **hō** means "emit, release," **san** means "spread," and **tsū** means "pain." It is well known that the signs of visceral disease are back pain and/or shoulder pain, and common signs of heart attacks are shoulder pain, back pain, and teeth pain.

4. The verb for "stitch" in Japanese is **nū/nui-masu**. It requires a counter, and the counter for "stitch" is -**hari** (needle). In the terms for one and two stitches, the number used is from the Japanese as opposed to the Chinese number system. To form the respective counters, take **hito-tsu** (one) and **futa-tsu** (two), drop the suffix -tsu, and replace it with -**hari**. From three stitches on, the counter uses the number from the Chinese system plus -**hari**.

one stitch	**hito-hari**	two stitches	**futa-hari**
three stitches	**san-hari**	four stitches	**yon-hari**
five stitches	**go-hari**	six stitches	**roku-hari**
ten stitches	**jyū-hari**	fifteen	**jyū-go hari**
twenty-five stitches	**nijyū-go hari**	thirty stitches	**sanjyū-hari**

Kōtsū-jiko no kanjya wa migi-ashi o ni-jyū-hari nuimashia.
The patient from the car accident had twenty stitches in his/her right leg.

5. The following are some expressions used to explain how an accident happened.

Kaidan o agarimashita.	I was going up to the stairs.
Kaidan o orimashita.	I was going down the stairs.
Kaidan o fumi-hazushi-mashita.	I missed the step on the stairs.
Kaidan ni tsumazuki-mashita.	I stumbled on the stairs.
Kaidan kara ochimashita.	I was falling down from the stairs.
Tesuri ni tsukamarimashita.	I was holding onto a handrail.

6. The word for "joint" is **kan-setsu**. Literally, **kan** means "between," and **setsu** means "connection." Spoken Japanese sometimes uses the term **fushi-bushi** (every joint). **Fushi** means "joint," and **bushi** is also "joint."

Ude no kan-setsu ga itai(n) desu.
I have pain in my elbow (*lit.*, arm joint).

Migi-hiza no kan-setsu o shirabemashō ka.
Shall we examine your right knee (*lit.* knee joint)?

Karada no fushi-bushi ga itai(n) desu.
My whole body's joints ache./Every joint in my body aches.

7. Japanese has a unique expression, **ne-chigaeru**, that means "sleep in an awkward position and wake with a crick in one's neck." **Ne-chigaeru** is a compound of the actions of **neru** (sleep) and **chigaeru** (change).

Kyō wa ne-chigae-te, kubi ga tottemo itai(n) desu.
I have a lot of pain in my neck due to an awkward position during sleep.

Ne-chigae-te, kata ga ugokanai(n) desu.
I slept awkwardly and could not move my shoulder.

8. Japanese has two expressions for sprains: **nenza** and **tsuki-yubi**. **Nenza** is a sprain caused by twisting, and **tsuki-yubi** (sprained finger) is sprain caused by jamming a finger.

Kodomo wa koronde ashi-kubi o nenza shimashita.
The child fell and twisted his ankle

Kaidan o fumi-hazushite, ashi-kubi o nenza shimashita.
I missed a step on the stairs, and I sprained my ankle.

Kono teido no nenza-nara, suguni naoru deshō.
A sprain like this one will probably heal soon.

Yakyū o shite, hidari-naka-yubi o tsuki-yubi shimashita.
I sprained the middle finger of my left hand while playing baseball.

9. In Lesson 18, we studied the passive ending **-rare-ru/-rare-masu**. The following chart lists more passive verbs. **-rare-ru/masu** is present tense, and **-rare-ta/mashita** is past tense.

ENGLISH	DICTIONARY FORM	PRESENT PASSIVE (-RARERU)	PAST PASSIVE (-RARE-TA)
cut	**ki-ru**	**ki-rareru**	**ki-rare-ta**
bump	**ata-ru**	**ata-rareru**	**ata-rare-ta**
swell	**hare-ru**	**hare-rareru**	**hare-rare-ta**
pinch	**hasa-mu**	**hasa-ma-rareru**	**hasa-ma-rare-ta**
scratch	**hikka-ku**	**hikka-ka-rareru**	**hikka-ka-rare-ta**
hit	**u-tsu**	**uta-rareru**	**uta-rare-ta**
stick	**sa-su**	**sasa-rareru**	**sasa-rare-ta**
bit	**ka-mu**	**kama-rareru**	**kama-rare-ta**
fall down	**koro-bu**	**koroba-rareru**	**koroba-sa-rare-ta**
scrape	**surimu-ku**	**surimuka-rareru**	**surimu-ka-sa-rare-ta**
stumble	**tsumazu-ku**	**tsumazu-ka-rareru**	**tsumazu-ka-sa-rare-ta**

10. Other useful expressions for diagnosis in orthopedics:

Kansetsu ga itami masu ka.	Do you have joint pain?
Nenza ga hidoi desu ne.	You have a bad sprain, don't you?
Ashi-kubi o nenza shita yō desu.	You have sprained your ankle.
Gibusu o torimasu ka.	Do you want your cast removed?
Migi-ashi ga mukun de imasu.	Your right leg is swollen.
Yoku te-ashi ga shibire masu ka.	Do you often have numbness in your limbs?

Koko no kansetsu-kō ga semaku natte imasu.
There is a narrowing of the joint cavity.

Shinkei ga appaku sarete imasu.
Your nerve is being pinched.

Sakotsu ni karui hibi ga haitte imasu.
You have a small fracture in your collarbone.

Hiza ni mizu ga tamatte iru yōdesu.
You may have fluid in your knee.

11. More useful expressions for the orthopedist:

Gibusu o maite kotei shimasu.	I will put a cast on you.
Shibaraku kono mama de ite kudasai.	Please keep it on for a while.
Nurasa-nai yōni shite kudasai.	Please keep it dry.
Undō ya, aruki-sugi ni ki o tsukete kudasai.	Please be careful not to exercise and walk too much
Shibaraku kyūyō shite kudasai.	You should rest for a while.
Kenin-ryōhō shita hō ga ii desu ne.	You should have traction therapy.
Mainichi rihabiri ni kayotte kudasai.	Please come to the physical therapy every day.
Korusetto ga hitsuyō desu ne.	You need to wear a corset.
Basuto-bando o tsukete kudasai.	Please put on the chest tape.
Yoru wa hazushite oyasumi kudasai.	Please take it off when you sleep at night.

12. The names of sports

A common explanation for an injury is "**Supōtsu de kega o shimashita**" "I was injured in sports," or "**Supōtsu o shite-ite kegao shimashita**" "While I was playing sports, I got hurt." The following are the names of some popular sports.

ENGLISH	JAPANESE	ENGLISH	JAPANESE
baseball	**yakyū**	tennis	**tenisu**
running, track	**rikujyō**	soccer	**sakkā**
swimming	**sui-ei**	volleyball	**barei-bōru**
gymnastics	**taisō**	basketball	**basukketo-bōru**
walking	**sanpo**	ice hockey	**aisu hokkei**

Language Roots

The word **kotsu** (骨) means "bone." It's also pronounced **hone**.

kotsu-ban	pelvis
ro-kkotsu	rib
daitai-kotsu	thighbone

The word **niku** (肉) indicates flesh, body, meat, muscle.

kin-niku	muscle
niku-tai	flesh, body
niku-gan	naked eye
niku-banare	torn muscle

The word **tsui** (椎) indicates the spine and vertebral column.

yō-tsui	lumbar spine
kei-tsui	cervical spine
seki-tsui	vertebral column
tsui-kanban	intervertebral disk

Seiki-Geka Yōhin (Orthopedic Supports)

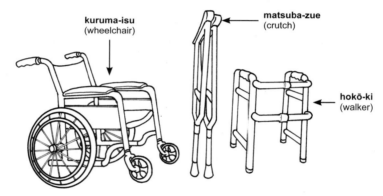

kuruma-isu
(wheelchair)

matsuba-zue
(crutch)

hokō-ki
(walker)

Culture Notes

Understanding and encouraging patients

Japanese health practitioners often say "**Sō-desu-ka, Sore wa taihen desu ne.**" "Is that so? I am sorry to hear that," while asking questions of patients. This expression suggests to the patient that the health practitioner has listened to the patient's complaints and understands the patient's hardship.

The origin of **matsuba-zue** (crutch)

Japanese call crutches **matsuba-zue**. Literally, **matsu** means "pine tree," -**ba(ha)** means "leaf," and **zue (tsue)** means "stick." Japanese pine needles are of a forked or bifurcated shape, and for that reason crutches are named after them.

The origin of **gibusu** (cast)

Japanese call casts **gibusu**. Japan was strongly influenced by Western medicine from the Netherlands during the Edo Period (1603–1868) and from Germany during the Meiji Period (1868–1912), and in Dutch and German casts are called Gips or Gibbs, respectively. For that reason, Japanese still use the word **gibusu** today.

Comprehension

Answer the following questions.

1. Which of the following does NOT belong with the others?
   a. **Hasamu**   b. **Sasareru**
   c. **Kanō**   d. **Utsu**

2. Which of the following could NOT be used to express a doctor's opinion?
   a. **Kossetsu mitai desu.**   b. **Kansetsu-en desu ka.**
   c. **Dakkyū ni chigai arimasen.**   d. **Nenza kamo shiremasen.**

3. Which of the following best completes the sentence below?
   Kanjya wa sensei (   ) migi-ashi no kensa o shite moraimashita.
   (The patient had his/her right leg examined by the doctor.)
   a. **kara**   b. **node**
   c. **made**   d. **ni**

4 You are trying to build trust with a patient. In order to understand the patient's complaint and suffering, which of the following expressions should you say to the patient?
   a. **Sore wa taihen desu ne.**   b. **So dewa arimasen.**
   c. **Soko ga chigai-masu.**   d. **Tsuki-yubi kamo.**

Select the appropriate meaning from the list below.

5. **Kenshō-en dewa naika to omoimasu.**   (   )
6. **Mita tokoro, migi-hiza ga orete iru yō desu.**   (   )
7. **Hi ni sawatta totan ni, migi-te o yakedo shimashita.** (   )
8. **Kanjya-san wa sensei kara shindan-sho o moraimashia.** (   )
9. **Hako o ageru dakede, koshi ga itai(n) desu.**   (   )

a. The patient received an excuse from the doctor.
b. I think you probably have tendonitis.
c. The moment I touched the fire, I burned my right hand.
d. I have back pain just when I lift the box.
e. In my estimation, you have broken your right knee.

Practice

Respond to the following in Japanese using the cues that have been provided.

1. Naming symptoms.
   (Patient)   (Healthcare professional)
   1. **Daboku shimashita.**   _____
                                          (You have a bruise mark.)
   2. **Hiza ga itai(n) desu.**   _____
                                          (You have a fracture on your left knee.)
   3. **Kata ga ugokimasen.**   _____
                                          (You probably have a dislocation.)
   4. **Ashi-kubi ga itakute ugokimasen.** _____
                                          (You have sprained your right ankle.)
   5. **Hito-sashi-yubi ga itai(n) desu.** _____
                                          (You have a splinter in your index finger.)

2. Instructing the patient.
   (Patient)   (Healthcare professional)
   1. **Hiza ga itai(n) desu.**   _____
                                          (Please bend your knee.)
   2. **Koshi ga itai(n) desu.**   _____
                                          (Please stretch your back.)
   3. **Kubi ga itai(n) desu.**   _____
                                          (Please turn your neck.)
   4. **Katakori ga shimasu.**   _____
                                          (Please move your shoulder up and down.)
   5. **Gikkuri-goshi mitai desu.**   _____
                                          (Please move your back slowly.)

3. Giving advice to the patient.
   (Patient)   (Healthcare professional)
   1. **Koshi ga itai(n) desu.**   _____
                                          (You should have traction therapy.)
   2. **Ashi ga mukun de imasu.**   _____
                                          (You need to apply a cold pack.)
   3. **Kossetsu shimashita.**   _____
                                          (Your need to have a cast.)

4. **Muchi-uchi-shō mitai desu.** _____

(You need to wear a corset.)

5. **Hiza ga itai(n) desu.** _____

(Please be careful of doing too much exercise.)

4. Dialogue comprehension. Based on the dialogue, answer the following questions.
   1. **Kato-san wa doko o itame mashita ka.** _____
   2. **Kato-san no ashi wa shibirete imasu ka.** _____
   3. **Kato-san wa itsu itami ga arimasu ka.** _____
   4. **Kato-san wa hōsan-tsū ga arimasu ka.** _____
   5. **Dochira no ashi o ageru to itai(n) desu ka.** _____
   6. **Kato-san no byōmei wa nan desu ka.** _____

5. Free response questions.
   (Questions)   (Answers)
   1. **Ima katakori ga shimasu ka.** _____
   2. **Kotsu-ban wa seijyō desu ka.** _____
   3. **Yōtsū wa itakatta desu ka.** _____
   4. **Akiresu-ken o kitta koto ga arimasu ka.** _____
   5. **Muchi-uchi-shō ni natta koto ga arimasu ka.** _____

Exercises

1. Say the following words in Japanese.
   A. Sprains _____
   B. Dislocate _____
   C. Bruise _____
   D. Broken _____
   E. Crack _____

2. Say the following in Japanese.
   A. I think you probably have sciatica. _____
   B. The patient had a cast put on by the doctor. _____
   C. At the moment of opening the door, I pinched my thumb. _____
   D. I got a fracture just by hitting here. _____
   E. In my estimation, you've torn a ligament in your right leg. _____

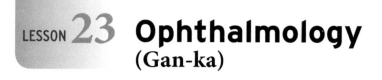

LESSON 23 Ophthalmology
(Gan-ka)

Basic Vocabulary (CD 23-1)

Listen to the CD and repeat the vocabulary.

1.	eyesight/vision/visual acuity	**shiryoku**	視力
2.	eye chart	**shiryoku kensa-hyō**	視力検査表
3.	damage to vision/impaired vision	**shiryoku shōgai**	視力障害
4.	visual correction	**shiryoku kyōsei**	視力矯正
5.	eyestrain	**gansei-hirō**	眼精疲労
6.	bloodshot	**jyū-ketsu**	充血
7.	mucous discharge from eyes	**me-yani**	目やに
8.	tear	**namida**	涙
9.	floaters	**hibun-shō**	飛蚊症
10.	dry eye	**gan-kansō**	眼乾燥
11.	bleary eyes	**kasumu**	翳む
12.	distort	**yugami**	歪み
13.	sty	**mono-morai**	ものもらい
14.	trichiasis	**sakasa matsuge**	逆さ睫毛
15.	blinking	**mabataki**	瞬き
16.	nearsighted/shortsighted/myopic	**kin-shi**	近視
17.	false nearsighted/pseudo myopia	**kasei-kin-shi**	仮性近視
18.	farsighted	**en-shi**	遠視
19.	presbyopia	**rō-gan**	老眼
20.	blepharitis	**ganken-en**	眼瞼炎
21.	conjunctivitis	**ketsumaku-en**	結膜炎
22.	color blind	**shiki-mō**	色盲
23.	lost vision/blindness	**shitsu-mei**	失明
24.	astigmatic	**ran-shi**	乱視
25.	cross-eyed/bad squint	**sha-shi**	斜視
26.	night blindness	**tori-me**	鳥目
27.	cataract	**hakuni-shō**	白内障
28.	glaucoma	**ryokunai-shō**	緑内障
29.	retinal detachment	**mōmaku-hakuri**	網膜剥離
30.	epidemic keratoconjunctivitis/pinkeye	**ryūkō-sei-kaku-ketsumaku-en/hayari-me**	流行性角結膜炎/はやり目

Gankyū (Eyeball)

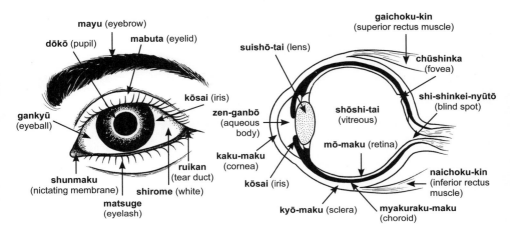

mayu (eyebrow)
dōkō (pupil)
mabuta (eyelid)
suishō-tai (lens)
gaichoku-kin (superior rectus muscle)
chūshinka (fovea)
kōsai (iris)
zen-ganbō (aqueous body)
shōshi-tai (vitreous)
shi-shinkei-nyūtō (blind spot)
gankyū (eyeball)
kaku-maku (cornea)
kōsai (iris)
mō-maku (retina)
naichoku-kin (inferior rectus muscle)
shunmaku (nictating membrane)
ruikan (tear duct)
shirome (white)
matsuge (eyelash)
kyō-maku (sclera)
myakuraku-maku (choroid)

Dialogue (CD 23-2)

Listen to the CD and repeat the dialogue.

At the Ophthalmology Clinic

Dr. Meyer (female doctor): **Kyō wa dō nasare mashita ka.**
Are you concerned about anything today?

Mr. Suzuki: **Sūjitsu-mae kara, me ga jyūketsu-shi, me mo harerushi, hikari ga mabushī node shinsatsu o onegaishimasu.**
Since a few days ago, my eyes have been red, my eyelids have been swollen, and the light is dazzling, I would like to have an examination.

Soreni, me-yani mo dete kimashita. Sarani, me ga gogo-gogo shimasu.
I have some discharge, too. And my eyes feel gritty.

Dr. Meyer: **Sō desu ka. Sore wa taihen desu ne.**
Is that so? I am sorry to hear that.

Dewa, kensa o shite mimashō ka.
Well, shall we examine you?

Kochira o yoku mite kudasai.
Please look to this side.

Mr. Suzuki: **Hai, kore de ii desu ka.**
Yes, is this all right (to look over here)?

Dr. Meyer:	**Me ga enshō o okoshite iru yō desu ne.**
	Your eyes looks like you have an inflammation, don't you?
	Dewa, sanpuru o totte, me no kensa o shite mimashō ka.
	Shall we test your eyes by taking a sample?
Mr. Suzuki:	**Hai, onegai shimasu.**
	Yes, thank you.

(After 20 minutes)

Dr. Meyer:	**Suzuki-san, kensa no kekka ga demashita. Ryūkōsei kaku ketsu-maku-en toiu uirusu-sei no ketsumaku-en desu. Iwayuru, haya-rime desu ne.**
	Mr. Suzuki, we have the test results. It's epidemic keratoconjunctivitis, which is a viral type of conjunctivitis. This is the so-called pinkeye.
Mr. Suzuki:	**Byōki wa naorimasu ka.**
	Can it (this illness) be cured?
Dr. Meyer:	**Osoraku, ni-san shū-kan teido de yokunaru to omoimasu.**
	I think you probably will be cured in two to three weeks.
	Kansen o yobō-suru tame ni kōkin-zai no tengan-yaku to, enshō o osaeru tame ni suteroido no tengan-yaku o dashimasu node, ichinichi ni shi-go kai, ten-gan shite kudasai ne.
	I will prescribe you an antibacterial eyedrop for preventing infections, and steroid eyedrops to reduce the inflammation, so please use both drops four to five times a day.
	Sorekara, kansen o fusegu tame ni, me ni sawattari, kosuttari shi-nai de kudasai.
	And then, in order to prevent further infection, you should avoid doing things like touching or rubbing your eyes.
	Yoku sekken nado de, te o aratte kudasai ne.
	Please wash your hands often with soap.
	Sarani, taoru nado o hokano hito to kyōyū shinai de kudasai ne.
	Furthermore, please don't share towels or things with other people.
	Saigo-ni, sūjitsu-kan, shigoto wa yasumu koto ni naru to omoimasu.
	I think you should stay away from work for few days.
	Jyūbun kyūyō shite kudasai.
	Please get plenty of rest.

Soredewa, i-sshū-kan-go ni mata kenshin ni kite kudasai ne.
Well then, please visit us for a checkup again in a week.

Odaiji ni.
(Please) Take care.

Grammar

1. ## The constructions VERB or i-ADJECTIVE + -shi and NOUN/na-ADJECTIVE + -dashi

The conjunction -**shi** means "and" in an emphatic way. It is usually translated as "not only . . . but also . . ; and what's more; so; and." -**shi** is placed just after a stem verb, i-adjective, or negative form in this construction. For nouns and **na**-adjectives, -**da** is affixed to **shi** to make -**dashi**.

> **Oishī gohan mo tabetashi, kusuri mo nondashi, chōshi ga iishi, genki ni natta.**
> I not only eat good meals but also take medicine and am in good condition, so I have become healthy.

> **Me no jyūketsu mo naishi, gan-sei-hirō mo naishi, shiryoku mo waruku nai desu.**
> I do not have bloodshot eyes, and what's more I do not have eyestrain or weakened vision

> **Shiryoku kensa o shitara, ran-shi dashi, shikimō-dashi, ketsumaku-en nimo kakatte imashita.**
> When I examined your eyes, you appeared to have an astigmatism, color blindness, and conjunctivitis.

2. ## The quote marker **toiu**

The quote marker **toiu** is a combination of **to** (and) and **iu** (say) that identifies the noun preceding it as what something or someone is called or named. Healthcare professionals could use this expression to rephrase or explain a phrase that follows it. It is often translated as "called, that says, that, which."

> **Kono kusuri wa shiryoku shōgai toiu fukusayō ga arimasu.**
> This medicine has a side effect that is called visual impairment.

> **Ryūkō-sei kaku ketsumaku-en toiu uirusu-sei no ketsumaku-en desu.**
> It's epidemic keratoconjunctivitis, which is a viral type of conjunctivitis.

> **Kanjya ga shitsu-mei shita toiu shirase o kikimashita.**
> I heard the news that the patient has lost his/her vision.

Kasei-kinshi toiu byōki ni natta koto ga arimasu ka.
Have you ever been affected an illness called false nearsightedness?

When **toiu** is used at the end of sentences, it is translated as "I heard that; they say; it is said that." When using a noun or **na**-adjective, **da** must be placed in front of **toiu**.

Kensa no kekka, kanjya wa hakunai-shō datoiu.
I heard that the patient has a cataract according to the test result.

Kanjya no hanashi ni yoruto, sensei no chiryō wa jyōzu datoiu koto desu.
According to the patient, the doctor's treatment is said to be skillful.

3. The expression **iwayuru**

The expression **iwayuru** specifies a rephrasing in the sentence that follows it. **Iwayuru** is translated as "what is called; as it is called; the so-called; so to speak."

So no enshō wa iwayuru kesumaku-en desu.
That inflammation is what is called conjunctivitis.

Sensei wa iwayuru mei-i dato omoimasu.
I think that doctor is what you call a great doctor.

Hayari-me ga iwayuru kansen-sei no tsuyoi kesumaku-en desu.
So-called pinkeye is actually a highly contagious form of conjunctivitis.

4. The adverb **osoraku (wa)**

The adverb **osoraku** expresses a range between possibility and probability and translates as "probably, likely, perhaps, possibly." Expressions with **osoraku** sometimes use **osoraku wa** as the grammatical subject when the actual subject is clear in order to avoid repeating it.

Kono shōjyō wa osoraku hakunai-shō desu ne.
This symptom is probably a cataract.

Osowaku wa mōmaku-hakuri no yōdesu.
It's likely retinal detachment.

Osoraku, kensa no kekka wa ashita okurarete kimasu.
Perhaps the test result will arrive tomorrow.

5. The verb **osoreru/osoremasu**

The verb **osoreru/osoremasu** means "worry, concern" and connotes a special seriousness or gravity. When a healthcare professional speaks of a patient's serious condition, she or he may do so using the constructions NOUN plus **no osore ga arimasu** or STEM VERB OF THE PRESENT TENSE plus **osore ga arimasu** (it is worrisome/a matter of concern that).

> **Kanjya wa hakunai-shō no osore ga arimasu.**
> It is worrisome that the patient probably has cataracts.

> **Kanjya wa shitsu-mei suru osore ga arimasu.**
> It is a matter of (grave) concern that the patient might lose his vision.

6. The constructions NOUN + **no tame(ni)** and VERB + **tame(ni)**

The constructions NOUN plus **no tame(ni)** and VERB plus **tame(ni)** express purpose, benefit, reason, and cause. In this construction, the dictionary form of the verb and **i**-adjective use **tame ni** only, but nouns and **na**-adjectives must use **no** with **tame ni**. The construction is usually translated as "for; for the purpose of; for the sake of; for the benefit of; for the good of; on behalf of; in order to; because of." To place more emphasis on the purpose, benefit, reason, and cause, the particle **ni** can be dropped.

> **Gan-atsu-kensa no tame (ni) migi-me o ōkiku akete kudasai.**
> For (the purpose of) the intraocular pressure test, please open wide your right eye.

> **Gantei kensa suru tame (ni) kengan-kyō o tsukaimasu.**
> To examine the fundus of your eye, I will use an ophthalmoscope.

> **In-nai kansen o fusegu tame (ni), shōdoku o shitahō ga ii to omoimasu.**
> I think it's better to sterilize hospital rooms in order to prevent nosocomial infection.

7. The phrase **-tari . . . -tari**

The phrase **-tari . . . -tari** is used to express a series of two or more actions or states. The phrase can be translated as "do things like; and; or sometimes X and sometimes Y." When placed after a stem verb that ends in **-mu**, **-tari** is pronounced and spelled **-dari**. If **-tari suru/shimasu** is not the final statement in a sentence, **suru** may be dropped.

> **Me ni sawattari, kosuttari shinai de kudasai.**
> You should not do things like touch and rub your eyes.

Me o aketari tojitari shite kudasai.
Please open and close your eyes.

Me ga kasundari, namida ga detari shimasu ka.
Are your eyes bleary and tearing up? (*lit.,* Do you have bleary and tearing up eyes?)

Soshite, me o aketari (shimasu).
And open your eyes.

8. The phrase **koto ni naru/narimasu**

The phrase **koto ni naru/narimasu** is used when some decision or arrangement is made by others, for example, when something happens because of circumstances beyond your control or something has been decided by others. It may be translated as "it will be decided that; come about; be arranged that; turn out that."

Byōki ga utsuru koto ni narimasu.
The illness turns out to be contagious.

Ashita kensa no kekka ga wakaru koto ni narimasu.
They've arranged for the test result to be available tomorrow.

Tengan-yaku no okage de, mono-morai ga naoru koto ni narimasu.
Thanks to the eyedrops, the sty will be cured.

Koto ni natte iru is used to express a custom, a scheduled event, or a rule or expectation in the sense of an ongoing arrangement. The ongoing arrangement might be for a one-time event, like an appointment, for example, or for a recurring event, The phrase **koto ni natte iru** reflects that some decision made by others took place in the past and is still in effect, so that it has becomes an arrangement, a rule, a custom, or part of a schedule.

Rai-shū, kensa o suru koto ni natte imasu.
I am scheduled to have an examination next week.

Kyō shigoto ni iku koto ni natte imashita.
It was arranged that I go to work today.

Mai-nichi, me-gusuri o sasu koto ni natte imasu.
I am scheduled to use eyedrops every day.

In contrast, **koto ni suru** indicates a decision, arrangement, desire, preference, or option made by oneself. **Koto ni suru** is translated as "decide to."

Me-gusuri no kawari ni nankō o tsukau koto ni shimasu.
Instead of eyedrops, I decided to use ointment.

Useful Expressions (CD 23-3)

Listen to the CD and repeat the sentences.

1. **Me ga jyūketsu shite imasu.** Your eyes are bloodshot.
2. **Me-yani ga demasu ka.** Do you have a mucous discharge from your eyes?
3. **Shiryoku ga dandan ochite imasu ne.** Your eyesight is getting worse, isn't it?
4. **Chīsai moji ga kasunde miemasu.** Small print looks bleary/dim.
5. **San-nen mae ni mōmaku-hakuri o okoshi mashita.** I had a retinal detachment three years ago.
6. **Migi me no hakunai-shō no shujyutsu o shimashita.** I had an operation for the cataract in my right eye.
7. **Shiryoku shōgai no kanōsei ga arimasu.** There is a possibility you may have damage to your vision.
8. **Mabataki o suru-to itai(n) desu ka.** Do you have pain when blinking?
9. **Mono ga ni-jyū ni miemasu ka.** Are you seeing double?
10. **Shiya ga semaku natta yō desu.** I am afraid my visual field has narrowed.

Key Sentences (CD 23-4)

Listen to the CD and repeat the sentences.

1. **Me ni jyūketsu mo nakunatta-shi, me-yani mo nakunatta-shi, kasumi mo nakunatta-shi, yoku narimashita yo.**
   Your eyes aren't bloodshot anymore, and what's more, you no longer have a mucous discharge or bleary vision, and (your eyes) seem healthy..
2. **Ganken-en to-iu byōki ni natta koto ga arimasu ka.** Have you ever had an illness called blepharitis?
3. **Kensa no tame(ni) ryō-me o ōkiku akete kudasai.** For (the purpose of) the examination, please open both your eyes wide.
4. **Me ni sawattari, kosuttari shinai de kudasai.** You should not do things like touch and rub your eyes.
5. **Ketsumaku-en wa utsuru koto ni narimasu.** The conjunctivitis turns out to be contagious.

Additional Words

arau/araimasu wash
kawaru/kawarimasu change/ substitute
boyakeru/boyakemasu dim
tojiru/tojimasu close (for eye, book, and curtain)
nai-shashi crossed eye
gai-shashi wall eye
shiro-me wandering eye (or wall eye)
ni-jyū double
san-jyū triple
moji letter
nan-jyū multiple vision
kyōyū share
sekken soap
kontakuto-renzu contact lens
mei-i good doctor; excellent physician
kyōsei-shiryoku corrected vision
rēshikku-shujyutsu lasik surgery

kakumaku-kansen-shō corneal infection
ganshin kensa nystagmus test
kakumaku kansō-shō corneal xerosis
ragan naked eye
shiryoku-kyōsei-shujyutsu vision correcting surgery
nijyū-shōten renzu bifocal lenses
fuku-shi double vision
shiryoku-shōgai-sha blind person/ visually impaired person
kengan-kyō ophthalmoscope
shiya-kensa visual field test
kyōsei renzu corrective lenses
enkin ryōyō renzu progressive lenses
gantei-kensa eye ground test
gan-atsu-kensa intraocular pressure
kussetsu-ritsu kensa refractive index test

Language Notes

1. The following are some expressions for complaints in ophthalmology. As usual, to make the statements into questions, add **ka** to the end of sentences. This is a handy way to check a patient's symptoms.

Me ga itai(n) desu.	My eyes are sore.
Me ga kayui(n) desu.	My eyes feel itchy.
Mabuta ga piku-piku shimasu.	My eyelid is twitching.
Me ga goro goro shimasu.	My eyes feel gritty/sandy.
Me ga chika chika shimasu.	My eyes feel like they are flickering.
Me ga hiri hiri shimasu.	My eyes sting.
Me ga chiku chiku shimasu.	I have a prickling sensation in my eyes.
Me ga atsui kanji desu.	My eyes feel hot.
Me ga jyūketsu shite imasu.	My eyes are bloodshot.
Me ga kasumi masu.	My vision is bleary.
Mono ga bonyari miemasu.	My sight seems dim.
Mono ga kasunde miemasu.	Distant things look blurry.
Namida ga tomarimasen.	My eyes tear/tear up constantly.
Me-yani ga demasu.	I have a (mucous) discharge from my eyes.

| **Mabuta ga keiren shite imasu.** | My eyelid is spasming/I have spasms in my eyelid. |
| **Mabataki ga shinikui desu.** | I am having trouble blinking. |

2. The Japanese language does not have many syllables or sound combinations, and therefore there are often two or more words that have the same sound and/or the same spelling but differ in meaning. The verb **sasu** represents eight of these homophones. It means: 1) raise an umbrella, 2) sandbank, 3) pierce/stab, 4) point/select, 5) shine, 6) insert, 7) pour, and 8) light (a fire). In the case of **megusuri o sasu**, the seventh meaning of the verb is the one that pertains: "pour (eye) drops into the eyes."

To ask how many objects the patients can see, you use the phrase **Nan-jyū ni miemasu ka** (How many can you see?). **Nan-jyū** means "how many times." Generally, the interrogative pronoun **nan** means "what." However, with numbers **nan** changes its meaning to "how many" when used interrogatively and "several" or "many" when it is not. The **jyū** becomes a counter for double or multiple (vision) and the number of images perceived.

| **ni-jyū** | double | **san-jyū** | triple |
| **nan-jyū** | how many (images) | **nan-byaku** | hundreds |

Mono ga ni-jyū ni miemasu.	I see it double (twice).
Moji ga san-jyū ni miemasu.	I see the letter triple (three letters).
Moji ga nan-jyū nimo miemasu ka.	Can you see the letter with many layers?
Yubi ga nanbon miemasu ka	How many fingers do you see?
Nan-jyū nimo miemasu.	I see several (images/visions).

3. Comparison of vision test scores used by the United States and Japan

(To convert, follows this rule: 20 divided by 20 = 1.0; 20 divided by 40 = 0.5)

Snellen Chart (USA)	Landolt Ring (Japan)	Snellen Chart (USA)	Landolt Ring (Japan)
20/10	2.0	20/100	0.2
20/13	1.53	20/200	0.1
20/16	1.25	20/250	0.08
20/20 or 30/30	1.0	20/400	0.05
20/25	0.8	20/500	0.04
20/30	0.67	20/800	0.025
20/40	0.5	20/1000	0.02
20/50	0.4	20/2000	0.01
20/70	0.28		

Japanese say **ten** for "point." "Equals" is pronounced **wa**. Some examples of measures of visual acuity are as follows:

20/16 = 1.5	**ni-jyū, jyū-roku wa ichi ten go desu.**
20/20 = 1.0	**ni-jyū, ni-jyū wa ichi ten zero desu.**
20/40 = 0.5	**ni-jyū, yon-jyū wa rei ten go desu.**

4. The following expressions are used frequently when checking the eyes.

Kono yubi o mite kudasai.	Please look at this finger.
Kono yubi o otte kudasai.	Please follow this finger.
Me o migi-hidari ni ugokashite kudasai.	Please move your eye to the left and right.
Ue o mite kudasai.	Please look up.
Shita o mite kudasai.	Please look down.
Migi o mite kudasai.	Please look to the right side.
Hidari o mite kudasai.	Please look to the left side.
Hikari ga miemasu ka.	Can you see the light?
Moji ga miemasu ka.	Can you see the letter?
Moji ga yomemasu ka.	Can you read the letter?
Ichi-ban shita no moji ga yomemasu ka.	Can you read the last line (of letters)?
Shita kara ni-ban-me no moji ga yomemasu ka.	Can you read the next-to-last line?

Language Roots

The word **shi** (視) relates to vision, sight, and the visual.

shi-ryoku	vision/ eyesight
kin-shi	nearsighted
en-shi	farsighted

The word **gan** (眼) means "eyeball" and in compounds indicates the eye.

gan-ka	ophthalmology
gan-sei-hirō	eyestrain
rō-gan	presbyopia

Culture Notes

Health professionals as intellectuals and paragons of politeness

Japanese was first a phonetic or spoken language; later the Japanese adopted Chinese characters for writing. Because of this history, Japanese has two ways of reading the Chinese characters, or kanji, that are used in the written language: **kun** and **on**. Kun-reading (**kun** literally means "reading") is so-called Japanese-style, in which only one kanji corresponds to a given word. **On**-reading (**on** literally means "sound reading") is so-called Chinese-style, in which more than one kanji correspond to a word, which makes for a more intellectual, or intellectually challenging, language. Because of this, Japanese usually has two expressions for the same thing, such as **megusuri** and **tengan-yaku** for "eyedrops," or **megane** and **gankyō** for "eyeglasses." In daily usage, **megane** is the customary term. Generally, only well-educated people or intellectuals would use the **On**-reading, **gankyō**, and so **gankyō** is considered formal. Similarly, **megusuri** is standard Japanese, but **tengan-yaku** is much more formal. Healthcare professionals in Japan commonly use the formal terms.

Health-related Japanese proverbs XI

Feed a cold and starve a fever.
Kaze niwa taishoku, netsu niwa zesshoku.
風邪には大食、熱には絶食

A disease known is half cured.
Yamai o shire-ba, iyuru-ni chikashi.
病を知れば癒ゆるに近し

Comprehension

Answer the following questions.

1. Which of the following does NOT belong with the others?
   a. **Mabataki**　　　b. **Monomorai**
   c. **Enshō**　　　d. **Jyūketsu**

2. Which of the following could NOT be used to say discomfort of the eyes?
   a. **Me ga goro-goro shimasu.**　b. **Me ga doki-doki shimasu.**
   c. **Me ga chika-chika shimasu.**　d. **Me ga hiri-hiri shimasu.**

3. Which of the following best completes the sentence below?
   Enshō o fusegu (　　), tengan-yaku o sashite kudasai.
   It is better to use eyedrops for the sake of preventing inflammation.
   a. **shika**　　　b. **toiu**
   c. **dake**　　　d. **tame**

4. The patient is telling you about a symptom. Which of the following means "My eyes are bleary?"
   a. **Me ga jyūketsu shite imasu.**
   b. **Me ga kasumi masu.**
   c. **Me ga kayui desu.**
   d. **Me ga itai desu.**

Select the appropriate meaning from the list below.

5. **Ketsumaku-en wa uturu kono ni narimasu.** ( )
6. **Me ni jyūketsu mo arimasu shi, me-yani mo arimasu shi,** ( )
   yokunai yō desu.
7. **Kakumaku-en toiu byōki ni natta koto ga arimasu ka.** ( )
8. **Tengan-yaku no tame(ni) migi-me o ōkiku akete kudasai.** ( )
9. **Me ni sawattari, kosuttari shinai de kudasai.** ( )

a. For the (purpose of) eyedrops, please open your right eye wide.
b. You have bloodshot eyes, and what's more, you have a mucous discharge, and it does not look good.
c. The conjunctivitis turns out to be contagious.
d. Have you ever had an illness called inflammation of the cornea?
e. You should not do things like touch and rub your eyes.

Practice

Respond to the following in Japanese using the cues that have been provided.

1. Asking questions about the symptoms.
   (Patient)   (Healthcare professional)
   1. **Me ga itai(n) desu.**   _____

                                       (Do you have pain when blinking?)
   2. **Me ga harete imasu.**   _____

                                       (Can you open both eyes wide?)
   3. **Me-yani ga demasu.**   _____

                                       (Did you take eyedrops?)
   4. **Me ga kayui(n) desu.**   _____

                                       (Did you touch and rub your eyes.)
   5. **Chīsai moji ga kasunde miemasu.** _____

                                       (Are you seeing double?)

2. Directing the patient's eye movement.
   (Patient)   (Healthcare professional)
   1. Need to look up.   _____
   2. Need to look down.   _____
   3. Need to look to the left side. _____
   4. Need to look to the right side _____
   5. Need to follow doctor's finger. _____

3. How do you say the following conditions in Japanese?
   (Conditions)   (Healthcare professional)
   1. Patient feels prickling sensation in eyes.   _____
   2. Patient's eyes see or experience a flickering. _____
   3. Patient's eyes feel gritty or sandy.   _____
   4. Patient's eyes sting.   _____
   5. Patient's eyelid is twitching.   _____

4. Dialogue comprehension. Based on the dialogue, answer the following questions.
   1. **Suzuki-san wa itsu kara me no chōshi ga warui(n) desu ka.**

   _____

   2. **Suzuki-san no me wa don-na yōsu desu ka.**

   _____

   3. **Suzuki-san no byōmei wa nan desu ka.**

   _____

   4. **Me ga yoku-naru made, donokurai kakari masu ka.**

   _____

   5. **Kansen o fusegu tame(ni), nani ga hitsuyō desu ka.**

   _____

   6. **Suzuki-san wa itsu mata shinsatsu ni kimasu ka.**

   _____

5. Free response questions.
   (Questions)   (Healthcare professional)
   1. **Saikin, shiryoku-kensa o ukemashita ka.**   _____
   2. **Gansei hirō ga arimasu ka.**   _____
   3. **Me ga kasun-dari, namida ga detari shimasu** _____
      ka.
   4. **Kinshi desu ka, enshi desu ka.**   _____
   5. **Megane o kakemasu ka.**   _____

Exercises

1. Say the following words in Japanese.
   A. Bad squint   _____
   B. Night blindness   _____
   C. Color blind   _____
   D. Astigmatic   _____
   E. Lost vision   _____

2. Say the following expressions in Japanese.
   A. For the checkup, please open wide your left eye first.
   B. You have a bloodshot eye, and what's more, you have a mucous discharge, and it does not look good.
   C. This inflammation turns out to be contagious.
   D. Have you ever had an illness called conjunctivitis?
   E. You should not do things like touch and rub your eyes.

3. How do you ask your patients the following questions in Japanese?
   A. Do you see the small print as bleary or dim?
   B. When did you have a detached retina (or retinal detachment)?
   C. Is there an operation to correct the cataract in my right eye?
   D. Do you have pain when blinking?
   E. Do you see double?

4. Answer the following questions in Japanese.

   Q: **Me ga tottemo harete iru no desu ga.**
   A: _____
       (I think you probably have an infection.)

   Q: **Me ga sukoshi itai(n) desu.**
   B: _____
       (For the checkup, please open your right eye wide.)

   Q: **Nanika ki o tsukeru koto ga arimasu ka.**
   C: _____
       (You should not do things like rub your eyes.)

LESSON 24 Otolaryngology: Ear, Nose, and Throat
(Jibi-inkō-ka)

Basic Vocabulary (CD 24-1)

Listen to the CD and repeat the vocabulary.

1.	pollen allergy/hay fever	**kafun-shō**	花粉症
2.	discharge from ear	**mimi-dare**	耳垂れ
3.	ear infection	**mimi-kabure**	耳かぶれ
4.	earwax	**mimi-aka**	耳垢
5.	inflammation of external ear/otitis external	**gaiji-en**	外耳炎
6.	inflammation of middle ear/otitis media	**chūji-en**	中耳炎
7.	inflammation of inner ear/otitis interna	**naiji-en**	内耳炎
8.	eardrum	**komaku**	鼓膜
9.	tympanostomy	**komaku-sekkai-jyutsu**	鼓膜切開術
10.	impaired hearing	**nan-chō**	難聴
11.	difficulty hearing high-pitched sound	**kō-on-sei nan-chō**	高音性難聴
12.	difficulty hearing low-pitched sound	**tei-on-sei nan-chō**	低音性難聴
13.	residual hearing	**zan-chō**	残聴
14.	nasal cavity	**bikō/hana no ana**	鼻腔/鼻の穴
15.	rhinitis/inflammation of nasal mucosa	**bi-en**	鼻炎
16.	head and neck cancer	**tō-kei-bu-gan**	頭頸部癌
17.	allergic rhinitis	**arerugī-sei bi-en**	アレルギー性鼻炎
18.	sinus trouble	**chikunō-shō**	蓄膿症
19.	snore	**ibiki**	鼾
20.	sense of smell/olfaction	**kyū-kaku/shū-kaku**	嗅覚/臭覚
21.	saliva	**da-eki**	唾液
22.	stuffed nose/plugged nose	**hana-zumari**	鼻詰まり
23.	nasal voice	**hana-goe**	鼻声
24.	nasal discharge	**hana-kuso**	鼻糞

25.	nose cosmetic surgery	**hana no seikei-shujyutsu**	鼻の整形手術
26.	balloon sinuplasty	**barūn kakuchō-jyutsu**	バルーン拡張術
27.	laryngitis	**kōtō-en**	喉頭炎
28.	vocal polyp	**seitai-porīpu**	声帯ポリープ
29.	physical balance	**heikō-kankaku**	平衡感覚
30.	caloric test	**ondo-ganshin kensa**	温度眼振検査

Dialogue (CD 24-2)

Listen to the CD and repeat the dialogue.

At the Ear, Nose, and Throat Clinic

Dr. Kim (male doctor): **Kyō wa dō sare mashita ka.**
How are you feeling today?

Mrs. Kato: **Hai, kesa, totsuzen(ni) miminari to memai ga shite, tatte irare masen.**
(Yes,) The ringing in my ears and dizziness started all of sudden this morning, and I could not stand up.

Dr. Kim: **Dewa, beddo ni yoko ni natte kudasai.**
Then would you lie down on this bed?

Hakike ya, karada no doko-ka ni shibire ga arimasen ka.
Do you have nausea or numbness in any parts of your body?

Mrs. Kato: **Kesa wa hakike-de kibun ga warukute tamarimasen-deshita ga, karada ni shibire wa arimasen deshita.**
I was extremely nauseous this morning, but I didn't feel any numbness in my hands or body.

Dr. Kim: **Me ya, karada no dokoka(ni) itami ga arimasu ka.**
Do you have any pain in your eyes or other parts of your body?

Mrs. Kato: **Iie, itami wa arimasen.**
There is no pain.

Mr. Kim: **Watakushi no koe ga hakkiri kikoe masu ka.**
Can you hear my voice clearly?

Mrs. Kato: **Hidari-mimi ni kō-on no miminari ga shite, oto ga kikoe nikui desu.**
I have a high-pitched ringing noise in my left ear, and it is difficult to hear.

Dr. Kim: **Soredewa, saikin karada no chōshi wa dōdeshita ka.**
If that is the case, how have you been feeling in general recently?

Mrs. Kato: **Karada no chōshi wa mā-mā desu.**
I have been feeling so-so.

Dr. Kim: **Tabun, naiji no kinō-shōgai darōto omoimasu.**
Then you probably have a functional disorder of your inner ear.

Memai ya, nanchō ya, mimi-nari wa naiji no kinō-teika ni ōi shōjyō desu.
Your dizziness, deafness, and tinnitus are in many cases caused by decreasing internal ear function.

Dewa mazu, ondo-ganshin kensa o shite mimahō ka.
Well, first of all, shall we try a caloric test?

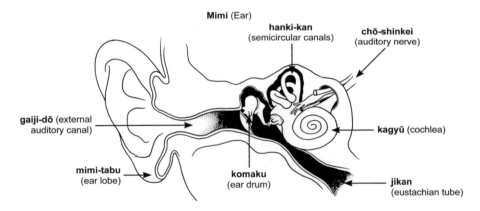

Mimi (Ear)

hanki-kan
(semicircular canals)

chō-shinkei
(auditory nerve)

gaiji-dō (external
auditory canal)

kagyū (cochlea)

mimi-tabu
(ear lobe)

komaku
(ear drum)

jikan
(eustachian tube)

Grammar

1. **The adverb totsuzen(ni)**

The adverb **totsuzen(ni)** indicates a sudden action and translates as "suddenly, abruptly, unexpectedly, all at once." **Kyū ni** also expresses sudden action, but **totsuzen(ni)** suggests a more unexpected suddenness than **kyū ni**.

Totsuzen(ni) mimi-nari ga hajimari mashita.
Suddenly, I've started to have tinnitus.

Totsuzen no nan-chō ni odorokimashita.
I was surprised to have impaired hearing all of a sudden.

(Watakushi wa) tō-kei-bu-gan ga totsuzen-de odorokimashita.
I was shaken when I unexpectedly developed a head and neck cancer.
(*lit.*, A head and neck cancer was developed unexpectedly, so I was shaken.)

2. The construction **te**-form + **iraremasen**

The construction **te**-form plus **iraremasen** means "not be able to do something." It uses both the present progressive form (**te**-form plus **iru/imasu**), which was introduced in Lesson 5, and the suffix -**rareru** that is often used to express patient views and actions and describe symptoms, which we studied in Lesson 18. **Te iraremasen** is the negative form of **te iraremasu**, which means "is able to do something."

> **(Watakushi wa) kuchi o akete iraremasen.**
> I could not open my mouth.
>
> **Mimi ga itakute, sakuban wa nete iraremsen deshita.**
> I had an earache, and because of it I could not sleep last night.
>
> **Kesa kara memai ga shite, tatte iraremasen.**
> My dizziness started this morning, and I could not stand up.
>
> **Sukoshi, tatte iraremasen ka.**
> Can you stand for a moment?

3. The idiomatic expression **tamaranai/tamarimasen**

The idiomatic expression **tamaranai/tamarimasen** can be translated as "terrible, severe, extreme, unbearable" or the related adverbs and conveys the notion of not being able to cope with a situation. **Tamaranai** is an adjective and informal expression, and **tamarimasen** is a verb and formal expression. When using these with a noun, add **de** to make **de tamaranai/tamarimasen**. For **i**-adjectives, drop the -**i** ending and replace it with -**kute tamaranai/tamarimasen**. For verbs, use VERB BASE plus -**takute tamaranai/tamarimasen**.

> **Bi-en de tamarimasen.**
> I have terrible rhinitis. (*lit.*, I cannot cope with rhinitis.)
>
> **Mimi ga itakute tamaranai desu ka.**
> Do you have a severe earache?
>
> **Kono kusuri o nomitakute tamaranai desu.**
> I really, really want to take this medicine.

4. The constructions VERB BASE + -**nikui** and VERB BASE + -**yasui**

The construction VERB BASE plus -**nikui** means "difficult to do (something)," and VERB BASE plus -**yasui** means "easy to do (something)."

Kafun-shō wa tokidoki gaman shi-nikui desu.
Pollen allergies are sometimes difficult to cope with.

Chikunō-shō wa naori-nikui desu.
Sinus trouble is difficult to cure.

Hana-zumari wa naori-yasui desu.
A stuffed-up nose is easy to remedy.

Oto ga kikitori-yasui desu ka, kikitori-nikui desu ka.
Is it easy or difficult to hear the sound?

5. The conjunction **sore-dewa**

In Lesson 8, we studied the conjunction **sore-kara** (and then). In Lesson 11, we saw that **sore-dewa** is used at the beginning of sentences to express the notion of "in that case." It can also be translated as "if so; then; well then." **Sore-dewa** is often shortened to **dewa**, which is further contracted to **jā** in informal usage. **Sore-dewa**, **dewa**, and **jā** are frequently used in Japanese conversation when expressing agreement or concluding a conversation.

Sore-dewa, migi-mimi wa itai(n) desu ka.
Well then, do you have pain in your right ear?

Sore-dewa, kensa o hajime mashō ka.
If so, shall we start the examination?

Dewa, odaiji ni (shite kudasai).
Then please take care.

6. The phrase **darō-to omoimasu**

In Lesson 11, we studied the phrase **to omoimasu** (I think that). **Darō-to omoimasu** expresses probability. Conjugation with **darō-to omoimasu** does not require any change in a noun, adjective, or stem verb.

Bi-en darō-to omoimasu.
I think you probably have rhinitis.

Kōtō-en wa itai(n) darō-to omoimasu.
I think your laryngitis is probably/must be painful.

Kanjya-san wa nan-chō desu ga, sukoshi kikoeru darō-to omoimasu.
The patient has impaired hearing, but I think probably she can hear a little.

7. The words ōi; ōku no; ōzei (many)

The **i**-adjective **ōi** is used to express quantity or number and translates as "many, a lot of, much." **Ōi** usually uses the subject marker **ga** in order to modify its subject.

> **Kodomo ni wa kafun-shō ga ōi desu.**
> There are many pollen allergies among children.

> **Otoshiyori ni wa nanchō-sha ga ōi desu.**
> There are many old people with impaired hearing (*lit.*, There are many impaired-hearing persons among old people).

Ōi is usually not placed in front of a noun, but **ōku no** can modify the noun in this way. It is formed by dropping the -i ending from **ōi** and replacing it with -**ku no** followed by the noun.

> **Ōku no kodomo ga kafun-shō desu.**
> There are many children who suffer from pollen allergies.

> **Ōku no otoshiyori ga nanchō desu.**
> There are many old people have impaired hearing.

Ōku no can be replaced by **takusan no** and **ōzei no** but only for human beings.

> **Byōin niwa ōzei no kanjya ga tsū-in shite imasu.**
> There are many patients who commute to the hospital.

> **Takusan no kanjya ga bi-en ni kakatte imasu.**
> There are many patients who suffer from rhinitis.

> **Byōin niwa takusan no kensa kigu ga arimasu.**
> There are many instruments for performing tests in hospitals.

Though it usually follows a noun (plus **ga**), **ōi** can be placed before the noun it modifies, but in this case it doesn't mark a subject and it usually translates as "typical."

> **Mimi-nari wa naiji no kinō teika ni ōi shōjō desu.**
> Tinnitus is a typical symptom of decreased inner ear function.

> **Ibiki wa chikunō-shō ni ōi shōjyō desu.**
> Snoring is a typical symptom of sinus trouble.

Finally, **ōi**'s antonym **sukunai** expresses the notion of "small in number or quantity" and is usually translated as "few; small number; little; small quantity of." **Sukunai** functions grammatically in the same way as **ōi** but has no form with **ku no**, and both subject markers **ga** or **wa** are acceptable.

Kanjya niwa naiji-en ga sukunai yō desu.
It seems that few people are affected by inflammation of the inner ear.

Seitai-porīpu o toranai hito wa sukunai desu.
A small number of people never have vocal polyps removed.

Useful Expressions (CD 24-3)

Listen to the CD and repeat the sentences.

1. **Mimi-nari ga shimasu ka.** Do you have ringing in your ear?
2. **Mimi-aka ga toremasen.** I can't remove your earwax.
3. **Yoku kushami ga demasu ka.** Do you sneeze a lot?
4. **Hidari-mimi kara mimi-dare ga dete imasu.** You have a discharge from your left ear.
5. **Mimi-aka ga kataku natte shimaimashita.** Your earwax got very hard.
6. **Migi-mimi ni nani-ka haitte imasu.** There is something in your right ear.
7. **Hana ni porīpu ga aruyō desu.** You may have a polyp in your nose.
8. **Hentōsen ga harete imasu.** Your tonsils are swollen.
9. **Sakana no hone ga nodo ni hikkakari mashita.** There is a fish bone stuck in my throat.
10. **Mimi no kansen-shō ni yoku kakarimasu ka.** Do you often have ear infections?

Key Sentences (CD 24-4)

Listen to the CD and repeat the sentences.

1. **Ōku no kanjya ga kafun-shō ni kakatte imasu.** There are many patients who suffer from pollen allergies.
2. **Kuchi o akete iraremasen ka.** Are you still able to open your mouth?
3. **Chikunō-shō de tamarimasen ka.** Do you have terrible sinus trouble?
4. **Kafun-shō wa naori nikui desu.** Allergies to pollen are difficult to cure.
5. **Soredewa, kensa o hajime mashō ka.** Well then, shall we start the examination?

Additional Words

hikkakaru/hikkakemaau stuck in
hairu/hairimasu enter/break into
mazu first of all
hakkiri clearly
kinō-shōgai functional disorder
heikō-kankaku physical balance
kigu tools
hochō-ki tekigō kensa hearing aid test
mimi-kansen-shō ear infection

fusagaru/fusakagimasu be closed/
  blocked
meiro labyrinth
bisoku nasal breathing
kinō-teika decreasing function
(o)toshiyori old people
hochō-ki hearing aid
gaman patience/tolerance
hana-no-ana nostrils

Language Notes

1. There are many expressions for complaints about ear-related symptoms. The onomatopoetic complaint of the patient in the following expressions may help you to understand what kind of pain the patient is suffering from. Adding **ka** at the end of the sentences makes them into questions.

Atama ga guru-guru mawatte imasu.	My head is spinning.
Atama ga furatsukimasu.	I feel dizzy.
Mimi-nari ga shimasu.	I have ringing in my ear.
Mimi ga zukin-zukin itamimasu.	I have a throbbing pain in my ear.
Mimi ga kiri-kiri itamimasu.	I have a tingling pain in my ear.
Mimi ga fusagatte iru kanji desu.	I feel like my ear is plugged up.
Mimi ga yoku kikoemasen.	I have trouble hearing.
Kizetu suru kanji ga shimasu.	I feel like I am about pass out.

2. The following are expressions for complaints related to the nose.

Hana-mizu ga demasu.	I have a runny nose.
Hana ga tsumarimasu.	I have a stuffed up nose.
Hana no naka ni haremono ga arimasu.	I have swelling in my nose.
Itsumo kushami ga demasu.	I am sneezing all the time.
Hana-ji ga demasu.	I have a nosebleed.
Takusan ibiki o shimasu.	I snore a lot.

3. The following are expressions for complaints related to the throat.

Hentōsen ga harete imasu.	My tonsils are swollen.
Nodo ga kawaita kanji desu.	My throat is dry. (*lit.*, I have the feeling of a dry throat.)
Nodo ga igarappoi kanji desu.	My throat is dry, raw, and scratchy.

Nodo ga tsumatta kanji desu.	My throat is clogged up.
Nodo ga gara-gara desu.	I have a raspy throat.
Nodo ga hiri-hiri desu.	I have a sore throat.
Nodo ga harete imasu.	My throat is swollen.
Koe ga demasen.	I lost my voice.
Koe ga karete imasu.	I'm hoarse.
Seki ga demasu.	I have a cough.
Tsuba o nomuto itai(n) desu.	I have pain when swallowing.
Muse masu.	I am choking.

Language Roots

The word **ji** (耳) means "ear" and "hearing" and in compounds indicates these meanings. The same character is also pronounced **mimi**.

chū-ji-en	inflammation of middle ear
ji-kō	ear hole
mimi-nari	tinnitus
mimi-aka	earwax

The word **bi** (鼻) means "nose" and indicates the nose in compounds. The same character is also pronounced **hana**.

bi-soku	nasal breathing
bi-en	rhinitis
hana-mizu	runny nose
hana-goe	nasal voice

Culture Notes

Japanese cannot say "no."

The adverb **mā-mā** expresses the idea of "not enough for satisfaction but almost; not quite; not exactly." Its equivalent in English is *so-so*. Japanese use the expression **mā-mā desu** (*lit.*, This is not enough for satisfaction) when they are not even almost satisfied. For Japanese people, expressing negative or uncomfortable feelings to others is difficult. The cultural values of self-negation and seeking to help others have been ingrained deeply in the Japanese since the arrival of Buddhism and Confucianism in Japan in the sixth century. When they encounter a difficult situation in daily life, Japanese can't say "no" but instead will say **mā-mā desu** and fix the situation by smiling. Most Japanese patients in healthcare facilities may well express their feelings and judgment frankly, but healthcare professionals should be aware of this cultural reticence in order to understand your patients better.

Health-related Japanese proverbs XII

Sickness is a matter of mind (*lit.*, Sickness come from mental weakness).
Yamai wa ki kara.
病は気から

Years know more than books.
Kame no kō yori, toshi no kō.
亀の甲より年の功

Comprehension

Answer the following questions.

1. Which of the following does NOT belong with the others?
   a. **Ibiki**   b. **Mimi-aka**
   c. **Bi-en**   d. **Chikunō-shō**

2. Which of the following could NOT be used to express a complaint about the throat?
   a. **Igarappoi kanji desu**   b. **Gan-gan itai(n) desu.**
   c. **Hiri-hiri itai(n) desu.**   d. **Gara-gara desu.**

3. Which of the following best completes the sentence below?
   Hana ga itakute, saku-ban wa (   ) iraremsen deshita.
   (I had pain in my nose, so I could not sleep last night.)
   a. **shite**   b. **nete**
   c. **kaku**   d. **dete**

4. The patient is telling you about her symptoms. Which of the following expressions means "My tonsils are swollen?"
   a. **Koe ga demasen.**   b. **Nodo ga kayui desu.**
   c. **Hentōsen ga harete imasu.**   d. **Nodo ga kara-kara desu.**

Select the appropriate meaning from the list below.

5. **Sukoshi, tatte iraremasen ka.**   (   )
6. **Ōku no kanjya ga bi-en ni kakatte imasu.** (   )
7. **Soredewa, kensa o hajime mashō ka.**   (   )
8. **Mimi-aka de tamarimasen ka.**   (   )
9. **Kuchi o akete iraremasen ka.**   (   )

a. Do you have excessive earwax?
b. There are many patients who are affected by rhinitis.
c. Are you still able to open your mouth?
d. Can you stand for a moment?
e. Well then, shall we start the examination?

Practice

Respond to the following in Japanese using the cues that have been provided.

1. Understanding the kind of pain from the onomatopoetic complaint of the patient.
   (Patient)   (Healthcare professional)
   1. I have a sore throat.   _____
   2. I have a raspy throat.   _____
   3. I have a throbbing pain in my ear.   _____
   4. I feel like my ear is plugged up.   _____
   5. I feel like my throat is clogged up.   _____

2. Instructing the patient.
   (Patient)   (Healthcare professional)
   1. **Nodo ga harete itai(n) desu.**   _____
                                         (Please open your mouth.)
   2. **Hana no naka ga itai(n) desu.** _____
                                         (Please show me your nostrils.)
   3. **Migi-mimi ga itai(n) desu.**   _____
                                         (Please turn your head to the left.)
   4. **Yoku mimi ga kikoemasen.**   _____
                                         (Then please show me your ears.)
   5. **Yoku kushami ga demasu.**   _____
                                         (Allergies to pollen are difficult to cure.)

3. Describing the symptoms.
   (Patient)   (Healthcare professional)
   1. **Hidari-mimi kara umi ga demasu.**   _____
                                                   (You have a discharge from your left ear.)
   2. **Mimi-aka ga toremasen.**   _____
                                                   (Your earwax is very hard.)
   3. **Hidari mimi ni nani-ka haitte iru yō desu.** _____
                                                   (You may have a polyp in your left ear.)

    4. **Hentōsen ga harete imasu.**

_____

(Your throat is red, and it must hurt when you swallow.)

    5. **Hana no oku ga itakute tamarimasen.**

_____

(You may have an irritation in your nostrils.)

4. Dialogue comprehension. Based on the dialogue, answer the following questions.

    1. **Kato-san wa kesa don-na shōjyō deshita ka.**

_____

    2. **Kato-san wa karada ni shibire ga arimasu ka.**

_____

    3. **Kato-san no hidari-mimi wa don-na shōjyō desu ka.**

_____

    4. **Saikin no Kato-san no karada no chōshi wa dōdesu ka.**

_____

    5. **Kim sensei wa don-na byōmei dato itte imasu ka.**

_____

    6. **Kato-san wa mazu don-na kensa o shimasu ka.**

_____

5. Free response questions.

(Questions)   (Healthcare professional)

    1. **Toki-doki mimi-nari ga shimasu ka.** _____

    2. **Saikin, chōryoku-kensa o ukemashita ka.** _____

    3. **Kafun-shō desu ka.** _____

    4. **Ibiki o kaki masu ka.** _____

    5. **Kaze no toki(ni) hana-goe ni narimasu ka.** _____

Exercises

1. Say the following words or phrases in Japanese.

    A. Snore _____

    B. Rhinitis _____

    C. Allergy to pollen _____

    D. Sinus trouble _____

    E. Impaired hearing _____

2. Say the following in Japanese.
   A. There are many patients who are affected   _____
      by inflammation of the middle ear.
   B. Are you able to stick out your tongue?   _____
   C. Do you have poor residual hearing?   _____
   D. Can you stand for a moment?   _____
   E. Well then, shall we start the checkup?   _____

3. How do you ask your patients the following questions in Japanese?
   A. Do you have ringing in the ear?   _____
   B. Do you sneeze a lot?   _____
   C. Do you have something in your right ear?   _____
   D. Do you often have eye infections?   _____
   E. Do you have a runny nose?   _____

4. Answer the following questions in Japanese.

   Q: **Sensei, nodo ga itai(n) desu ga.**
   A: _____.
      (I want to examine your throat, so would you open your mouth?)

   Q: **Kensa o onegai shimasu.**
   B: _____.
      (Well then, let's start the examination.)

   Q: **Hentō-sen ga harete kurushii(n) desu.**
   C: _____.
      (Do you have difficulty breathing?)

Dermatology
(Hifu-ka)

Basic Vocabulary (CD 25-1)

Listen to the CD and repeat the vocabulary.

1.	dermatitis	**hifu-en**	皮膚炎
2.	skin cancer	**hifu-gan**	皮膚癌
3.	herpes	**herupesu/hō-shin**	ヘルペス/疱疹
4.	drug rash/pustules from drug reaction	**yaku-shin**	薬疹
5.	hives/urticaria	**jinma-shin**	蕁麻疹
6.	wheal	**bō-shin**	膨疹
7.	frostbite	**tō-shō**	凍傷
8.	erosion of skin/mucous membrances	**biran/tadare**	びらん/ただれ
9.	chilblain	**shimo-yake**	霜焼け
10.	sunburn/suntan	**hi-yake**	日焼け
11.	dry skin	**kansō-hada**	乾燥肌
12.	corn	**uo-no-me**	魚の目
13.	bed sore/pressure sore	**toko-zure**	床ずれ
14.	freckles	**sobakasu**	雀斑
15.	rough skin	**hada-are**	肌荒れ
16.	blots/age spot	**shimi**	シミ
17.	wart	**ibo**	疣
18.	bruise	**aza**	痣
19.	mole	**hokuro**	黒子
20.	athlete's foot	**mizu-mushi**	水虫
21.	pityriasis	**hatake**	ハタケ
22.	ringworm/tinea	**tamushi**	タムシ
23.	insect bite	**mushi-sasare**	虫さされ
24.	body odor	**tai-shū**	体臭
25.	dandruff	**fuke**	フケ
26.	alopecia/hair loss	**datsu-mō-shō**	脱毛症
27.	hair fall	**nuke-ge**	抜け毛
28.	impetigo contagiosa	**tobihi/densen-sei nōka-shin**	トビヒ/伝染性膿痂疹
29.	underarm odor	**waki-ga**	腋臭
30.	keloid	**keroido**	ケロイド

Dialogue (CD 25-2)

Listen to the CD and repeat the dialogue.

At the Dermatology Department

Dr. Young (female doctor): **Kyō wa dō nasai-mashita ka.**
Are you concerned about anything today?

Mr. Tanaka: **Kinō kara mune ya waki-no-shita ni hasshin ga dekite, kaitara kaette kayukute kayukute tamarimasen.**
Since yesterday, my chest and underarms have broken out in a rash, and it itches more than I can stand when I scratch it.

Dr. Young: **Soredewa, uwagi o nuide, jō-hanshin o misete kudasai.**
Would you take off your shirt, and let's see your upper body?

Nani-ka, tabeta mono de omoi-ataru tebemono wa arimasen ka.
Can you think of anything you ate that might have caused it?

Mr. Tanaka: **Kinō wa sakana o tabemashita.**
I ate fish yesterday.

Sakana wa shinsen na-node tabereru to omoimashita.
The fish was fresh, so I thought it was all right to eat.

Dr. Young: **(Go)kazoku no naka ni onaji-yōna shōjyō no kata ga oraremasu ka.**
Do any members of your family have similar symptoms?

Mr. Tanaka: **Iie, watakushi wa hitori gurashi desu.**
No, but I live alone.

Dr. Young: **Shōjyō kara mite, kore wa densen-sei nōkashin dato omoware-masu. Iwayuru, tobihi desu.**
The symptoms suggest that this is probably impetigo. This is the so-called tobihi.

Saikin, nani-ka ni sesshoku shita kanōsei ga arimasu.
You probably came into contact with the germs that cause it recently.

Mr. Tanaka: **Tottemo kayui node, kayumi dake demo nantoka shite itadake-masen ka.**
It's very itchy, so can you do something to stop the itching?

Dr. Young: **Wakarimashita. Saikin o osaeru tameni kōsei-bushitsu no nankō to, kayumi o tomeru tameni kō-hisutamin no nomi-gusuri o dashimasu.**

I understand. I will give you an antibiotic ointment to kill the germs and an oral antihistamine for the itch.

Soshite, te-aria ya, tsume o mijikaku kittari, karada o seiketsu ni tamotte kudasai.

And you need to keep your body clean by washing your hands and cutting your nails short.

Soredewa, shibaraku yōsu o mimashō.

Well then, let's see what happens in a little while.

Grammar

1. ### The construction VERB BASE + **-tara, kaette**

The adverb **kaette** is used to characterize a situation or event that occurs contrary to one's expectation in the construction VERB BASE plus **-tara**. The suffix **-tara** expresses expectation. **Kaette** is translated as "and (instead) . . . more . . . ."

Nankō o tsuketara, kaette hada-are shimashita.
I applied the ointment, and my skin got rougher (contrary to my expectation).

Hikkaitara, kaette kizu ga kayuku narimasu.
I scratched (my skin), and the spot got itchier (contrary to my expectation).

Ude ni rōshon o nuttara, kaette itai(n) desu.
I put lotion on my left arm and had more pain (contrary to my expectation).

Shisshin o kosuttara, kaette waruku narimashita.
I scrubbed the eczema, and it only got worse (contrary to my expectation).

To form the construction with **ru**-verbs, drop the **-ru** ending from stem verb and replace it with **-tara**. If the last syllable of verb base ends with **-ri**, the suffix **-tara** requires a change in pronunciation to **-ttara**.

Ru-verbs

ENGLISH	MASU-FORM/ VERB BASE	STEM VERB	TARA (SUPPOSITION)
bend	**mage-masu**	**mage-ru**	**mage-tara**
lift up/raise	**mochiage-masu**	**mochiage-ru**	**mochiage-tara**
bind/harden	**katame-masu**	**katame-ru**	**katame-tara**
close (eye, book)	**toji-masu**	**toji-ru**	**toji-tara**

ENGLISH	MASU-FORM/ VERB BASE	STEM VERB	TARA (SUPPOSITION)
swell	hare-masu	hare-ru	hare-tara
develop skin rash	kabure-masu	kabure-ru	kabure-tara
bitten	kamare-masu	kamare-ru	kamare-tara
sting/pierce	sasare-masu	sasare-ru	sasare-tara
change/substitute	kawari-masu	kawa-ru	kawa-ttara
cut	kiri-masu	ki-ru	ki-ttara
slip	suberi-masu	sube-ru	sube-ttara
enter/break into	hairi-masu	hai-ru	hai-ttara
apply/paint	nuri-masu	nu-ru	nu-ttara

For **u**-verbs, the construction is formed from the verb base, to which the supposition suffix -**tara** is added. However, if the last syllable of the verb base is -**ki**, the -**ki** is dropped and replaced by the supposition suffix, which changes to -**i-tara**. If the last syllable of the verb base is -**bi** or -**mi**, the -**bi** or -**mi** is dropped and replaced by -**n-dara**. If the last syllable ends with -**chi** or -**i**, the -**chi** or, -**i**, is dropped and replaced by -**ttara**.

U-verbs

ENGLISH	MASU-FORM/ VERB BASE	STEM VERB	TARA (SUPPOSITION)
push	oshi-masu	o-su	oshi-tara
sting	sashi-masu	sa-su	sashi-tara
stretch	nobashi-masu	noba-su	nobashi-tara
live in	kurashi-masu	kura-su	kurashi-tara
unfasten/remove	hazushi-masu	hazu-su	hazushi-tara
move	ugoki-masu	ugo-ku	ugo-itara
scratch	hikkaki-masu	hikka-ku	hikka-itara
fall down	korobi-masu	koro-bu	koro-ndara
tie	musubi-masu	musu-bu	musu-ndara
bite	kami-masu	ka-mu	ka-ndara
drink	nomi-masu	no-mu	no-ndara
keep/hold	tamochi-masu	tamo-tsu	tamo-ttara
hit	uchi-masu	u-tsu	u-ttara
wash	arai-masu	ara-u	ara-ttara
stitch	nui-masu	nu-u	nu-ttara

2. The noun **mono** following a verb

Adding the noun **mono** after a verb forms a noun phrase that can be translated as "things to (action)." Moreover, when **mono** is attached to the verb base, it forms a new noun.

taberu mono	(things to be eaten)
tabeta mono	(things that [someone] ate)
tabemono	(things to eat = foods)

Tabeta mono de, kibun ga waruku narimashita ka.
Did you become sick from something you ate?

Nonda mono de, nikibi ga fuemashita ka.
Do you get more pimples because of what you drink?

Nutta mono de, hiyake shimashia ka.
Did you get sunburn from something you applied on your skin?

3. The compound verb **omoi-ataru**

Unlike English, Japanese can make compound verbs consisting of two different verbs to create a new meaning. The compound verbs stretch the limitations of the language in order to describe a kind of action. For example, **omoi-ataru**:

omoi-ataru = **omoi-masu** (think) + **ataru/atari** (hit) = come to mind; recall; think of

omoi-kaesu = **omoi-masu** (think) + **kaesu** (return) = re-think; think back; change mind

Yakushin no genin o omoi-atari-mashita.
I recalled that pustules were caused by the reaction to a drug.
(*lit.*, The cause of the pustules from the reaction to a drug, I recalled.)

Dōshite, aza ga dekitaka omoi-atara-nai.
I could not think of why I have a birthmark.

Kono hifu-en ni tsuite omoi-atari ga arimasu ka.
Did something come to your mind about this dermatitis?

4. Adding **-rareru/-rare** to the **te**-form to form honorific expressions

In Lesson 3, we studied the verb **iru/imasu** (there is, I have, be located). **Iru/ imasu** is used for living beings (animate subjects) such as people, dogs, fish, birds, and so on. The polite form of **imasu** is **irasshai-masu**. However, the super polite form of **imasu** is **oraremasu/iraremasu**. Adding **-rareru/-rare** to the **te**-form makes the passive as well as an honorific expression.

Yangu sensei ga oraremasu.	There is Dr. Young.
Kango-shi-san ga oraremasu.	There is a nurse.
Shisshin no kanjya ga oraremasu ka.	Is the eczema patient there?
Sensei wa kanjya o mite oraremasu.	The doctor is examining the patient.

5. The construction VERB BASE + -reru/-remasu

The construction VERB BASE plus **-reru/-remasu** expresses the possibility of doing something or that something can be done. It is similar in meaning to **koto ga dekimasu.**

Sakana wa atarashii node, tabereru to omoimasu.
I think that fish is fresh, so it can be eaten.

Kono aza wa sū-jitsu de toreru yo.
This bruise will have disappeared in a few days.

Jinmashin no kanjya-san wa suguni uchi ni kaereru deshō.
The patient with hives can probably go home soon.

6. Counters indicate singular or plural in Japanese.

Japanese requires counters for counting nouns/objects. This is a unique feature of the language. Japanese nouns themselves do not have singular or plural forms or endings but require counters to convey this information. We've met the following counters so far: in Lesson 2, for cylindrical objects (**pon**), floors (**kai**), and animals (**hiki**); in Lesson 3, for years, as in "years old" (**sai**); in Lesson 15, for tablets (**jyō**), capsules (**kapuseru**), liquids/drops (**teki**), and powder (**fukuro**); in Lesson 22, for stitches (**hari**).

The counters in the table below are also used in frequently:

NO.	PERSON (**NIN**)	FLAT OBJECT (**MAI**)	SHOES (**SOKU**)	MACHINE (**DAI**)
1	hitori*	ichi-mai	i-ssoku*	ichi-dai
2	futari*	ni-mai	ni-soku	ni-dai
3	san-nin	san-mai	san-soku	san-dai
4	yo-nin*	yon-mai	yon-soku	yon-dai
5	go-nin	go-mai	go-soku	go-dai
6	roku-nin	roku-mai	roku-soku	roku-dai

* Irregular pronunciation

7. The adverb **nantoka**

The adverb **nantoka** expresses the notion of doing something by any means, doing anything, in order to achieve a seemingly impossible result or outcome. The word **nantoka** comes from two words: **nani** (what) and **toka** (and the like/and so on). It can be translated "somehow; anyhow; something; anything; one way or another."

> **Nantoka, hifi-gan o naoshite agetai desu.**
> I wish I could cure your skin cancer somehow.

> **Tottemo itai no de, nantoka shite itadakemasen ka.**
> It's very painful, so is there anything you can do to stop it?

> **Nantoka shite kudsai.**
> Please do something, anything.

8. The verb **omowareru/omowaremasu**

The verb **omowareru/omowaremasu** is the passive form of **omou/omoimasu**, which means "to think." However, though it is passive in form, **omowareru/omowaremasu** doesn't have the meaning of the passive voice. Rather, it indicates what is manifest or apparent and may be translated as "apparently, in fact, it appears that." **Omowareru/omowaremasu** takes **dato** for nouns or **na**-adjectives and **to** for verbs and **i**-adjectives.

> **Kore wa tamushi dato omowaremasu.**
> This is apparently ringworm.

> **Hifu wa mō kirei dato omowareru.**
> It appears that the skin is already clean.

> **Keroido ni natteiru to omowaremasu.**
> This is apparently becoming keloid tissue.

> **Sono mizu-mushi wa tottemo kayui to omowaremasu.**
> It seems that athlete's foot is extremely itchy.

9. The construction STEM VERB + **tame(ni)** and the conjunction **node**

In Lesson 23, we studied the constructions STEM VERB (PRESENT TENSE) plus **tame(ni)** and NOUN plus **no tame(ni),** meaning "to ; in order to; for; for the sake of."

> **Saikin o osaeru tameni kōsei-bushitsu o nonde kudasai.**
> Please take an antibiotic (in order) to kill the germs.

Hiyake-dome no tameni san-oiru o nutte kudasai.
Please apply suntan lotion for sunburn.

The construction STEM VERB + **tame(ni)** expresses a causal link similar to **node** (because).

Hiyake o shita tame(ni), shimi ni narimashita.
Because of my sunburn, I got a blot.

Hiyake o shita node, shimi ni narimashita.
I got blots because of sunburn.

Useful Expressions (CD 25-3)

Listen to the CD and repeat the sentences.

1. **Shimi ni nayande imasu.** I am worried about my blots.
2. **Hasshin ni komatte imasu.** I am troubled by this rash.
3. **Kubi ni shisshin ga dekite imasu.** You have eczema on your neck.
4. **Oshiri ni odeki ga dekite imasu.** You have a boil on your buttocks.
5. **Fuke ga hidoi desu ne.** You have severe dandruff.
6. **Keshō-hin de kabure te imasu.** You have a skin rash caused by cosmetics.
7. **Oyu de yakedo o shimashita ka.** Were you burned by boiling water?
8. **Mizu-mushi no ato [wa] kayui(n) desu ka.** Do you itch from athlete's foot?
9. **Karada-jyū ni fukidemono ga arimasu.** You have eruptions all over your body.
10. **Koko-ni aru hifu-gan ga ki-ni narimasu.** I am nervous about skin cancer in this area.

Key Sentences (CD 25-4)

Listen to the CD and repeat the sentences.

1. **Kusuri o nondara, kaette shimi ni narimashita.** I took the medication and got a blot [contrary to my expectation].
2. **Sawatta mono de, shisshin ga demashita ka.** Can you get eczema by touching something?
3. **Kono hasshin ni tsuite omoi-atari ga arimasu ka.** Has anything come to mind about this rash?
4. **Nantoka, shuyō o naoshite agetai desu.** I wish I could cure your tumor somehow.
5. **Kore wa fukide-mono dato omowaremasu.** This is apparently an eruption.

Additional Words

tamotsu/tamochimasu keep
kurasu/kurashimasu live in
kamu bite
kui-chigiru bite off
sesshoku contact
mijikai short
keshō-hin cosmetics
uo-no-me tako corn
nomi flea
dani tick
nezumi mouse
doku-mushi poison insect
urushi poison ivy
oyu hot water
eda-ge split ends
senzai detergent

kabureru/kaburemasu develop skin rash
sasu sting
kami-kizu bite wound
fukide-mono eruption
seiketsu clean
atarashii new
rōshon lotion
raimu-byō Lyme disease
shirami louse
kumo spider
ke-mushi caterpillar
ki-ni naru worry/concern
mizu-bukure blister
nettō boiled water
hachi bee

Language Notes

1. Japanese tend to repeat adjectives twice in a phrase or sentence to express wishes, feelings, and emotions, and i-adjectives may be used in this way. In order to conjugate i-adjectives, drop the -i ending and replace it with -kute. Verbs in the sentence also need to be changed from the verb base, and take the ending -takute (see Lessons 17 and 19). Another way to express a wish, want, or desire is the tai form. The tai form is made by adding -tai to the verb base: for example, mi-tai (wish/want to see), tabe-tai (wish/want to eat), nomi-tai (wish/want to drink), ne-tai (wish/want to sleep). Verbs in the sentence also can change from the tai form by dropping the final -i and replacing it with -kute. These expressions are usually associated with shikataga nai (it can't be helped; I can't stand it) or tamaranai (intolerable, unbearable), or are used without any verbs at the end of a sentence.

i-adjectives

MEANING	I-ADJECTIVE	-KUTE (-I DROPPED)
painful	ita-i	ita-kute
itchy	kayu-i	kayu-kute
tired	daru-i	daru-kute
cold	tsumeta-i	tsumeta-kute
hot	atsu-i	atsu-kute

Verbs

MEANING	VERB BASE/**MASU** FORM	**TAI** FORM (WISH)	**-KUTE** (DROP **-I** AND ADD **-KUTE**)
see/look/watch	**mi-masu**	**mi-tai**	**mi-ta-kute**
eat	**tabe-masu**	**tabe-tai**	**tabe-ta-kute**
drink	**nomi-masu**	**nomi-tai**	**nomi-ta-kute**
do/play	**shi-masu**	**shi-tai**	**shi-ta-kute**
buy	**kai-masu**	**kai-tai**	**kai-ta-kute**
scratch	**kaki-masu**	**kaki-tai**	**kaki-ta-kute**
heal/cure	**naoshi-masu**	**naoshi-tai**	**naoshi-ta-kute**

Kata no hifu ga itakute itakute shikataga-nai desu.
I can't stand the pain in the skin on my shoulder.

Koko ga kayukute kayukute tamarimasen.
I have an intolerable itch here.

Nikibi ga itakute itakute.
I have a very painful pimple.

Sushi ga tabetakute, tabetakute.
I really want to eat sushi.

2.   One sign of good command of Japanese is in the use of polite expressions. Japanese culture emphasizes politeness for yourself and others. Polite expressions reflect one's family, educational, and social background, which all can be easily evaluated by the way one handles the language.

Dare-ka imasu ka	Is anybody here? (standard)
Donata-ka irasshai-masu ka.	Is anybody here? (polite)
Donata-ka oraremasu ka.	Is anybody here? (super polite)

Gokazoku no naka ni onaji yōna shōjyō no kata ga imasu ka.
Gokazoku no naka ni onaji yōna shōjyō no kata ga irasshai masu ka.
Gokazoku no naka ni onaji yōna shōjyō no kata ga oraremasu ka.
Do any members of your family have similar symptoms?

3.   There are many expressions for dermatological complaints.

Hasshin ga mizu-bukure ni narimashita.	My rash has started to blister.
Senzai de te ga kabure mashita.	I got a skin rash on my hand from detergent.
Urushi ni kabure mashita.	I got a rash from poison ivy.

Hada-are ga hidoi(n) desu.	I have seriously rough skin.
Hada ga kansō shite imasu.	I have dry skin.
Hada ga aburappoi desu.	I have greasy/oily skin.
Mansei hifu-en ga arimasu.	I have chronic dermatitis.
Tōshō ni kakarimashita.	I have frostbite.
Eda-ge ni nayande imasu.	I am bothered by split ends.
Hachi ni sasaremashita.	I was stung by a bee.
Atama ni enkei datsumō-shō ga arimasu.	I have a round bald spot on my head.

Language Roots

The word **shō** (焼) indicates a burn. It is also pronounced **yake**.

shō-shin	burning oneself to death
yake-do	burnt
shimo-yake	chilblain
hi-yake	sunburn

The word **shō** (傷) indicates a wound, cut, scrape, or scratch, and the wound may be physical or not. The character is also pronounced **kizu**.

fu-shō	wound/injury/assault
daboku-shō	bruise
suri-kizu	scratch, abrasion
kiri-kizu	cut, incision

Culture Notes

The origin of **jinma-shin**

Jinma is the Chinese name for the herb the stinging nettle (*Urtica dioica*). The nettle has tiny thorns on its stem and leaves that cause pain, swelling, and rashes on the skin. Hives are a common symptom when one has touched a nettle. For this reason, Japanese call hives **jinma**'s rash (**jinma-shin**). Traditionally, nettles are used as an herbal tea to cure or ameliorate hay fever.

The origin of **ibo**

The Japanese word for warts is **ibo**. Ibo derives from **i-ibo**, the literal meaning of which is "grain of boiled rice." For the ancient Japanese, warts were seen as similar in shape to a grain of rice, hence the word **ibo**.

The origin of **aza**

The Japanese word for bruise is **aza**. The word **aza** derives from **aza-yaka**, which means "brilliant." For the ancient Japanese, bruises must have seemed brilliant compared to ordinary skin tone. For Japanese, black bruises (as in the English phrase "bruised black and blue") are **ao-aza** (literally, blue bruise).

> **Tsuyoku koronde, hiji ni ao-aza ga dekimashita.**
> I fell down hard and got a black bruise on my elbow.

Comprehension

Answer the following questions.

1. Which of the following does NOT belong with the others?
   a. **Yakushin** b. **Zenshin**
   c. **Hosshin** d. **Hasshin**

2. Which of the following could NOT be used to express a complaint about skin problems?
   a. **Kabure desu** b. **Aburappoi desu**
   c. **Doki-doki desu.** d. **Hada-are desu.**

3. Which of the following best completes the sentence below?
   Tottemo itai (   ), nantoka shite itadake-masen ka.
   (It's very painful, so can you do something to stop it?)
   a. **node** b. **shiro**
   c. **made** d. **dake**

4. The patient is telling you about a symptom. Which of the following means "I have dry skin"?
   a. **Hada ga kansō shite imasu.**
   b. **Hada ga aburappoi desu.**
   c. **Hada ga hiyake shite imasu.**
   d. **Hada ga tadarete imasu.**

Select the appropriate meaning from the list below.

5. **Nantoka, hifu-gan o naoshite agetai(n) desu.** (   )
6. **Kusuri o nondara, kaette fukidemono ga demashita.** (   )
7. **Sawatta mono de, hasshin ga demashita ka.** (   )

8. **Kono nioi wa wakiga dato omowaremasu.**   (   )
9. **Kono aza ni tsuite omoiatari ga arimasu ka.**   (   )

a. Has anything come to mind about this bruise?
b. I wish I could cure you of skin cancer somehow.
c. It seems that this smell is body odor.
d. When I take the medication, I get eruptions (contrary to my expectation).
e. Do you have a rash from touching things?

Practice

Respond to the following in Japanese using the cues that have been provided.

1. Confirming the patient's symptoms.
    (Symptom)   (Healthcare professional)
    1. A blister   _____ (You have a blister.)
    2. Frostbite   _____ (You have frostbite.)
    3. A skin rash   _____ (You have a skin rash.)
    4. Dry skin   _____ (You have dry skin.)
    5. Oily skin   _____ (You have oily skin.)

2. Instructing the patient.
    (Patient)   (Healthcare professional)
    1. **Hasshin ga demashita.**   _____
                                 (Please cut your nails short.)
    2. **Uo-no-me ga itai(n) desu.**   _____
                                 (Please show me your foot.)
    3. **Mizumushi ga kayui(n) desu.**   _____
                                 (Please clean your feet.)
    4. **Kao no shimi ga ki-ni-narimasu.**   _____
                                 (I will give you an ointment.)
    5. **Kao ni fukide-mono ga demashita.**   _____
                                 (Please wash your face.)

3. Describing the symptoms.
    (Patient)   (Healthcare professional)
    1. **Oshiri ga itai(n) desu.**   _____
                                 (You have a boil on your buttocks.)
    2. **Atama ga kayui(n) desu.**   _____
                                 (You have severe dandruff.)

3. **Kao ga tsuppari-masu.** _____

(You have a skin rash caused by cosmetics.)

4. **Karada-jyū ga kayukute, kayukute.** _____

(You have eruptions all over your body.)

5. **Kubi ga kayui(n) desu.** _____

(You have eczema on your neck.)

4. Dialogue comprehension. Based on the dialogue, answer the following questions.

1. **Tanaka-san wa kinō kara don-na shōjyō desu ka.** _____

2. **Tanaka-san wa kinō nani o tabemashita ka.** _____

3. **Shōjyō kara mite, Tanaka-san no byōmei wa nan desu ka.** _____

4. **Tanaka-san wa don-na kusuri o nomimasu ka.** _____

5. **Tanaka-san wa nani ni, ki o tsukemasu ka.** _____

5. Free response questions.

(Questions)   (Healthcare professional)

1. **Toki-doki hasshin ga demasu ka.** _____

2. **Hiyake o shite imasu ka.** _____

3. **Nuke-ge ga ki ni narimasu ka.** _____

4. **Karada ni aza ga arimasu ka.** _____

5. **Kao ni ōkii hokuro ga arimasu ka.** _____

Exercises

1. Say the following words in Japanese.
   A. Dandruff   _____
   B. Wart   _____
   C. Blots   _____
   D. Mole   _____
   E. Athlete's foot   _____

2. Say the following in Japanese.
   A. When I take a medicine, I got pustules from the reaction to a drug (contrary to my expectation).

   _____

   B. Do you have impetigo contagiosa from touching germs?

   _____

   C. Has anything come to your mind about these hives?

   _____

    D. I wish I could cure your sunburn somehow.

    _____

    E. It seems that this is athlete's foot.

    _____

3. How do you ask your patients the following questions in Japanese?
    A. Are you bothered by blots? _____
    B. Do you have a rash on your chest? _____
    C. Do you have severe dandruff? _____
    D. Were you burned by boiling water? _____
    E. Do you have an itch from the sunburn? _____

4. Answer the following questions in Japanese.

    Q: **Kusuri o nondara, kaette shimi ni narimashita.**
    A: _____ .
    (I wish I could cure your blots somehow.)

    Q: **Kinō kara hasshin ga dete, kayui(n) desu ga.**
    B: _____ .
    (Has anything come to mind about this rash?)

    Q: **Kono fukidemono wa nan-deshō ka.**
    C: _____ .
    (This is apparently pimples.)

LESSON 26 Neurology and Psychiatry
(Seishin-ka)

Basic Vocabulary (CD 26-1)

Listen to the CD and repeat the vocabulary.

#	English	Romaji	Japanese
1.	psychotherapy	**seishin-ryōhō**	精神療法
2.	psychological examination/ mental test	**shinri-kensa**	心理検査
3.	neuritis	**shinkei-en**	神経炎
4.	epilepsy	**tenkan**	癲癇
5.	personality disorder	**jinkaku-shōgai**	人格障害
6.	senile dementia	**rōjin-sei-chihō-shō**	老人性痴呆症
7.	schizophrenia	**sōgō shichō-shō**	総合失調症
8.	manic depression/bipolar disorder	**sō-utsu-byō**	躁うつ病
9.	depression	**utsu-byō**	うつ病
10.	obsessive-compulsive disorder	**kyōhaku-shinkei-shō**	強迫神経症
11.	mysophobia	**fuketsu-kyōfu-shō**	不潔恐怖症
12.	anthropophobia/fear of people	**taijin-kyōfu-shō**	対人恐怖症
13.	autism	**jihei-shō**	自閉症
14.	stammering symptom	**kitsuon-shō**	吃音症
15.	insanity	**sēshin-ijyō**	精神異常
16.	suicide	**jisatsu**	自殺
17.	pharmacotherapy	**yakubutsu-ryōhō**	薬物療法
18.	medical poisoning	**yaku-butsu chūdoku**	薬物中毒
19.	drug abuse	**yaku-butsu ranyō**	薬物乱用
20.	cognitive disease	**ninchi-shō**	認知症
21.	hallucination; illusion	**gen-kau**	幻覚
22.	auditory hallucination	**gen-chō**	幻聴
23.	delusion	**mōsō**	妄想
24.	anxiety attack	**fuan-hossa**	不安発作
25.	powerlessness	**muryoku-kan**	無力感
26.	addiction	**izon-shō**	依存症
27.	hopelessness	**zetsubō-kan**	絶望感
28.	mental irritation	**ira-ira**	イライラ

29. professional ethics **shokugyō rinri** <ruby>職<rt>しょく</rt>業<rt>ぎょう</rt>倫<rt>りん</rt>理<rt>り</rt></ruby>
30. paranoid personality disorder **mōsō-sei jinkaku-shōgai** <ruby>妄<rt>もう</rt>想<rt>そう</rt>性<rt>せい</rt>人<rt>じん</rt>格<rt>かく</rt>障<rt>しょう</rt>害<rt>がい</rt></ruby>

Shinkei Kei (Nervous System)

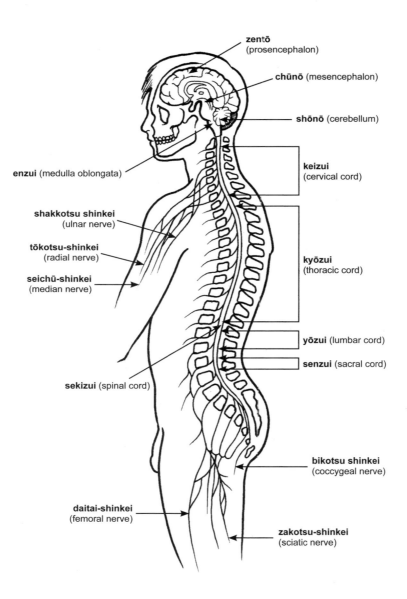

zentō (prosencephalon)

chūnō (mesencephalon)

shōnō (cerebellum)

enzui (medulla oblongata)

keizui (cervical cord)

shakkotsu shinkei (ulnar nerve)

tōkotsu-shinkei (radial nerve)

seichū-shinkei (median nerve)

kyōzui (thoracic cord)

yōzui (lumbar cord)

senzui (sacral cord)

sekizui (spinal cord)

bikotsu shinkei (coccygeal nerve)

daitai-shinkei (femoral nerve)

zakotsu-shinkei (sciatic nerve)

Dialogue (CD 26-2)

Listen to the CD and repeat the dialogue.

At the Psychiatric Clinic

Dr. Goldberg (male doctor): **Kyō wa dō sare mashita ka.**
Is there anything you're concerned about today?

Mrs. Kato: **Koko san-ka-getsu (kan) hodo, karada no chōshi ga yokunai mitai desu.**
It seems to me that I haven't been in good health for about the past three months.

Yoru mo yoku nemure-naishi, karada ga itsumo tsukare-gimi desu.
I also haven't been able to sleep well and am always feeling tired.

Dr. Goldberg: **Sō desu ka. Shoku-yoku wa arimasu ka.**
Is that so? Do you have a good appetite?

Mrs. Kato: **Amari arimasen. Nandaka saikin wa tsukarete hotondo taberaremasen.**
No, (am) not really. For some reason, recently I'm tired and can't eat much.

Dr. Goldberg: **Dewa, hokani chōshi ga okashii tokoro wa arimasen ka.**
Well, has there been anything else unusual with your health?

Mrs. Kato: **Tonikaku, karada ga tsukare-yasuku, yatara(ni) kuchi ga kawaite, benpi-gachi ni natte imasu.**
Generally, I get lethargic, my mouth becomes unexpectedly dry, and I tend to have some constipation.

Dr. Goldberg: **Naruhodo (wakarimashita). Dawa, kibun wa dō desu ka. Ochikondari, meitteiru to omoimasu ka.**
I see. Then, how about your feelings? Do you feel that you are in a slump or depressed?

Mrs. Kato: **Hai. Tonikaku, ki ga meitte, tsukarete yoko ni narazu-niwa iraremasen.**
Yes. In any case, I am depressed, and I can't keep going without lying down because of being so tired.

Tokidoki, jibun wa inai-hō ga (ii) to omottari, shini-tai to omottari shimasu.
Sometimes, I think I shouldn't exist, and I want to die.

Dr. Goldberg: **Sō desu ka. Tabun anata wa utsu-jyōtai ni arimasu. Fumin-shō mo sore ga genin deshō.**

Is that so? You probably have a depressive disorder. Perhaps your insomnia is because of that.

Utsu-byō no chiryō niwa kyūyō to yakubutsu-ryōhō ga kakase-masen.

The treatment for depression emphasizes the necessity of rest and pharmacotherapy.

Mazu, kyūyō o (o)susume shimasu.

First of all, I recommend you take some time off.

Sorekara, shōjyō no tameni kōutsu-zai to suimin dōnyū-zai o shohō shimasu kara, kanarazu nonde kudasai.

And to help your symptoms, I'll prescribe you an antidepressant and sleeping pills, so please be sure to take them.

Odaiji ni.

Please take care.

Grammar

1. ### The construction **koko** + DURATION OF TIME + **hodo**

    The construction **koko** plus DURATION OF TIME plus **hodo** is often used in conversation to express a very recent time period that continues to the speaker's present. Sometimes **kono** can substitute for **koko**, and **gurai** can substitute for **hodo** to express less urgency. Also, **hodo** may be omitted in order to express urgency.

    Koko ni-shū-kan hodo, taijyū ga hette imasu.
    I have been losing weight for the last two weeks.

    Koko san-ka-getsu gurai, taijyū ga fuete imasu.
    You have been gaining weight for the last three months (*lit.*, In the last three months, you are gaining weight).

    Kono han-toshi hodo, itsu mo nemui kanji ga shimasu.
    For the last half year, I've been feeling sleepy all the time.

    Koko i-shū-kan [hodo], kyū ni yase dashimashita.
    I have suddenly been losing weight for the last week.

2. The construction VERB BASE + -renai/-remasen

In Lesson 25, we studied how to express affirmative possibility using a verb base plus -**reru/-remasu**. The construction VERB BASE plus -**renai/-remasen** is used to express the impossibility of doing something or that something can be done. In meaning, it is similar to **koto ga dekimasen**.

Yoru mo yoku nemu-renai.	It has been impossible for me to sleep at night.
Gohan mo yoku tabe-remasen.	I have not been able to eat the meals.
Kibun ga warukute, tatte ira-remasen.	I cannot stand up because of feeling sick.

3. The noun suffixes -gimi and -gachi

In Lesson 8, we saw that the noun suffix -**gimi** can mean "feel, feel like," as in **Kaze-gimi desu** "I feel like I have a cold." -**gimi** also expresses the idea of "looking like" or "appearing to be" but with a negative or undesirable connotation. It is often translated as "look like; show a tendency to or a sign or touch of; seem; appear." With a similar negative or undesirable connotation, the noun suffix -**gachi** describes a general tendency in someone or something, and can be translated as "tend to; apt to; often; a tendency." When the suffixes -**gimi** and -**gachi** are conjugated with verbs, the construction is VERB BASE plus -**gimi/-gachi**.

Watakushi wa konran-gimi desu.	I feel slightly confused.
Anata wa konran-gimi no yō desu.	You look like you are a little confused.
Watakushi wa magotsuki-gimi desu.	I have a tendency to get disoriented.
Anata wa magotsuki-gimi no yō desu.	You look like you are disoriented.
Watakushi wa tsukare-gimi desu.	I feel a little exhausted.
Anata wa tsukare-gimi no yō desu.	You look like you are feeling exhausted.
Watakushi wa hirō-gimi desu.	I get a little worn out/weary.
Anata wa hirō-gimi no yō desu.	You look like you are worn out/weary.
Watakushi wa kaze-gimi desu.	I have a slight cold.
Anata wa kaze-gimi no yō desu.	You seem to be showing signs of a cold.
Watakushi wa byōki-gachi desu.	I have a tendency to get sick.
Anata wa byōki-gachi no yō desu.	You look like you have a tendency to get sick.
Watakushi wa futori-gimi desu.	I feel like I'm gaining weight.
Watakushi wa futori-gachi desu.	I have a tendency to gain weight.

4. The NEGATIVE SHORT FORM OF THE VERB + **ni(wa) irarenai/iraremasen**

The construction NEGATIVE SHORT FORM OF THE VERB plus **ni(wa) irarenai/ iraremasen** means "I cannot stand (action) without . . ." In this construction, the particle **wa** in **ni(wa)** can sometimes be omitted for urgency. The procedure for making the negative short form is, as usual, different for the **u**-verbs and **ru**-verbs. (See Lesson 6 and 13 for the negative verb form.)

For **u**-verbs, drop the -**masu** ending to reveal the verb base and replace the -**i** (-**hi**) with -**a**, -**chi** with -**ta**, or, if a vowel precedes the -**i**, with -**wa**. Then add -**zu** to make the negative short form. Another way to make the negative short form is to first drop the -**u** ending from the stem verb and replace it with -**a**; drop -**tsu** and replace it with -**ta**; or if what is left is a vowel, replace it with -**wa**. Then add -**zu** to make the negative short form.

ENGLISH	MASU-FORM/ VERB BASE	NEGATIVE FORM	STEM VERB	NEGATIVE SHORT FORM
drink	nomi-masu	noma-nai	nomu	noma-zu
read	yomi-masu	yoma-nai	yomu	yoma-zu
go	iki-masu	ika-nai	iku	ika-zu
speak	hanashi-masu	hanasa-nai	hanasu	hanasa-zu
return	kaeri-masu	kaera-nai	kaeru	kaera-zu
listen	kiki-masu	kika-nai	kiku	kika-zu
pull down	oroshi-masu	orosa-nai	orosu	orosa-zu
cool	hiyashi-masu	hiyasa-nai	hiyasu	hiyasa-zu
scratch	kaki-masu	kaka-nai	kaku	kaka-zu
smell/sniff	kagi-masu	kaga-nai	kagu	kaga-zu
become	nari-masu	nara-nai	naru	nara-zu
start/go out	dashi-masu	dasa-nai	dasu	dasa-zu
live in	kurashi-masu	kurasa-nai	kurasu	kurasa-zu
worry	nayami-masu	nayama-nai	nayamu	nayama-zu
be depressed	ochikomi-masu	ochikoma-nai	ochikomu	ochikoma-zu
wait	machi-masu	mata-nai	matsu	mata-zu
keep/hold	tamochi-masu	tamota-nai	tamotsu	tamota-zu
wash	arai-masu	arawa-nai	arau	arawa-zu
laugh	warai-masu	warawa-nai	warau	warawa-zu

For **ru**-verbs, in general just add -**zu** for the negative short form for both verb base or stem verb. If the verb base ends with -**ri**, first change it to -**ra**, and then add -**zu** for the negative short form. Using the stem verb, first drop -**ru** and add -**zu**, or, if the verb base ends with -**ri**, add -**razu** to make the negative short form.

ENGLISH	MASU FORM/ VERB BASE	NEGATIVE FORM	STEM VERB	NEGATIVE SHORT FORM
sleep	ne-masu	ne-nai	ne-ru	ne-zu
eat	tabe-masu	tabe-nai	tabe-ru	tebe-zu
warm, warm up	atatame-masu	atatame-nai	atatame-ru	atatame-zu
manifest/ appear	araware-masu	araware-nai	araware-ru	araware-zu
inform/notify	shirase-masu	shirase-nai	shirase-ru	shirase- zu
shiver	furue-masu	furue-nai	furue-ru	furue-zu
go out/appear	de-masu	de-nai	de-ru	de-zu
allow/make to do	sase-masu	sase-nai	sase-ru	sase-zu
see/look/ examine	mi-masu	mi-nai	mi-ru	mi-zu
tighten	shime-masu	shime-nai	shime-ru	ssime-zu
leak	more-masu	more nai	more-ru	more-zu
open	ake-masu	ake-nai	ake-ru	ake-zu
recommend	susume-masu	susume-nai	susume-ru	susume-zu
wear (clothes)	ki-masu	ki-nai	ki-ru	ki-zu
feel	kanji-masu	kanji-nai	kanji-ru	kanji-zu
wake up	oki-masu	oki-nai	oki-ru	oki-zu
slump	meiri-masu	meira-nai	mei-ru	mei-razu
become	nari- masu	nara-nai	na-ru	na-razu
apply/paint	nuri-masu	nura-nai	nu-ru	nu-razu
mix	majiri-masu	majira-nai	maji-ru	maji-razu
empty/die/ use up	nakunari-masu	nakunara-nai	nakuna-ru	nakuna-razu
choke	tsumari-masu	tsumara-nai	tsuma-ru	tsuma-razu
measure	hakari-masu	hakara-nai	haka-ru	haka-razu

ENGLISH	MASU FORM/ VERB BASE	NEGATIVE FORM	STEM VERB	NEGATIVE SHORT FORM
anger	okori-masu	okora-nai	oku-ru	oko-razu
transmit/ move	utsuri-masu	utsura-nai	utsu-ru	utsu-razu
stand up	tachiagari-masu	tachiagara-nai	tachiaga-ru	tachiaga-razu
paint/put/ spread	nuri-masu	nura-nai	nu-ru	nu-razu
cut	kiri-masu	kira-nai	ki-ru	ki-razu
sit down	suwari-masu	suwara-nai	suwa-ru	suwa-razu
roll up	makuri-masu	makura-nai	maku-ru	maku-razu
not speak/ be silent	damari-masu	damara-nai	dama-ru	dama-razu
do/play*	shi-masu	shi-nai	su-ru	se-zu
come*	ki-masu	ko-nai	ku-ru	ko-zu (not use)

* Irregular

Nezu ni(wa) iraremasen.
I cannot stand going without sleep.

Tabezu ni(wa) iraremasen.
I cannot stand going without eating.

Shōjyō o hanasazu niwa iraremasen.
I cannot stand going without telling someone about my symptom.

Tenkan no kusuri o nomazu niwa iraremasen.
I cannot stand going without taking my epilepsy medication.

5. The construction X niwa Y ga hitsuyō/kakasenai/taisetsu desu

In Lesson 14, we studied the compound particle **ni(wa)** (in which **wa**, when used with **ni**, places emphasis on a subject) and the construction STEM VERB plus **niwa** to express the idea of "in order to, for the purpose of." In the health-care fields, this construction with **niwa** is often associated with predicates that express the necessity or importance of doing something and with such words as **ga hitsuyō desu** (necessary), **kakasemasen** (essential, indispensable, necessary), and **taisetsu desu** (most important).

Sōgō-shichō-shō niwa yakuji-ryōhō ga kakasemasen.
It is essential to treat schizophrenia with pharmacotherapy.

Utsu-byō no chiryō niwa kyūyō ga hitsuyō desu.
It is necessary to treat depression with rest.

Shinri-ryōhō niwa kyūyō ga taisetsu desu.
The most important treatment for psychotherapy is rest.

Seishin-ka-i niwa shokugyō-rinri ga taisetsu desu.
Professional ethics is important for psychiatrists.

6. The verb **susumeru/susumemasu**

The verb of command **susumeru/susumemasu** means "recommend, advise, encourage." The verb base **susume** can be made into a noun by putting **o** before **susume**, to form the polite expression **osusume**, meaning "recommendation, advice, encouragement."

Shibaraku no aida, ryōyō o susumemasu.
I will recommend that you receive medical treatment for a while.

Kono kusuri wa osusume desu.
This medicine is recommended.

Mazu, kyūyō o (o)susume shimasu.
First of all, I recommend that you get some rest. (polite)

Tabako ya, osake wa susume masen.
I will not encourage smoking and drinking.

Tabako ya, osake o susume-naide kudasai.
Please don't encourage smoking and drinking.

7. The adverbs **tonikaku, yatara-ni, muishiki-ni,** and **muyami-ni**

Japanese use adverbs a lot to change topics or to fill a gap in conversation. Using adverbs correctly is a way to demonstrate command of the Japanese language. The adverb **tonikaku** means "anyway, anyhow, at any rate, in any case, generally speaking." **Yatara-ni** means "unexpectedly, uncontrollably, recklessly, incredibly." **Muishiki-ni** means "unintentionally, unconsciously." **Muyami-ni** has almost the same meaning and translates as "unreasonably, carelessly." **Muyamini** is used with the negative form of the verb.

Tonikaku, kensa o shimashō.
Anyway, let's do a test.

Tonikaku, sugu ni kusuri o nonde, hayaku naoshite kudasai.
In any case, please take the medication immediately, and it will be cured soon.

Kyō wa yatarani atamaga itai(n) desu.
Unexpectedly, I have a headache today.

Konogoro, yatarani kuchi ga kawakimasu.
I've been incredibly thirsty these days.

Kanjya wa muishiki-ni hanashite imasu.
The patient is speaking unnconsciously.

Muyamini kusuri o nomanai de kudasai.
Please don't be careless about taking your medication.

Muyamini yōryō ijyō no kusuri o nomanai de, hayaku yasunde kudasai.
Please do not (uncontrollably) take more than the prescribed amount of medicine, but get rest immediately.

8. The adverb **naruhodo**

The adverb **naruhodo** expresses agreement, as in "I see, that's right, indeed." When **naruhodo** is used alone, it implies **wakarimashita** "I understand," which can also replace it.

Naruhodo ketsuatsu ga takai desu ne.
I see you have high blood pressure, don't you?

Kore wa naruhodo warui shōjyō desu.
This is indeed a bad symptom.

Naruhodo, (wakarimashia).
Yes, I understand indeed.

Useful Expressions (CD 26-3)

Listen to the CD and repeat the sentences.

1. **Saikin, hidoi hen-zutsū ga arimasu ka.** Recently, have you been having terrible migraines?
2. **Zutsū ga suru-to, yokoni narazu niwa iraremasen ka.** Do you have to lie down when you have a headache?
3. **Tachi-agaru to, memai ga shimasu ka.** Do you feel dizzy when you stand up?
4. **Saikin, tokidoki kizetsu shite imasu ka.** Have you been passing out occasionally recently?
5. **Shoku-yoku ga zenzen arimasen.** I have no appetite at all.
6. **Don-nani tsukarete itemo yoku nemuremasen.** I cannot sleep no matter how tired I am.
7. **Nemurō to suruto, masu-masu neraremasen ka.** Do you have a hard time sleeping when you try it?
8. **Fumin-shō ni nayande imasu ka.** Have you been suffering from insomnia?

9. **Karada ga omoku(te), darui kanji ga shimasu ka.** Do you have a heavy and dull feeling?

10. **Anata no shōjyō wa sutoresu kara kite imasu.** Your symptoms come from your stress.

Key Sentences (CD 26-4)

Listen to the CD and repeat the sentences.

1. **Koko i-kka-getsu-hodo, kyūni yase dashimashita.** I have suddenly lost weight in the last month.

2. **Anata wa fumin-shō-gimi no yōdesu.** You look like you have insomnia.

3. **Sō-utsu-byō no kusuri o nomazu-niwa iraremasen.** I cannot stand going without taking my medication for bipolar disorder.

4. **Ira-ira niwa yakuji ryōhō ga kakasemasen.** The necessary treatment for mental irritation is pharmacotherapy.

5. **Nyū-in o (o)susume shimasu.** I recommend you be hospitalized.

Nō (Brain)

dai-nō (cerebrum)

nō-ryō (corpus callosum)

shishō (optic thalamus)

shishō-kabu (hypothalamus)

kyō (pons)

shō-nō (cerebellum)

enzui (medulla oblongata)

sekizui (spinal cord)

Additional Words

tachiagaru/tachiagarimasu stand up
meiru/meirimasu slump
damaru/damarimasu not speak/be silent
nayamu/nayamimasu worry
arutsuhaimā-byō Alzheimer's disease
kaishō reduce/eliminate
jishō-kōi self-mutilation

dasu/dashimasu start/go out
ochikomu/ochikomimasu depress
suwaru/suwarimasu sit down
susumeru/susumemasu recommend
utsu-jyōtai depressed condition
kyōsei restrain/forced
jinken human rights

jinken shingai violation of human rights	**jinken-yōgo** protection of human rights
kioku memories	
kaihō-byōtō open ward	**heisa-byōtō** closed ward
kizetsu faint/swoon	**han-toshi** half year
hidoi terrible	**hisuterī** hysteria
hontō truth	**uso** lying
muishiki-ni unconsciously	**kō-seishin-yaku** psychotropic drug

Language Notes

1. The adjective **okashii** has three meanings, "funny, doubtful, problematic." Its usage depends on the context and situation, as does the meaning. To change to the negative form **okashiku-nai** (not funny, not doubtful, not problematic), drop the -**i** and add -**kunai**.

   Sensei no hanashi wa okashii desu.
   The doctor's speech is funny.

   Sensei no hanashi wa chotto okashii desu.
   The doctor's speech is a little dubious.

   Karada no chōshi ga okashii desu.
   My health is problematic.

   Kensa no kekka wa okashiku-nai desu.
   The test result is not problematic.

2. There are several expressions for speaking about one's health or physical condition. In the following, **karada** means "body" and **chōshi** means "condition."

   Karado no chōshi ga ii desu.   I am in good health (condition).
   Karada no chōshi wa yokunai desu.   I am not in good health (condition).

   Karada no chōshi ga okashii desu.
   There is something wrong with (the condition of) my/your health.

   Karada no chōshi wa okashikunai desu.
   There is nothing wrong with (the condition of) my/your health.

   Karada no chōshi ga warui desu.
   I am in poor health (condition).

   Karada no chōshi wa warukunai desu.
   I am not in poor health (condition).

3. There are several expressions for asking about someone's health or physical or athletic condition:

    Karada no chōshi wa ii desu ka.
    Are you in good condition?

    Karada no chōshi wa warui desu ka.
    Are you in bad condition?

    Karado no chōshi wa ikaga desu ka.
    How is about your health (condition)?

    Karada no chōshi wa yokunai desu ka.
    Are you not in good health (condition)?

    Karada no chōshi wa okashikunai desu ka.
    Is there something wrong with your health (condition)?

    Karada no chōshi wa warukunai desu ka.
    Aren't you in poor health (condition)?

4. The idiom **ki ga meiru** is a common way to say, "I am depressed." **Ki** is a noun of feeling or emotion, and the verb **meiru** means "depressed." **Meiru** is sometimes replaced by **ochikomu** (feel down, in a slump) to express more unfavorable or stressful conditions. In ordinary conversation, Japanese often drop **ki** and use the verbs alone. Since **meiru** and **ochimoku** are used only for expressing a depressive or "down in the dumps" state of mind, the subject **ki** isn't felt to be necessary.

[Ki ga] meitte imasu ka.	Are you depressed?
[Ki ga] ochikonde imasu ka.	Are you feeling down?

    The informal way to say the same thing uses the **te**-form plus **iru-yo**, which is a present progressive. A still more informal way drops the **-i**, to make **-te** plus **[i]-ru-yo**.

(Ima ki ga) meitte imasu.	(I am) depressed (now). (formal)
(Ima kibun ga) ochikonde imasu.	(I am) feeling down (now). (formal)
Meitte (i)ru yo.	(I am) depressed. (informal)
Ochikonde (i)ru yo.	(I am) feeling down. (informal)
Meitte-ru.	Depressed. (very informal)
Ochikonde-ru.	Feeling down. (very informal)

Language Roots

The word **shin** (神) indicates spirit and psyche.

shin-kei	nerve
sei-shin-byō	mental illness/psychosis
shin-kei-shō	nervous disorder/neurosis
shin-kei-shitsu	nervousness, neurotic
shi-shin	faint

The word **nō** (脳) indicates brain and memory.

nō-socchū	brain stroke
nō-hinketsu	cerebral anemia
nō-shukketsu	brain hemorrhage
nō-ri	one's mind

Culture Notes

The new terminology for schizophrenia

The German word *schizophrenia* was translated into Japanese as **Seishin-bunretsu-byō** (literally, "mental break apart disease") in the Meiji Period (1868–1912). However, this name is now perceived as pejorative and disrespectful to the patients, and the Japanese Society of Psychiatry and Neurology changed the name of the disease to **Sōgō shichō-shō** (literally, "total lost of harmony disease") in 2002.

Morita therapy

The Japanese psychotherapy known as Morita Therapy was developed by Morita Shoma (1874–1938) in 1919. Morita Therapy is not only intended as a cure for neuroses but also offers a method for being aware of and understanding the patient's sensory systems and behavioral patterns. Through awareness and understanding of the self, the patients is able to recover his or her original state of being.

The word **okashii** and understanding the Japanese view of natural beauty

Today, the word **okashii** conveys the sense of "funny, strange, wrong." In the Heian Period (794–1185), however, the meaning of **okashii** was very different: "tasteful, attractive, excellent." According to the *Pillow Book* (**Makura-no-shōshi**) by Sei-shō-nagon, Japanese felt the beauty of nature in each season and accepted it as it was, neither rejecting it nor seeking to conquer it. They especially prized moments of wonder. According to the introduction of the *Pillow Book*, the most interesting, tasteful, attractive, and excellent moments in nature are as follows:

> Spring is for the moment when the sun rises above the skyline, with rays shining and clouds turning purple.

> Summer is for midnight. The full moon is so marvelous. No moon but many fireflies is also fascinating. One or two fireflies left wandering are still graceful. Night rain is also so special.

> Autumn is for twilight. At sunset, the skyline is illuminated and birds hurry back to their roosts. Wild geese receding in flight make excellent scenery. After sundown, the sound of the wind and crickets in the breeze is wonderful, too.

> Winter is for early morning. Snow falling is incomparable. The flare of charcoal lighting in the cold morning, whether the ground was coated white with frost or not, is attractive.

Comprehension

Answer the following questions.

1. Which of the following does NOT belong with the others?
   a. **Utsubyō**   b. **Jiheishō**
   c. **Tenkan**   d. **Yakubutsu-chūdoku**

2. Which of the following could NOT be used to express a complaint about one's health?
   a. **Karado no chōshi ga okashii desu.**
   b. **Sono hanashi wa okashii desu.**
   c. **Zutsū ga shimasu.**
   d. **Karada ga darui(n) desu.**

3. Which of the following best completes the sentence below?
   Kō-utsu-zai o nomazu (   ) iraremasen.
   (I can't stand not taking my antidepressant.)
   a. **niwa**   b. **node**
   c. **demo**   d. **kara**

4. The patient is telling you about a symptom. Which of the following could NOT be used to say, "I am depressed?"
   a. **Utsu-byō desu.**   b. **Ki ga ii desu.**
   c. **Ki ga meitte imasu.**   d. **Ki ga ochikonde imasu.**

Select the appropriate meaning from the list below.

5. **Anata wa fuketsu-kyōfu-shō-gimi no yōdesu.**   (   )
6. **Rōjinsei-chihō niwa yakuji ryōhō ga kakasemasen.**   (   )
7. **Tsūin o (o)susume shimasu.**   (   )
8. **Koko san-ka-getsu hodo, kyū ni yase dashimashita.**   (   )
9. **Fuan-hossa no kusuri o nomazu niwa iraremasen.**   (   )

a. I cannot stand going without taking my medication for anxiety attacks.
b. I recommend you visit a hospital.
c. I have suddenly lost weight in the last three months.
d. You seem to be showing signs of mysophobia.
e. The necessary treatment for senile dementia is pharmacotherapy.

Practice

Respond to the following in Japanese using the cues that have been provided.

1. Offering suggestions.
   (Symptom)   (Healthcare professional)
   1. **Fumin-shō mitai desu.**   _____ (Please take a sleeping pill.)
   2. **Sōgō shichō-shō mitai desu.** _____ (Please hospitalize yourself.)
   3. **Sugoi henzutsū ga shimasu.** _____ (Please get some rest.)
   4. **Shoku-yoku ga arimasen.**   _____ (You look like you are worn out.)
   5. **Ochikomi gimi desu.**   _____ (Please relax.)

2. Offering opinions.
   (Patient)   (Healthcare professional)
   1. **Tabe-sugi mitai desu.**   _____
                                     (You have a tendency to gain weight.)
   2. **Tsukarete-iru mitai desu.** _____
                                     (You have a tendency to get exhausted.)
   3. **Byōki gachi desu.**   _____
                                     (You have a tendency to get depressed.)
   4. **Atama ga tottemo itai(n) desu.** _____
                                     (You have a tendency to insomnia.)

5. **Taorete kioku ga arimasen.** _____
(You have a tendency to drug abuse.)

3. Asking about symptoms.
(Patient) (Healthcare professional)
1. **Tsukare-gimi desu.** _____
(Do you have stress?)
2. **Neru koto ga dekimasen.** _____
(Do you have auditory hallucinations?)
3. **Hitori de sabishii desu.** _____
(Do you have bipolar disorder?)
4. **Saikin, ira-ira shite imasu.** _____
(Do you have schizophrenia?)
5. **Hito to hanashi ga dekimasen.** _____
(Do you have anthropophobia?)

4. Dialogue comprehension. Based on the dialogue, answer the following questions.
1. **Kato-san wa itsu kara karada no chōshi ga okashii desu ka.**

_____

2. **Kato-san wa don-na shōjyō desu ka.**

_____

3. **Kato-san no kibun wa dō desu ka.**

_____

4. **Kato-san wa don-na jyōtai desu ka.**

_____

5. **Kato-san wa nani ga hitsuyō desu ka.**

_____

5. Free response questions.
(Questions) (Healthcare professional)
1. **Saikin, ki ga meiru koto ga arimasu ka.** _____
2. **Chika-goro, datsuryoku-kan o kanji masu ka.** _____
3. **Sō-utsu-byō-gachi ni narimasu ka.** _____
4. **Tonikaku anata wa fuketsu-kyōfu-shō desu ka.** _____
5. **Taijin kyōfushō-gimi dato omoimasu ka.** _____

Exercises

1. Say the following words in Japanese.
A. Epilepsy _____
B. Schizophrenia _____

      C. Obsessive-compulsive neurosis   _____

      D Suicide   _____

      E. Personality disorder   _____

2. Say the following in Japanese.

    A. I cannot stand going without taking my neuritis medication.

    _____

    B. You seem to show signs of depression.

    _____

    C. I have suddenly gained weight in the last month.

    _____

    D. I recommend you to get some rest.

    _____

    E. The necessary treatment for schizophrenia is pharmacotherapy.

    _____

3. How do you ask patients the following in Japanese?

    A. Do you feel dizzy when you stand up?   _____

    B. Recently, have you been having terrible neuritis?   _____

    C. Do you have a feeling of heaviness and weakness?   _____

    D. Is it harder for you to sleep when you try to?   _____

    E. Do you suffer from bipolar disorder?   _____

4. Answer the following questions in Japanese.

    1. Q: **Koko ni-ka-getsu hodo de, kyū ni yase dashi-mashita.**

       A: _____

       (I will recommend that you take this medicine for a while.)

    2. Q: **Watakushi wa sō-utsu-byō no yōdesu.**

       A: _____

       (The necessary treatment for bipolar disorder is pharmacotherapy.)

    3. Q: **Don-nani tsukarete ite-mo yoku nemure-masen.**

       A: _____

       (I recommend you see a specialist.)

Obstetrics & Gynecology
(Sanfujin-ka)

Basic Vocabulary (CD 27-1)

Listen to the CD and repeat the vocabulary.

#	English	Romaji	Japanese
1.	vagina	**chitsu**	膣
2.	pelvic inflammatory disease	**kotsuban-nai-enshō**	骨盤内炎症
3.	endometrial cancer	**shikyū-taigan**	子宮体癌
4.	endometriosis	**shikyū-naimaku-shō**	子宮内膜症
5.	fibroid tumors/uterine fibroids	**shikyū-kinshu**	子宮筋腫
6.	uterine cancer, cancer of the uterus	**shikyū-gan**	子宮癌
7.	cervical cancer; cancer of the cervix	**shikyū-kei-gan**	子宮頸癌
8.	ovary	**ransō**	卵巣
9.	ovarian tumors	**ransō-shuyō**	卵巣腫瘍
10.	vaginitis/vagina infections	**chitsu-en**	膣炎
11.	vaginal itching	**chitsu no kayumi**	膣の痒み
12.	laparoscopy	**shikyū-naishi-kyō**	子宮内視鏡
13.	menstrual cycle	**gekkei shūki**	月経周期
14.	menstrual irregularity	**seiri-fujyun**	生理不順
15.	menopause	**heikei**	閉経
16.	vaginal discharge	**ori-mono**	下り物
17.	ova	**ran-shi**	卵子
18.	genital organ	**sei-ki**	性器
19.	breast cancer	**nyū-gan**	乳癌
20.	mammary gland	**nyūsen**	乳腺
21.	breast self examination	**nyū-gan jiko-kenshin**	乳癌自己検診
22.	menopausal symptoms	**kōnenki-shōgai**	更年期障害
23.	abnormal vaginal bleeding	**fusei shukketsu**	不正出血
24.	basal body temperature	**kiso-taion**	基礎体温
25.	ovulation	**hairan**	排卵
26.	infertile	**funin-shō**	不妊症
27.	pregnancy test	**ninshin-kensa**	妊娠検査
28.	birth control	**hinin**	避妊
29.	abortion	**jinkō-chūzetsu**	人工中絶
30.	artificial insemination	**jinkō-jyusei**	人口受精

Jyosei-seishoku-ki (Woman's Reproductive System)

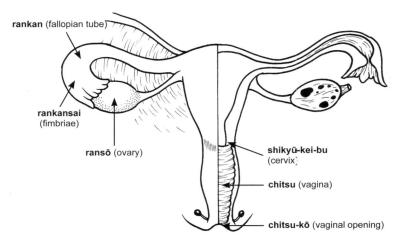

rankan (fallopian tube)

rankansai
(fimbriae)

ransō (ovary)

shikyū-kei-bu
(cervix)

chitsu (vagina)

chitsu-kō (vaginal opening)

Dialogue (CD 27-2)

Listen to the CD and repeat the dialogue.

At the Obstetrics & Gynecology Clinic

Dr. Chen (male doctor):   **Kyō wa dō nasare mashita ka.**
Is there anything you're concerned about today?

Mrs. Tanaka: **Saikin yoku tsukarete, ikigire o kanjiru koto ga airmasu.**
I have been feeling tired and short of breath recently.

Soreni, hinketsu-gimi desu.
And I feel a little anemic.

Dr. Chen: **Mazu, shitsumon o sasete itadakimasu. Seiri wa jyunchō desu ka.**
First of all, I have a question for you. Have your periods been regular?

Mrs. Tanaka: **Hai, ichiō, jyunchō dato omoimasu.**
Yes, I think my period is normal for the most part.

Tada, koko sū-ka-getsu hodo, seiri no ryō ga ōkattari, fusei-shukketsu ga attari shimashita.
However, I sometimes have heavy periods, and sometimes abnormal vaginal bleeding in recent months.

Dr. Chen: **Soredewa, naishin to chō-onpa de shinstau shite mimashō.**
Well then, let's do a pelvic exam and an ultrasound exam.

Mrs. Tanaka:	**Hai, onegai-shimasu.**
	Yes, please. . . .
Dr. Chen:	**Chō-onpa kensa dewa, shikyū ga ōkiku-natte iru no ga wakari-masu.**
	According to the ultrasound examination, we can see your uterus is enlarging.

Futsū no shikyū wa tamago no ōkisa kuraina hazu nanoni, ana-ta no baai wa futsū no yaku ni-bai no ōkisa desu.
Usually the size of uterus is like a hen's egg, but in your case it is twice as large.

Chō-onpa kensa de, chokkei ni-senchi hodo no kinshu ga mitsu-kari-mashita.
In the ultrasound exam, we found a myoma about two centimeters in diameter.

Tabun, kore ga tairyō no gekkei to hinketus no genin dato kangae-raremasu.
This is perhaps the cause of your heavy periods and anemia.

Mrs. Tanaka:	**Shujyutsu ga hitsuyō desu ka.**
	Do I need surgery?
Dr. Chen:	**Iie, anata nowa tekishutsu-shujyutsu o suru hodo wa ōkikunai node, shujyutsu wa ima-no-tokoro hitsuyō-nai to omoimasu.**
	No, I don't think it is necessary to have surgery because your my-oma is not big enough to be removed.

Mazu, kanō na kagiri hinketus ya shukketsu o osaeru chiryō o shimashō.
Anyway, we will try to control your anemia and stop your bleeding as much as possible with treatment.

Sorekara, keika-kansatsu o suru yōni shimashō.
Then let's be sure to monitor your illness carefully.

Grammar

1. The adverbs ichiō and **toriaezu**

The adverb **ichiō** expresses tentativeness and is used to mark a determination or decision. It can be translated as "just in case; tentatively; for the time being. the most part." The adverb **toriaezu** has the same meanings but in addition may mean "first of all; for now; at once."

Ichiō kōnenki-shōgai no kensa o shimashō.
Just in case, let's examine your menopausal troubles.

Kensa no kekka wa ichiyō mondai nai desu yo.
The results of the examination tentatively show no problem.

Shikyū kei-gan ga shinpai nanode, ichiō kensa shite mimasu ka.
I am worried about cervical cancer, so would you like to examine me, just in case?

Toriaezu, kensa o shimashō.
Let's take a look just in case.

2. The conjunction **tada** expresses a change in topic.

In Lesson 8, we studied the conjunctions **soshite** (and), **sorekara** (and then), **shikashi** (but), and **demo** (but). **Tada** is an abbreviation of **tada(shi)**, which indicates a change in topic that is conditioned on something and means "however, nevertheless, but." **Tada** can also have other meanings, such as "just, only, only just, merely, simply" and, as a noun, "free of charge."

Tada, kono shujyutsu wa muzukashii desu.
However, this operation is difficult.

Tada, asa okita toki(ni) kafukubu ga itakatta dake desu.
Nevertheless, I felt lower abdominal pain when I woke up in the morning.

Sensei ni tada hanashita dake desu.
I only just talked to the doctor.

Watakushi wa tada kensa o ukeru dake desu.
I will just have an examination.

Kyō no chiryōdai wa tada desu.
Today's treatment is free of charge.

Kusuri wa tada dewa arimasen.
The medicine is not free of charge.

3. The constructions NOUN **na**-ADJECTIVE + **dattari**, and **i**-ADJECTIVE + **kattari**

In Lessons 12 and 23, we discussed the verb **tari** and saw how the phrase **tari . . . tari . . .** can be used to string together two or more actions or states. When **tari . . . tari . . .** is used in a construction with a noun or **na**-adjectives, **da** must be inserted between the noun and **tari** to make **dattari**. In a construction with an **i**-adjective, you must drop the -**i** ending and replace it with **kattari**. The English translation for both constructions is "like A and

B; sometimes A and sometimes B." For **i**-adjectives, the negative is based on the negative adjective ending, **-kunai**. To make the negative **i**-adjective, drop the **-i** ending and replace it with **-kattari** to make **ku-nakattari**. For negative nouns and **na**-adjectives, add **de (mo)** for "also" or **de(wa)** for the subject marker plus **nakattari**.

Seiri no ryō ga ōkattari, fusei-shukketsu ga attari shimashita.
I sometimes had heavy periods, and sometimes abnormal vaginal bleeding.

Kanjya no byōki wa nyū-gan dattari, shukyū-gan dattari desu.
The patients' illnesses are things like breast cancer and cancer of the uterus.

Seiri-fujyun no shōjyō wa yōtsū dattari, kurushi-kattari desu.
The symptoms of menstrual irregularity are something like back pain and suffering.

Byōki wa itakattai, itaku-nakattari shimasu ka.
Do you have pain or not (pain) from your illness?

Kensa no kekka wa shikyū-kinshu de(mo) nakkatari, ranshō-shuyō de(mo) nakkari desu.
Your test results showed neither a fibroid tumor nor an ovarian tumor.

Nyū-gan no shujyutsu wa kantan de(wa) nakattari shimasu.
The operation for breast cancer is not easy.

The following are examples of **i**-adjectives conjugated in this way.

ENGLISH	I-ADJECTIVE	NEGATIVE FORM Drop -i, add **kunai**	**TARI** FORM Drop -i, add **kattari**	NEGATIVE **TARI** Drop i, add **kuna-kattari**
many	ōi	ō-kunai	ō-kattari	ō-ku-nakattari
big	ōkii	ōki-kunai	ōki-kattari	ōki-ku-nakattari
painful	itai	ita-kunai	ita-kattari	ita-ku-nakattari
itchy	kayui	kayu-kunai	kayu-kattari	kayu-ku-nakattari
sufferable	kurushii	kurushi-kunai	kurushi-kattari	kurushi-ku-nakattari

4. The suffix -sa

Like the English suffixes -*ness* and -*ty*, the suffix **-sa** is used to makes nouns out of adjectives and conveys the notion of current status, condition, situation, circumstances, degree, amount, grade, and quality. Adding **-sa** to an adjective stem also changes the meaning. For the suffix **-mi** added to adjectives, please see Lesson 6.

> **Kono shikori niwa katasa ga arimasu.**
> This lump has hardness.
>
> **Kono chiryō niwa muzukashisa garimasu.**
> This surgery has difficulty/some difficulty.
>
> **Ransō-shuyō no ōkisa ga shinpai desu.**
> I am worried about the size of the ovarian tumors.

ENGLISH	ADJECTIVE	NOUN	NOUN MEANING
big	**ōki-i**	**ōki-sa**	size
high	**taka-i**	**taka-sa**	height
wide	**hiro-i**	**hiro-sa**	size of space
difficult	**muzukashi-i**	**muzukashi-sa**	difficulty
long	**naga-i**	**naga-sa**	length
heavy	**omo-i**	**omo-sa**	weight

5. The phrase hazu nano ni

In the phrase **hazu nano ni**, **hazu nano** expresses expectation and confidence, but **ni** is similar to "on the contrary" and may be translated as "but, however." All together, **hazu nano ni** means "I am fairly certain that . . . , but; I expected . . . , but; I can say with confidence . . . , but."

> **Kafukubu-tsū wa tottemo itai hazu nano ni, itaku nai rashii desu.**
> I am fairly certain that low abdominal pain is very painful, but it does not seem painful (*lit.*, The low abdominal pain is very painful, but you look like you have no pain).
>
> **Hi-nin o shita hazu nano ni, ninshin o shimashita.**
> I can say with confidence that I used birth control, but I became pregnant.

6. The construction NUMBER + -bai

The suffix **-bai** is a counter for quantity or amount, and in the construction NUMBER plus **-bai** can mean "times, -fold, twice, double, triple, thrice."

Kusuri wa futsū no yaku ni-bai no ryō o shohō shimasu.
I will prescribe twice as much as the usual amount of medicine (*lit.*, I will prescribe medicine about two times more than the usual amount).

Ori-mono ga futsū no ni-bai arimashita ka.
Did you have two times more vaginal discharge than normal?

Hoken ga nai-node, shinsatsu-ryō wa san-bai da sō desu.
Since you don't have insurance, it looks like your doctor's fee will triple.

7. Understanding the transitive verb **o mitsukeru/mitsukemasu** and intransitive verb **ga mitsukaru/mitsukarimasu**

The transitive verb **mitsukeru** means "find, find out (something)." As a transitive verb, it can take a direct object, which usually is a person or animate being and is signaled by the object marker **o** that follows it. Transitive verbs are also used to make the passive voice, which is done by adding the suffix -**rareru**, as in this case with **mitsuke-rareru**. They also form the present progressive, using the **te**-form plus -**iru/-imasu**. In contrast, the intransitive verb **mitsukaru** (be found/turn up) cannot take a direct object or -**iru/-imasu**.

Sensei wa nyū-gan o mitsuke-mashita.
The doctor found breast cancer. (transitive verb)

Sensei wa nyū-gan o mitsuke-raremashita.
Breast cancer was found by the doctor. (transitive, passive form)

Sensei wa nyū-gan o mitsukete-imasu.
The doctor is finding breast cancer. (transitive, present progressive)

Nyū-gan ga mitsukari-mashita.
Breast cancer was found. (intransitive verb)

8. The expression **ima-no-tokoro**

The expression **ima-no-tokoro** means "for now; for the moment; so far; for the time being," and can be used to convey the progress of treatment. For example:

Kanjya wa ima-no-tokoro daijyōbu desu yo.
The patient is all right for now.

Shikyū-kei-gan kensa no kekka, ima-no-tokoro wa nantomo ie-masen.
For the moment, I cannot tell anything from the cervical cancer examination results.

Shujyutsu-go no keika wa ima-no-tokoro jyunchō desu.
The status after surgery is good so far.

Ima-no-tokoro wa funin-shō kensa no kekka o matsu tsumori desu.
For the time being, I intend to wait for the results of the infertility test.

9. The phrase **kanō na gakiri/dekiru kagiri**

The phrase **kanō na gakiri** conveys the idea of "(by) every possible means" and is equivalent to "whatever you can; whenever you can; as often as possible; as much as possible" in English. The phrase **dekiru kagiri** has the same meaning.

Kanō na kagiri, funin-shō no chiryō o shimashō.
Let's do whatever we can to treat your infertility.

Kanō na kagiri, kensa o ukete kudasai.
Please have an examination whenever you can.

Dekiru kagiri, kiso-taion o kiroku shite kudasai.
Please record your basal body temperature as often as possible.

10. The construction STEM VERB + **yōni suru**

In Lesson 17, we studied **yōni**, meaning "to be like, similar to." The construction STEM VERB plus **yōni suru** expresses the idea of making efforts or performing an action to make sure that something will happen.

Neru-mae ni kusuri o nomu-yōni shite kudasai.
Before you sleep, be sure to take (your) medicine.

Hinin o suru yō ni shite imasu ka.
Do you have birth control? (*lit.*, Are you making efforts to have birth control?)

Seiri-fujyun o chiryō suru yōni shimasu.
I intend to make sure that you will treat dysmenorrheal.

Useful Expressions (CD 27-3)

Listen to the CD and repeat the sentences.

1. **Saigo no seiri wa itsu deshita ka.** When was your last period?
2. **Ima, seiri-chū desu ka.** Are you having your period now?
3. **Seiri ga roku-shū-kan hodo okurete imasu.** My period is about six weeks late.
4. **Chibusa ni shikori ga arumitai desu.** You may have a lump in your breast.
5. **Chikubi kara bunpitsu-butsu ga dete imasu ka.** Do you have discharge from your nipple?
6. **Izen ni nyūsen-en o wazurai mashita ka.** Have you have mastitis before?

7. **Seiri ga arimasen.** I don't menstruate.
8. **Seiri ga ichi-do nukemashita.** I missed one period.
9. **Seiri ga fukisoku desu.** My period is irregular.
10. **Seiri-tsū ga hidoi desu ka.** Do you have terrible period pain?

Key Sentences (CD 27-4)

Listen to the CD and repeat the sentences.

1. **Ichiō, shikyū-kinshu no kensa o shimashō.** Just in case, let's examine you for fibroid tumors.
2. **Kyonen, gan-kensa o shita hazu nano ni, nyū-gan ni narimashita.** I can say with confidence that you had a cancer screening in the last year, but you got breast cancer.
3. **Nyū-gan no saihatsu wa ima-no-tokoro daijyōbu desu yo.** A recurrence of breast cancer is not a problem at the moment.
4. **Kanōna kagiri, seiri-fujyun no chiryō o ukete kudasai.** Please have treatments for menstrual irregularity whenever you can.
5. **Mai-asa, okiru mae ni kiso-taion o tsukeru yōni shite kudasai.** Before you get up in the morning every day, be sure to take your basal body temperature.

Additional Words

hiraku/hirakimasu open
tojiru/tojimasu close
kumu/kumimasu cross/put together
nukeru/nukemashita skip/fall out
okureru/okuremasu delay/behind
seishoku-ki reproductive organ
wazurau/wazuraimasu worry and suffer
tsukeru/tsukemasu record/attach
mitsukeru/mitsukemasu find (transitive verb)
mitsukaru/mitsukarimasu be found (intransitive verb)
shojyo-maku hymen
seishi sperm
tekishitsu-shujyutsu removal surgery
kanō-na possible
shochō first menstruation
kazoku keikaku family planning

horumon-zai hormone active drugs
naishin pelvic examination
hairan yūhatsu-zai ovulation-inducing drug
hairan yotei-bi ovulation day
chō-onpa ultrasound
keika progress
junchō favorable/doing well
fumei unknown
tairyō large quantity
manzoku-kan feeling of satisfaction
fukan-shō sexual frigidity
bunpitsu-butsu discharge
mata crotch
kinshu myoma
saihatsu recurrence
gekkei-zen shōkō-gun PMS/premenstrual syndrome

Language Notes

1. The expression DISEASE (NOUN) **no genin** means "the cause of DISEASE."

Byōki no genin wa fumei desu.	The cause of the illness is unknown.
Byōki no genin ga wakarimashita.	The cause of the illness was known.
Uirusu wa shikyū-gan no genin ni narimasu.	A virus may be the cause of uterine cancer.
Kono byōki no genin wa uirusu desu.	This illness is caused by a virus.

    Sutoreu ga funin-shō no genin ni natte iru baai ga ōi desu.
    There are many cases of infertility caused by stress.

2. The noun **chokkei** means "diameter." **Chokkei**, in the context of this chapter's topic, can be used to express the size of a tumor. **Hankei** is radius.

    MRI kensa-de, chokkei go-miri-hodo no shuyō ga mitsukari mashita.
    Through the MRI examination, we found a tumor about five millimeters in diameter.

    Nyū-gan kensa de, chokkei ni-senchi no gan ga mitsukari mashita.
    From the breast examination, we found a cancer about two centimeters in diameter.

    Chokkei donokurai no shuyō ga arimasu ka.
    What diameter tumor do you have?

3. Expressions for sexual-related complaints:

Sei-yoku ga arimasen.	I don't have any sexual desire.
Fukan-shō no yō desu.	I am afraid that I am sexually frigid.
Manzoku-kan ga arimasen.	I cannot get sexual satisfaction.
In-bu ga kayui(n) desu.	I have an itch in my pubic area.
Seikō suru to shukketsu ga arimasu.	I bleed while having sex.

4. Instructions that can be used during the physical examinations:

Kutsu o nuide kudasai.	Please take off your shoes.
Shinsagtsu-dai ni agate kudasai.	Please get up on the examination table.
Ashi o ashi-dai ni nosete kudasai.	Please put your legs on the leg rests.
Te wa mune no ue de kunde kudasai.	Please hold your hands on your chest.
Karada no chikara o nuite kudasai.	Please relax your body.
Ashi no chikara o nuite kudasai.	Please relax your legs.
Mata o hirai te kudasai.	Please open your crotch.
Mō-sukoshi sagatte kudasai.	Please move down a little.
Mō-sukoshi agate kudasai.	Please move up a little.

Language Roots

The word **kyū** (宮) indicates a holy place or womb.

shi-kyū	womb
shi-kyū-gai ninshin	ectopic pregnancy
shi-kyū-gan	uterus cancer

The word **ri** (理) indicates a principle, rule, and reason.

sei-ri	periods
ri-gaku ryōhō	physical therapy
ri-gaku ryōhō-shi	physiotherapist
ri-yū	reason

Culture Notes

Hot springs and healing illnesses

There are many hot springs throughout Japan. Each hot spring has different water quality and chemical elements that are good for many kinds of diseases, including female disorders, rheumatism, neuralgia, chronic digestive disease, allergies, joint pain, muscle pain, diabetes, gout, obesity, cardiovascular failure, gallstones, etc.

Health-related Japanese proverbs XIII

Labor is a seed of comfort.
Ku wa raku no tane.
苦は楽の種

Faith will move the mountain.
Shin-nen wa yama omo ugokasu.
信念は山をも動かす

Comprehension

Answer the following questions.

1. Which of the following does NOT belong with the others?
   a. **Seiki**   b. **Nyū-gan**
   c. **Shikyū**   d. **Chitsu**

2. Which of the following could be used to say "vaginal discharge"?
    a. **Ransō**   b. **Shochō**
    c. **Orimono**   d. **Funin-shō**

3. Which of the following best completes the sentence below?
    Hinin wa shita hazu nano (   ), ninshin o shimashita.
    (I can say with confidence that I took birth control, but I still became pregnant.)
    a. **ni**   b. **de**
    c. **to**   d. **ga**

4. You are asking a patient about a sexual disorder. Which of the following means "Do you have no sexual desire?"
    a. **Inbu ga kayui desu ka.**   b. **Sei-yoku ga arimasen ka.**
    c. **Fukan-shō no yō desu ka.**   d. **Manzoku-kan ga arimasen ka.**

Select the appropriate meaning from the list below.

---

5. **Dōki ga shitari, ikigire ga shitari shimasu ka.**   (   )
6. **Kanō na kagiri, gekkei-zen shōkō-gun no kensa o ukete kudasai.** (   )
7. **Kensa no kekka wa ichiyō mondai nai desu ne.**   (   )
8. **Nyū-gan jiko-kenshin o shita hazu nano ni, nyū-gan ni natte**   (   )
    shimaimashita.
9. **Shussan-go no keika wa ima-no-tokoro jyunchō desu ka.**   (   )

a. The examination result tentatively shows no problem.
b. Do you sometimes have palpitations or shortness of breath?
c. I can say with confidence that I did the breast self-examination, but I still developed breast cancer.
d. Is the status after the delivery good so far?
e. Let's do whatever you can test for premenstrual syndrome.

Practice

Respond to the following in Japanese using the cues that have been provided.

---

1. Giving the patient your opinion.
    (Symptom)   (Healthcare professional)
    1. **Shikyū-kei-gan mitai desu.**   _____
                                           (The cause of the illness is unknown.)

2. **Sei-kansen-shō mitai desu.** _____

(The cause of the illness was known.)

3. **Kafukubu-tsū no genin wa nan desu ka.** _____

(This illness resulted from endometriosis.)

4. **Shikyū-gan no genin wa nan desu ka.** _____

(This illness resulted from a virus.)

5. **Funin-shō no genin wa nan desu ka.** _____

(Stress is responsible for many cases of infertility.)

2. Answer the following questions.

(Patient)   (Healthcare professional)

1. **Chokkei donokurai no shikori ga arimasu ka.** _____ (1/4 inch)

2. **Chokkei donokurai no ransō-shuyō ga arimasu ka.** _____(3/4 inch)

3. **Chokkei donokurai no shuyō ga arimasu ka.** _____ (2 mm.)

4. **Inbu ga kayui(n) desu.** _____

(I will prescribe antibiotic medicine for you.)

5. **Sei-yoku ga demasen.** _____

(You should got some rest.)

3. Giving instructions.

(Patient)   (Healthcare professional)

1. **Kutsu wa dō-shimasu ka.** _____

(Please take off your shoes.)

2. **Shinsatsu-dai ni agarimasu ka.** _____

(Yes, please get up on the examination table.)

3. **Te wa dō shimasu ka.** _____

(Please hold your hands on your chest.)

4. **Kinchō shite imasu.** _____

(Please relax on your body.)

5. **Tai-i wa korede ii-desu ka.** _____

(Please move down a little.)

4. Dialogue comprehension. Based on the dialogue, answer the following questions.

1. **Tanaka-san wa don-na shōjyō desu ka.**

_____

2. **Tanaka-san no seiri wa jyunchō desu ka.**

_____

3. **Tanaka-san wa itsu kara fusei-shukketsu ga arimasu ka.**

_____

    4. **Tanaka-san wa don-na kensa o shimashita ka.**

    _____

    5. **Tanaka-san no kensa kekka wa dō-deshita ka.**

    _____

5. Free response questions.

    (Questions)   (Healthcare professionals)

    1. **Mainen, kenkō-shindan o shimasu ka.** _____

    2. **Kyō no chiryō-dai wa tada de ii desu ka.** _____

    3. **Kanjya no shōjyō wa itagattari shite imasu ka.** _____

    4. **Kanjya-san wa ima-no-tokoro daijyōbu desu ka.** _____

    5. **Sei-kansenshō ga shinpai desu ka.** _____

    6. **Hinin o suru yō ni shite imasu ka.** _____

Exercise

1. Say the following terms in Japanese.

    A. Endometrial cancer

    B. Cervical cancer   _____

    C. Breast cancer   _____

    D. Uterine cancer   _____

    E. Ovarian cancer   _____

2. Say the following in Japanese.

    A. The test result tentatively shows no problem at the moment.

    _____

    B. I can say with confidence that you have been treated with artificial insemi-
nation, but you have not become pregnant

    _____

    C. The patient is all right for the moment.   _____

    D. An ovarian tumor was found.   _____

    E. Let's do whatever we can treat your itchiness.   _____

3. How do you ask patients the following questions in Japanese?

    A. Do you have discharge from your vagina?   _____

    B. When was your last period?   _____

    C. Do you have terrible pain during your period? _____

    D. Have you had artificial insemination before? _____

    E. Do you have a lump in your breast?   _____

LESSON 28 Pregnancy & Childbirth
(Ninshin to Shussan)

Basic Vocabulary (CD 28-1)

Listen to the CD and repeat the vocabulary.

1.	childbirth	**shussan**	出産
2.	pregnant	**ninpu**	妊婦
3.	fetus	**taiji**	胎児
4.	due date	**shussan yotei-bi**	出産予定日
5.	morning sickness	**tsuwari**	つわり
6.	fetal heart sound	**shin-on**	心音
7.	fetal movement	**taidō**	胎動
8.	cervix of the uterus	**shikyū-kō**	子宮口
9.	delivery unit	**bunben-dai**	分娩台
10.	contractions/labor pains	**jintsū**	陣痛
11.	labor-inducing drugs	**jintsū-sokushin-zai**	陣痛促進剤
12.	pushing	**ikimi**	息み
13.	leg cramp	**komura-gaeri**	こむら返り
14.	membrane rupture	**hasui**	破水
15.	premature rupture (of the membranes)	**sōki-hasui**	早期破水
16.	delivery	**bunben**	分娩
17.	placenta	**taiban**	胎盤
18.	miscarriage	**ryū-zan**	流産
19.	cesarean section/C-section	**teiō-sekkai**	帝王切開
20.	early birth/premature birth	**sō-zan**	早産
21.	stillbirth	**shi-zan**	死産
22.	breech presentation	**saka-go**	逆子
23.	premature baby	**mijyuku-ji**	未熟児
24.	umbilical cord	**heso-no-o**	臍の緒
25.	newborn baby	**shinsei-ji**	新生児
26.	mother	**haha-oya**	母親
27.	breast feeding	**bonyū-eiyō**	母乳栄養
28.	bottle feeding	**jinkō-eiyō**	人工栄養
29.	twins	**futago**	双子
30.	tocodynamometer	**bunben kanshi-sōchi**	分娩監視装置

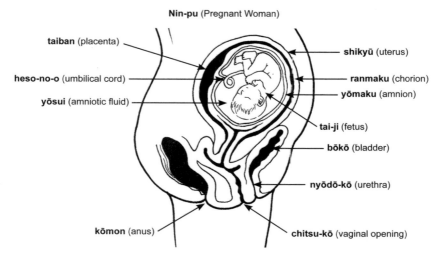

Nin-pu (Pregnant Woman)

taiban (placenta)

heso-no-o (umbilical cord)

yōsui (amniotic fluid)

shikyū (uterus)

ranmaku (chorion)

yōmaku (amnion)

tai-ji (fetus)

bōkō (bladder)

nyōdō-kō (urethra)

kōmon (anus)

chitsu-kō (vaginal opening)

Dialogue (CD 28-2)

Listen to the CD and repeat the dialogue.

At the Obstetrics & Gynecology Clinic

Dr. Chen:	**Ohayō gozaimasu. Kyō wa dō nasare mashita ka.** Good morning. Are you concerned about anything today?
Mrs. Yamada:	**Jitsu-wa seiri ga nai node, ninshin kensa o onegai shimashita.** Frankly speaking, I missed my period, so I asked to have a pregnancy test.
Dr. Chen:	**Sō desu ka. Saigo no seiri wa itsu deshita ka.** Is that so? When was your last period?
Mrs. Yamada:	**(Saigo no seiri wa) yon-ka-getsu gurai mae-ni arimashita.** (My last period was) About four months ago.
Dr. Chen:	**Sō desu ka. Kiso-taion wa tsukete imasu ka.** Is that so? Are you keeping track of your basal body temperature? **Shukketsu (ka) mata wa, onaka ga hattari shimasu ka.** Do you have either bleeding or bloating in your lower abdomen?
Mrs. Yamada:	**Iie, tokuni kiso-taion mo tsukete naishi, shukketsu mo naishi, onaka no hari mo arimasen.** No, I am not keeping special records of my basal body temperature, and I don't have either bleeding or bloating in my lower abdomen.

Shikashi, asa okita toki(ni) kibun ga hakike to onaji kurai mu-ka-muka shimasu.

However, I feel sick when I wake up in the morning.

Sorekara, suppai mono ga tabetaku-narimashita.

And also, I have a yen for sour foods.

Dr. Chen: **Moshi ninshin shita koto ga areba oshiete kudasai.**

Can you tell me if you have been pregnant before?

Mrs. Yamada: **Hai. masaka-towa omoimashita ga, ni-nen mae ni ichido ryū-zan o shimashita.**

Yes. I never expected to, but I had a miscarriage two years ago.

Dr. Chen: **Sō desu ka. Ima, ninshin kensa no kekka o mitara, anata wa nin-shin san-ka-getsu desu yo.**

Is that so? I just looked at the results of your pregnancy test, and it shows you are three months pregnant.

Shussan yotei-bi wa shi-gatsu jyō-jun gurai desu. Omedetō go-zaimasu.

Your due date is approximately in early April. Congratulations.

Grammar

1. The conjunction **jitsu-wa**

The conjunction **jitsu-wa** shifts topics to get to the truth of the matter and can be translated as "frankly speaking; in fact; the fact is that; actually; by the way; to tell you the truth; to be honest." It can also be used with the copula **nan/nan(o) desu** or **da** (informal) for nouns and **no desu** for verbs.

Jitsuwa, onegai ga aru-no desu ga.

Frankly speaking, I have a favor to ask of you.

Jitsuwa, (watakushi wa) ninshin-chū nan desu.

The fact is that I am pregnant.

Kare wa bijinesu-man no yōni mieru ga, jitsuwa kango-shi da.

He looks like a businessman, but in fact he is a nurse.

Jitsuwa, mijyuku-ji nano desu.

Actually, that baby was premature.

2. **The constructions** NOUN + **no mae-ni,** STEM VERB + **mae-ni, and** TIME + **mae-ni**

The constructions NOUN plus **no mae-ni,** STEM VERB plus **mae-ni,** and TIME plus **mae-ni** are all used to express an event or action that occurred earlier in time. The literal meaning of **mae** is "front/ahead," and the English equivalent of the particle **ni** is *at*. The first two constructions are often translated as "before (action)." TIME plus **mae-ni** can be translated as "before (time)" or "(time) ago." For ways to express a duration of time, see Lesson 8. The construction NOUN **no ato** (after) plus **de** is used to express an action or event that happens first.

> **Shussan no mae-ni kensa ga hitsuyō desu ne.**
> You need an examination before you give birth (*lit.*, Before you give birth, you need an examination).

> **Ikimu mae-ni, shinkokyū o shite kudasai.**
> Before pushing, please take a deep breath.

> **Saigo no seiri wa san-ka-getsu gurai mae-ni arimashita.**
> My last period was about three months ago.

> **Hasui wa go-fun mae-ni arimashita.**
> The membrane rupture happened five minutes ago.

> **Bunben no ato-ni taiban ga demashita.**
> The placenta came out after the delivery (*lit.*, After the delivery, the placenta came out).

3. **The conjunction mata wa**

The conjunction **mata wa** connects two possibilities or options expressed by noun phrases or sentences and is translated as "either . . . or . . . ; or." When **mata wa** connects two noun phrases, the **ka** after the first noun phrase is optional, or **mata wa** may be abbreviated and only **ka** remains in the sentences. Be careful not to confuse the conjunction **mata wa** (or), the adverb **mata** (again), and the noun **mata** (crotch). The adverb **mata** is used in such sentences as: **Mata kensa o shimasu.** "I will examine you again."

> **Mukumi ka, mata wa itami ga onaka ni arimasu ka.**
> Do you have either edema or pain in your abdomen?

> **Orimono (ka), mata wa seiri ga airmasu ka.**
> Do you have a discharge or are you menstruating?

> **Jintsu ka, (mata wa) hasui ga suguni aru-to omoimasu.**
> I think that you may have either contractions or a membrane rupture soon.

4. The idiom **mo nai(desu)shi . . . mo nai(desu)/arimasen**

The phrase **mo naishi . . . mo nai/arimasen** translates as "neither . . . nor; not either . . . or" and serves to link a list of elements belonging to the same part of speech. The conjunction **shi** that is part of **naishi** indicates repetition and translates as "and; and what's more; not only . . . but also . . . ; so." In polite expression, add **desu** (present tense)/**deshita** (past tense) before -**shi**.

> **Ima wa itaku-mo naishi, kayuku-mo naishi, shukketsu mo nai-desu.**
> There is neither pain, nor itchiness, nor bleeding now.

> **Mada, jintsū mo naishi, hasui mo arimasen.**
> Neither contractions nor the membrane rupture have happened yet.

> **Ninshin san-ka-getsu desu ga, onaka no hari mo nai-desu-shi, shukketsu mo nai-desu-shi, tsuwari mo arimasen.**
> She has neither bloating nor bleeding nor morning sickness, but she is three months pregnant.

5. The idiom **moshi . . . ga areba**

In Lesson 17, we studied the conjunction -**ba** (if), and in Lesson 18 we saw that the idiom **dō sureba ii(n) desu ka** (What shall I do?) is used to ask how or what to do to resolve questions or problems in connection with a conditional statement using **no toki wa** (when) and **no baai wa** (in case of). The expression **moshi . . . ga areba** is another way of expressing a hypothetical or conditional action conveyed in English by *if*.

> **Moshi ninshin shita koto ga areba oshiete kudasai masen ka.** (polite)
> Won't you tell me if you have been pregnant?

> **Moshi jintsū no toki wa oshiete kudasai.**
> Please tell me if you have contractions.

> **Moshi ryūzan ga areba suguni teiō-sekkai o shimasu.**
> In case of miscarriage, we will do a cesarean section immediately.

6. The interjection **masaka**

The interjection **masaka** expresses when a person's expectations are or may be contradicted by reality and may be translated as "never thought; never expected; don't tell me that; surely not; absolutely not; never; you don't say."

> **Masaka sōzan dato wa omowana katta desu.**
> I never thought it would be a premature birth.

Masaka ryūzan ga okoru towa omoimasen-deshita.
I never expected a miscarriage would happen.

Akai kao o shite iru kedo, masaka ninshin dewa naideshō ne.
You look red faced, but surely you're not pregnant, are you?

The expression **masaka no toki** is translated as "in case of emergency."

Masaka no toki wa denwa o kudasai.
In case of emergency, please call me.

7. The verb ending -tara

The verb ending **-tara** is used to express a conditional action or a supposition and translates as "when; if X, then Y." It's also used to express informal advice or suggestions In addition, **-tara** may indicate exasperation or mild frustration, dissatisfaction, or anger when placed after someone's name. There are two ways to change a verb to the **tara** form: VERB BASE plus **-tara**, or STEM VERB OF THE PAST TENSE plus **-ra**. The following **ru**-verb and **u**-verb charts give some examples of verbs with these endings. The stem verb past tense is only used in informal expression.

For **ru**-verbs, 1) find the verb base and add **-tara**, or 2) add **-ra** to the past tense of the stem verb. To make the past tense of the stem verb, drop the stem verb present tense ending **-ru** and add **-ta/-tta**.

Ru-verbs

ENGLISH	VERB BASE	STEM VERB −PRESENT TENSE	STEM VERB − PAST TENSE	TARA (IF)
sleep	**ne(masu)**	**ne-ru**	**ne-ta**	**ne-tara**
eat	**tabe(masu)**	**tabe-ru**	**tabe-ta**	**tabe-tara**
warm	**atatame(masu)**	**atatame-ru**	**atatame-ta**	**atatame-tara**
be visible/ appear	**araware(masu)**	**araware-ru**	**araware-ta**	**araware-tara**
inform/notify	**shirase(masu)**	**shirase-ru**	**shirase-ta**	**shirase-tara**
shiver	**furue(masu)**	**furue-ru**	**furue-ta**	**furue-tara**
go out/appear	**de(masu)**	**de-ru**	**de-ta**	**de-tara**
allow/make to do	**sase(masu)**	**sase-ru**	**sase-ta**	**sase-tara**
anger/be angry	**okori(masu)**	**oko-ru**	**oko-tta**	**oko-ttara**

ENGLISH	VERB BASE	STEM VERB –PRESENT TENSE	STEM VERB – PAST TENSE	**TARA** (IF)
infect/ transmit	**utsuri(masu)**	utsu-ru	utsu-tta	utsu-ttara
see/look	**mi(masu)**	mi-ru	mi-ta	mi-tara
tighten	**shime(masu)**	shime-ru	shime-ta	shime-tara
open	**ake(masu)**	ake-ru	ake-ta	ake-tara
wear (clothes)	**ki(masu)**	ki-ru	ki-ta	ki-tara
feel	**kanji(masu)**	kanji-ru	kanji-ta	kanji-tara
become	**nari(masu)**	na-ru	na-tta	na-ttara
apply/paint	**nuri(masu)**	nu-ru	nu-tta	nu-ttara
mix	**majiri(masu)**	maji-ru	maji-tta	maji-ttara
empty/die/ use up	**nakunari(masu)**	nakuna-ru	nakuna-tta	nakuna-ttara
choke	**tsumari(masu)**	tsuma-ru	tsuma-tta	tsuma-ttara
measure	**hakari(masu)**	haka-ru	haka-tta	haka-ttara
wake up*	**oki(masu)**	oki-ru	oki-ta	oki-tara
do/play*	**shi(masu)**	su-ru	shi-ta	shi-tara
come*	**ki(masu)**	ku-ru	ki-ta	ki-tara

* Irregular

For **u**-verbs, the stem verb past tense is used to make the **-tara** form, and there are different rules for four groups of verbs defined by the ending of the verb base: 1) If the verb base ends with -**mi** and the stem verb present tense ending is -**mu**, form the past tense by substituting -**nda** for -**mu** and add the -**ra** ending. 2) If the verb base ends with -**ri**, -**chi**, or -**i** and stem verb present tense ending is -**ru**, -**tsu**, -**u**, form the past tense by substituting -**tta** for the present tense ending and add -**ra**. 3) If the verb base ends with -**ki** or -**gi** and the stem verb present tense ending is -**ku** or -**gu**, form the past tense by substituting -**ita** for the present tense ending and add -**ra**. 4) If the verb base ends in -**shi** and the stem verb present tense ending is -**su**, form the past tense by substituting -**shita** for the present tense ending and add -**ra**.

U-verbs

ENGLISH	VERB BASE	STEM VERB – PRESENT TENSE	STEM VERB – PAST TENSE	TARA (IF)
drink	nomi (masu)	nomu	nonda	nonda-ra
read	yomi(masu)	yomu	yonda	yonda-ra
rub	momi(masu)	momu	monda	monda-ra
push down	ikimi(masu)	ikimu	ikinda	ikinda-ra
say/tell	ii (masu)	iu	itta	itta-ra
measure	hakari(masu)	hakaru	hakatta	hakatta-ra
stand up	tachi(masu)	tatsu	tatta	tatta-ra
buy	kai(masu)	kau	katta	katta-ra
wash	arai(masu)	arau	aratta	aratta-ra
inhale/smoke	sui(masu)	sū	sutta	sutta-ra
listen	kiki(masu)	kiku	kiita	kiita-ra
write	kaki(masu)	kaku	kaita	kaita-ra
vomit	haki(masu)	haku	haita	haita-ra
open	hiraki(masu)	hiraku	hiraita	hiraita-ra
smell/sniff	kagi(masu)	kagu	kaita	kaita-ra
speak	hanashi(masu)	hanasu	hanashita	hanashita-ra
pull down	oroshi (masu)	orosu	oroshita	oroshita-ra
cool	hiyashi (masu)	hiyasu	hiyashita	hiyashita-ra
throw up	hakidashi(masu)	hakidasu	hakidashita	hakidashita-ra
try	tameshi(masu)	tamesu	tameshita	tameshita-ra
stretch	nobashi(masu)	nobasu	nobashita	nobashita-ra
push	oshi(masu)	osu	oshita	oshita-ra

Ninshin kensa o shitara, ninshin wa mada desu ne.
When you do the pregnancy test, it shows whether you are not yet pregnant, doesn't it?

Jintsū ga okitara, suguni renraku shite kudasai.
If contractions occur, then please inform us immediately.

Ima ikindara, dame desu yo.	If you push now, it's not good.
Omizu o non-dara.	I advise you to drink water. (informal advice)
Yasundara.	You should rest. (informal advice)
Okitara.	Wake up, please. (exasperation)
Sensei-tara.	(mild frustration toward a doctor)
Kangoshi-san-tara.	(mild frustration toward a nurse)

Useful Expressions (CD 28-3)

Listen to the CD and repeat the sentences.

1. **Ninshin shite iru node, rentogen wa toranai de kudasai.** I am pregnant, so please do not take an X-ray.
2. **Ninshin nan-shū-me desu ka.** How many weeks have you been pregnant?
3. **Anata wa ninshin sanjyū-shū-me desu.** You are thirty weeks pregnant.
4. **Mada ikima-naide kudasai.** Don't push yet.
5. **Tsuyoku ikinde kudasai.** Please push harder.
6. **Hā-hā-hā to itte, itami o chirashite kudasai.** Say haa-haa-haa when you breathe out, and you will get some relief from pain.
7. **Nan-pun kan-kaku de jintsū ga kiteimasu ka.** How far apart are the contractions?
8. **Taidō ga arimasu ka.** Did your baby kick?
9. **Shussan yotei-bi wa itsu desu ka.** When is your date of confinement?
10. **Aka-chan wa genki desu yo.** Your baby is fine.

Key Sentences (CD 28-4)

Listen to the CD and repeat the sentences.

1. **Jitsuwa, [anata wa] teiō-sekkai ga hitsuyō desu.** The fact is that a cesarean section is required.
2. **Tsuwari ka, mata wa mukumi ga arimasu ka.** Do you have either morning sickness or swelling?
3. **Mada, itami mo naishi, jintsū mo arimasen.** There are neither pains nor contractions yet.
4. **Masaka sōzan dato wa omowana katta desu.** I never thought that it would be a premature birth.
5. **Jintū ga okitara, suguni renraku shite kudasai.**
   If contractions are happening, please inform us immediately.

Additional Words

okoru/okorimasu happen
ikimu/ikimimasu push down/strain
nuiawaseru/nuiawasemasu saw together
toridasu/toridashimasu take out/ pull out
kazoku-keikaku family planning

shussei-shōmei-sho birth certificate
jyunyū lactation period
san-go postpartum/afterbirth
koshitsu private room/LDRP room
shūki-teki periodically
bonyū breast milk
ninshin-shoki early pregnancy

ui-zan first childbirth
shosan-pu woman who has first childbirth/primipara
jyutai-bi date of conception/D.O.C
keisan-pu woman who has given birth/multipara

jyu-nyū nursing/suckling
chirasu disperse
kawaii cute
shinsei-ji tokutei shūchū chiryō shitsu NICU-neonatal intensive care unit

Language Notes

1. In Japanese conversation, there are male and female types of expressions defined by the sentence ending. **Nano** is a female type of expression and is used by females or by males to say something in a gentle (informal) way. The intonation rises on **nano**. Sometimes, ending sentences with **nano** will make it a question. **Nano** can substitute for **desu ka**, which is used for formal expression.

Byōki wa dō nano.	How is your illness? (informal)
Byōki wa dō nan desu ka.	How is your illness? (with feeling/sympathy)
Byōki wa dō desu ka.	How is your illness? (formal)

2. Delivery-related complaints by patients often concern the chest, abdomen, and legs. The expression **muka-muka** has the same meaning as "vomiting." Leg cramps can be expressed in three different ways in Japanese, but all have the same meaning.

    Chest:

Mune ga doki-doki shimasu.	I feel my heart beating hard.
Mune ga muka-muka shimasu.	I feel like vomiting.
Mune ga zukin-zukin shimasu.	I feel a throbbing pain.

    Abdomen:

Onaka ga zukin-zukin shimasu.	I feel a throbbing pain.
Onaka ga shiku-shiku shimasu.	I have a prolonged dull pain.
Onaka ga pan-pan ni hatte imasu.	My stomach is bloating/has gas/is gassy.
Onaka ga peko-peko desu.	I'm hungry.

    Legs:

Komura-gaeri ga arimasu.	I have a leg cramp.
Ashi ga piku-piku shimasu.	I have a leg cramp
Ashi ga tsuri masu.	I have a leg cramp.
Ashi ga pan-pan ni hari masu.	I have a leg cramp. (*lit.*, My leg has muscle pain.)

3. The time expressions **jyō-jun**, **chū-jyun**, **ge-jun** are used for months or terms. **Jō-jun** is for the early part, **chū-jun** is the middle part, and **ge-jun** is the later part of the month or term.

    > **Kon-getsu jyō-jun ni shussan suru yotei desu.**
    > Your date of confinement is expected to be early this month.

    > **Aka-chan wa sōzan de sen-getsu chū-jun ni umare-mashita.**
    > The baby was premature (*lit.*, a premature birth) and was born in the middle of last month.

    > **Shussan wa kon-getsu ge-jun no yotei desu.**
    > Delivery is expected in the latter part of this month.

4. Delivery-related expressions:

Jintsū wa mada desu ka.	Have you had contractions yet?
Jintsū ga hajimarimashita.	The contractions (have) started.
Jintsū ga yaku 5 fun tsuzuki masu.	Your contractions are lasting about five minutes.
Jintū ga 25 fun okini okimasu.	You have contractions every twenty-five minutes.
Jintsū ka hayaku natte kimashita.	Your contractions are becoming faster.
Iki o ōkiku sutte (kudasai).	Inhale deeply.
Iki o fukaku haite (kudasai).	Exhale deeply.
Iki o yukkuri sutte (kudasai).	Inhale slowly.
Iki o yukkuri haite (kudasai).	Exhale slowly.
Iki o su-ttari, hai-tari shite (kudasai).	Please inhale and exhale.
Ikinde kudasai.	Please push.
Motto ikinde kudasai.	Please push more.
Tsuyoku ikinde kudasai.	Please push harder.
Motto tsuyoku ikinde kudasai.	Please push even harder.
Ikima-nai de kudasai.	Please do not push.
Ikimu no o yamete kudasai.	Please stop pushing.
Hasui shimashita.	Your water broke.

5. Delivery-related words:

sō-zan	premature birth
mijiku-ji	premature baby
nan-zan	difficult delivery
an-zan	easy delivery
shi-zan	stillbirth
ryū-zan	miscarriage

ui-zan	first childbirth
shizen-bunben	natural childbirth
teiō-sekkai	cesarian section
shikyū-gai ninshin	ectopic pregnancy
saka-go	breech delivery
iden-byō	hereditary disease

6. Types of delivery (**bunben**):

mutsū bunben	painless childbirth
suichū bunben	water birth, underwater birth
tachiai shussan	birth attendance

7. Types of anesthesia (**masui**):

When speaking of anesthesia in Japanese, use the verb **kakeru/kakemasu** (put, start). The following are some simple sample sentences.

Masui o kakemasu.	I will give (you) anesthesia.
Masui o kakemashō ka.	Shall I give you anesthesia?

The following are types of anesthesia in Japanese.

kyokusho-masui	local anesthesia
zenshin-masui	general anesthesia
sekitsui-masui	spinal anesthesia
yōtsui-kōmaku-gai masui	lumbar epidural anesthesia

Language Roots

The word **san/zan** (産) indicates produce, confinement, delivery, and childbirth.

an-zan	easy delivery
san-go	afterbirth.
san-kyū	maternity leave

The word **nyū** (乳) indicates breasts and milk. It's also pronounced **chi**.

bo-nyū	breast milk
nyū-yō-ji	newborn baby
chi-busa	breast/nipple

Culture Notes

Hospitalization for the delivery

Japanese have a general consensus that women should stay in the hospital for about a week for delivery and follow-up in the days afterward. First-time childbirth usually requires staying in the hospital for seven days, while subsequent births require six days. This consensus is based in traditional values and the strong belief that giving birth is one of the most important tasks for women in order to prolong the family name. As well, it gives the mother a chance to rest in the hospital and be free from housework.

Lamaze and Zen meditation

People are apt to forget the importance of breath and the function of oxygen in the human body. To counter this, the Lamaze method promotes a dynamic experience of breathing and mental visualization during delivery. The purpose of Lamaze is to support an easy and painless childbirth. The focus of Zen, on the other hand, is on realizing the inner self and the nonduality through meditation, with great emphasis on breathing. A person who practices both Lamaze and Zen meditation may find similarities between them in technique, especially in the importance of focused breathing.

Circumcision (**hōhi-setsudan**) in Japanese society and culture

In the West, circumcision right after delivery or shortly thereafter is customary. Japanese, however, understand the body to be a gift from the parents and their ancestors that should not be cut. Cutting would defile this gift and therefore lead to dishonor of their family. In recent years, ear piercing has becomes popular among Japanese females. This demonstrates a changing Japanese social norm. Healthcare professionals should inform Japanese parents in advance about the institution's policy regarding circumcision, so that they will be able to decide whether their baby should be circumcised or not. **Hōhi** means foreskin (literally, **hō** means "cover," and **hi** means "skin"), and **setsudan** means cutting. Circumcision is called **katsu-rei** in religious ritual.

Comprehension

Answer the following questions.

1. Which of the following does NOT belong with the others?
    a. **Ikimi**   b. **Ryūzan**
    c. **Sōzan**   d. **Shizan**

2. Which of the following could be used to say "menstrual cycle"?
   a. **Shinseiji**   b. **Kiso taion**
   c. **Hasui**   d. **Seiri shūki**

3. Which of the following best completes the sentence below?
   Ima wa itakumo naishi, kayukumo naishi, shukketsu (   ) nai desu.
   (There is neither pain, nor itchiness, nor bleeding now.)
   a. **ni**   b. **to**
   c. **de**   d. **mo**

4. You are in the delivery room with a patient who is giving birth. Which of the following can you use to ask the patient to please push harder?
   a. **Yukkuri ikin de kudasai.**
   b. **Tsuyoku ikin de kudasai.**
   c. **Ikima nai de kudasai.**
   d. **Ikimu no o yamete kudasai.**

Select the appropriate meaning from the list below.

---

5. **Masaka shizan dato wa omowana-katta.**   (   )
6. **Jintū ga okitara, suguni renraku shite kudasai.**   (   )
7. **Jitsuwa, [anata wa] futago o shussan shimashita.** (   )
8. **Tsuwari ka, mata wa fusei shukketsu ga airmasu ka.** (   )
9. **Mada, jintsū mo naishi, bunben mo arimasen.**   (   )

a. The fact is that you gave birth to identical twins.
b. I never thought that it would be a stillbirth.
c. Do you have either morning sickness or abnormal vaginal bleeding?
d. There are neither contractions, nor has labor started yet.
e. If contractions are happening, please inform us immediately.

Practice

Respond to the following in Japanese using the cues that have been provided.

1. Asking the patient to breathe.
   (Patient's requirements)   (Healthcare professional)
   1. Needs to inhale slowly.   _____
   2. Needs to exhale slowly.   _____
   3. Needs to inhale a deep breath.   _____
   4. Needs to exhale a deep breath.   _____

   5. Needs to inhale and exhale.   _____

2.   Giving instructions on pushing.
     (Patient's requirements)   (Healthcare professional)
     1. Please push.   _____
     2. Please push more.   _____
     3. Please push harder.   _____
     4. Please do not push.   _____
     5. Please stop pushing.   _____

3.   Conveying the symptoms.
     (Patient)   (Healthcare professional)
     1. **Kimochi ga warui(n) desu.** _____ (Do you feel like vomiting?)
     2. **Onaka ga itai(n) desu.** _____ (Do you feel a throbbing pain?)
     3. **Onaka ga hatte imasu.** _____ (Your stomach is bloating.)
     4. **Ashi ga itai(n) desu.** _____ (You have a leg cramp.)
     5. **Ashi ga hatte imasu.** _____ (Your leg muscles are fully stretched.)

4.   Dialogue comprehension. Based on the dialogue, answer the following questions.
     1. **Yamada-san wa nan no kensa o shimashita ka.**
        _____
     2. **Yamada-san no saigo no seiri wa itsu deshita ka.**
        _____
     3. **Yamada-san no asa no kibun wa dō deshita ka.**
        _____
     4. **Yamada-san wa don-na mono ga tabetai desu ka.**
        _____
     5. **Yamada-san wa ni-nen mae-ni nani o shimashita ka.**
        _____
     6. **Yamada-san no shussan yoteibi wa itsu goro desu ka.**
        _____

5.   Free response questions.
     (Questions)   (Healthcare professional)
     1. **Jitsuwa anata wa futago nan desu ka.** _____
     2. **Anata no byōin ni NICU ga arimasu ka.** _____
     3. **Tsuwari wa hidokatta desu ka.** _____
     4. **Saikin, komura-gaeri ga arimasu ka.** _____
     5. **Heso no o wa tottearimasu ka.** _____

Exercise

1. Say the following words in Japanese.
   A. Morning sickness   _____
   B. Fetal movement   _____
   C. Contractions   _____
   D. Pushing   _____
   E. C-section   _____

2. Say the following in Japanese.
   A. I never thought that it would be a miscarriage.

   _____

   B. If a premature rupture happens, please inform us immediately.

   _____

   C. The fact is that you need a cesarean section.

   _____

   D. There are neither pains nor contractions yet.

   _____

   E. Do you have either morning sickness or lack of appetite?

   _____

3. How do you ask patients the following questions in Japanese?
   A. Have you had contractions yet?   _____
   B. Have the contractions started?   _____
   C. Do your contractions last about five minutes?   _____
   D. How often do you have contractions?   _____
   E. Are your contractions are becoming faster?   _____

4. Answer the following questions in Japanese.

   Q: **Ninshin nan-shū-me desu ka.**
   A: _____
   (You are fifteen weeks pregnant.)

   Q: **Jintsū ga hajimatta mitai desu.**
   B: _____
   (Say haa-haa-haa with your breath, and you will relieve the pain.)

   Q: **Ninshin no guai wa dō desu ka.**
   C: _____
   (Please tell me if you have contractions.)

Pediatrics
(Shōni-ka)

Basic Vocabulary (CD 29-1)

Listen to the CD and then repeat the vocabulary.

1.	gait disturbance/dysbasia	**hokō-shōgai**	歩行障害
2.	baby	**aka-chan**	赤ちゃん
3.	convulsion	**hikitsuke**	ひきつけ
4.	dandle	**ayasu**	あやす
5.	temper/bad mood	**kanshaku**	かんしゃく
6.	dehydration	**dassui-shōjyō**	脱水症状
7.	diaper rash	**omutsu-kabure**	オムツ被れ
8.	prickly heat	**asemo**	汗疹
9.	tuberculosis test	**tsuberukurin-kensa**	ツベルクリン検査
10.	tuberculosis reaction	**tsuberukurin-hannō**	ツベルクリン反応
11.	atopic dermatitis	**atopī-sei hifu-en**	アトピー性皮膚炎
12.	MMR vaccine	**emu-emu-āru wakuchin**	エム・エム・アール・ワクチン
13.	polio vaccine	**porio-wakuchin**	ポリオ・ワクチン
14.	rolled-back eye	**shirome**	白眼
15.	congenital	**senten-sei**	先天性
16.	weak constitution	**kyojyaku-taishitsu**	虚弱体質
17.	postnatal	**seigo**	生後
18.	developmental disorders	**hattatsu-shōgai**	発達障害
19.	hearing impairment	**chōkaku-shōgai**	聴覚障害
20.	learning disabilities	**gakushū-shōgai**	学習障害
21.	speech impediment	**gengo-shōgai**	言語障害
22.	normal development	**seijō-hattatsu**	正常発達
23.	cerebral palsy	**nō-sei-mahi**	脳性麻痺
24.	muscular dystrophy	**kin-jisutorohī**	筋ジストロフィー
25.	infantile asthma	**shōni-zensoku**	小児喘息
26.	weaning period	**rinyū-ki**	離乳期
27.	infant	**nyūyō-ji**	乳幼児
28.	enema	**kan-chō**	浣腸
29.	child abuse	**yōji-gyakutai**	幼児虐待
30.	dyslexia	**shitsu-doku-shō**	失読症

Dialogue (CD 29-2)

Listen to the CD and repeat the dialogue.

At the Pediatric Clinic

Dr. Simon: **Kyō wa dō shimashita ka.**
               Are you concerned about anything today?

Mrs. Yamada: **Musume wa mōsugu san-sai ni naru no desu ga, ni-san nichi mae-kara hatsu-netsu shi (ta ato), hana-mizu ya seki ga deha-jime mashita.**
               My daughter will be three years old soon, and she has had a fever since a couple of days ago, and she also has a runny nose and a cough.

Dr. Simon: **Dewa, chotto, (chōshinki de) mune-no-oto o kiite mimashō.**
               Well, let's listen to her chest sounds (with the stethoscope).

               Tashika ni, zei-zei itte iru yō desu.
               I can definitely hear a wheezing sound.

               Aān, kuchi o akete kudasai. Nodo mo harete akaku natte im-asu.
               Say, "Aaah." Please open your mouth. Her throat also looks red and inflamed.

               Kokyū kon-nan no shōjyō wa arimasen ka.
               Is she not having any difficulty breathing?

Mrs. Yamada: **Yoru mo amari yoku nemurete inai yōde, nan-kai mo seki de okite, guzutte naite imashita.**
               She seems not to be able to sleep well, and she wakes up several times in the night, coughing and whimpering.

Dr. Simon: **Shōjyō kara, osoraku uisuru-sei no kikanshi-en dato omoimasu.**
               Based on the symptoms, I think this is most likely viral bronchi-tis.

               Sakuban, shoku-yoku wa dō deshita ka.
               How was her appetite last night?

Mrs. Yamada: **Gohan mo tabe-naku-narimashita.**
               She didn't want any meal.

               Hayaku sensei ni mite moraeba yokkata to omoimasu.
               I feel like I wish I'd shown you earlier.

Dr. Simon:	**Tokorode, kao no akai hasshin wa itsu goro kara dete imasu ka.**
	By the way, tell me, how long has she had a reddish rash on cheek?
Mrs. Yamada:	**Kore wa, seigo ni-nen-me goro kara deteite, naka-naka naori masen.**
	She's had this reddish rash since she was two years old, and it hasn't gone away yet.
Dr. Simon:	**Sō desu ka. Soredewa, kyōbu-rentogen o totte, hai-en ni natte inaika tashikamete mimashō.**
	Is that so? Then, I would like to take an X-ray and rule out pneumonia.
	Sorekara, ketsueki-kensa mo shite, hakkekyū to CRP de enshō o shirabemasu.
	And then I would like to do a blood test to get the white blood cell count and a CRP to check for inflammation.
	Soredewa, kensa o onegai shimasu.
	Well, please have the test.

Grammar

1. The conjunction suffix **-shi**

The conjunction suffix -**shi** usually translates as "and" in English and is used to connect two sentences, as studied in Lesson 23. However, -**shi** may also mean "and what's more" or "and then" and emphasize the sense of a sequence or cumulation.

> **Ni-san nichi mae kara hatsu-netsu-shi, seki ga demashita.**
> I had a fever a couple of days ago, and what's more I started coughing.

> **Hikitsuke-shi (ta ato de), shirome ni narimashita.**
> You had convulsions, and (then) your eyes rolled back.

> **Gutari-shi (ta ato de), dassui-shōjyō ni narimashita.**
> You became weak, and this was followed by dehydration.

2. The compound verb **de-hajimeru** and the construction VERB BASE + hajimeru

The compound verb **de-hajimeru** is composed of two verbs: **deru** (go out) and **hajimaru** (begin). Note that the first verb is the **masu** form of the verb base. The verb **de-hajimeru** is usually used for the beginning or onset of symptoms. Other compounds formed this way are: **naori-hajimeru (naoru** means "cure, heal"), which is used when the healing process starts; and **-tore-hajimeru** (**toreru** means "come off, remove"), which is for when something begins to come off. To change the verb base, drop **-masu** from the **masu** form and add **-hajimeru/-hajime-masu**. Please note that the verb for "take" has two forms: **torimasu** (transitive) and **toremasu** (intransitive). The transitive verb **torimasu** takes a direct object with an animate/person subject. The intransitive verb **toremasu** (be taken) is used to make the passive voice. See Lesson 27 for transitive and intransitive verbs.

Hana-mizu ga de-hajime-mashita.	My nose has begun to run.
Seki ga naori-hajime-mashita.	My cough has begun to get better.
Asa-gohan o tabe-hajimemasu.	I will begin to eat breakfast.
Kasabuta ga tore-hajimeta.	The scabs have begun to come off.

Tori-hajimeru has many meanings based on the first verb, **tori**. For example, the verb **toru** can mean "collect, record, photograph, reduce, disappear, take off, etc."

Ketsueki o tori-hajime-masu.	I have begun to collect blood.
Kusuri de netsu o tori-hajime-mashō.	Let's begin to reduce the fever with medication.
MRI de gazō o tori-hajime-masu.	We will begin to record the image with an MRI.

3. **Nemureru/nemurenai** and the auxiliary verb **-reru/-rareru**

In Lesson 20, we saw that the verb base plus the auxiliary verb **seru/saseru** expresses the idea of an order or command (to make/order someone to do something). For example, **ne-seru/ne-saseru** is "make/order someone to sleep." On the other hand, **-reru/-rareru** expresses the ability to do something, as in the English *can do, can be done, is able to do*. For example, **ne-reru/ne-rareru** is "be able to/can sleep." **Ne-reru** is active and **ne-rareru** is spontaneous sleep and a polite expression.

Sakuban wa yoku nemure-mashita ka.	Were you able to sleep well last night?
Shin-on ga kikoenai desu ka.	Can you hear the sound of the heart?
Kodomo ga nemu-rete inai yō desu.	It seems that the child is not able to sleep.

For the **u**-verb negative form, change the **-i** (**hi**) ending of the the verb base or the **-u** ending of the stem verb to **a**, and add **-reru**. To make the negative form, drop the **-ru** ending from **-rareru** and replace it with the negative suffix **-nai**.

U-verbs

ENGLISH	**MASU** FORM/ VERB BASE	STEM VERB	SPONTANE- OUS FORM/ POLITE FORM	NEGATIVE FORM
drink	nomi-masu	no-mu	noma-reru	noma-re-nai
read	yomi-masu	yo-mu	yoma-reru	yoma-re-nai
go	iki-masu	i-ku	ika-reru	ika-re-nai
speak	hanashi-masu	hana-su	hanasa-reru	hanasa-re-nai
return	kaeri-masu	kae-ru	kaera-reru	kaera-re-nai
listen	kiki-masu	ki-ku	kika-reru	kika-re-nai
pull down	oroshi-masu	oro-su	orosa-reru	orosa-re-nai
cool	hiyashi-masu	hiya-su	hiyasa-reru	hiyasa-re-nai
take out/pull out	toridashi-masu	torida-su	toridasa-reru	toridasa-re-nai
scratch	kaki-masu	ka-ku	kaka-reru	kaka-re-nai
beat	tataki-masu	tata-ku	tataka-reru	tataka-re-nai
smell/sniff	kagi-masu	ka-gu	kaga-reru	kaga-re-nai
prevent	fusegi-masu	fuse-gu	fusega-reru	fusega-re-nai
become	nari-masu	na-ru	nara-reru	nara-re-nai
wait	machi-masu	ma-tsu	mata-reru	mata-re-nai
keep/hold	tamochi-masu	tamo-tsu	tamota-reru	tamota-re-nai
start/go out	dashi-masu	da-su	dasa-reru	dasa-re-nai
live in	kurashi-masu	kura-su	kurasa-reru	kurasa-re-nai
worry	nayami-masu	naya-mu	nayama-reru	nayama-re-nai
push down/ strain	ikimi-masu	iki-mu	ikima-reru	ikima-re-nai
depress	ochikomi-masu	ochiko-mu	ochikoma-reru	ochikoma-re-nai
wash	arai-masu	ara-u	arawa-reru	arawa-re-nai

For the **ru**-verb negative form, drop the -**ru** ending from the stem verb and add -**rareru**. For the negative form, drop the -**ru** ending from -**rareru** and replace it with the negative suffix -**nai**.

Ru-verbs

ENGLISH	MASU FORM/ VERB BASE	STEM VERB	SPONTANE- OUS FORM/ POLITE FORM	NEGATIVE FORM
sleep	ne-masu	ne-ru	ne-rareru	ne-rare-nai
eat	tabe-masu	tabe-ru	tabe-rareru	tebe-rare-nai
warm, warm up	atatame-masu	atatame-ru	atatame-rareru	atatame-rare-nai
manifest/ appear	araware-masu	araware-ru	araware-rareru	araware-rare-nai
inform/notify	shirase-masu	shirase-ru	shirase-rareru	shirase-rare-nai
shiver	furue-masu	furue-ru	furue-rareru	furue-rare-nai
frighten	obie-masu	obie-ru	obie-rareru	obie-rare-nai
go out/appear	de-masu	de-ru	de-rareru	de-rare-nai
allow/make do	sase-masu	sase-ru	sase-rareru	sase-rare-nai
see/look/ examine	mi-masu	mi-ru	mi-rareru	mi-rare-nai
tighten	shime-masu	shime-ru	shime-rareru	shime-rare-nai
leak	more-masu	more-ru	more-rareru	more-rare-nai
open	ake-masu	ake-ru	ake-rareru	ake-rare-nai
recommend	susume-masu	susume-ru	susume-rareru	susume-rare-nai
wear (clothes)	ki-masu	ki-ru	ki-rareru	ki-rare-nai
feel	kanji-masu	kanji-ru	kanji-rareru	kanji-rare-nai
wake up	oki-masu	oki-ru	oki-rareru	oki-rare-nai
slump	meiri-masu	mei-ru	mei-rareru	mei-rare-nai
become	nari-masu	na-ru	na-rareru	na-rare-nai
apply/paint	nuri-masu	nu-ru	nu-rareru	nu-rare-nai
mix	majiri-masu	maji-ru	maji-rareru	maji-rare-nai
empty/die/ use up	nakunari-masu	nakuna-ru	nakuna-rareru	nakuna-rare-nai
choke	tsumari-masu	tsuma-ru	tsuma-rareru	tsuma-rare-nai
measure	hakari-masu	haka-ru	haka-rareru	haka-rare-nai
anger	okori-masu	oku-ru	oko-rareru	oko-rare-nai
transmit/move	utsuri-masu	utsu-ru	utsu-rareru	utsu-rare-nai
stand up	tachiagari-masu	tachiaga-ru	tachiaga-rareru	tachiaga-rare-nai

ENGLISH	**MASU** FORM/ VERB BASE	STEM VERB	SPONTANE- OUS FORM/ POLITE FORM	NEGATIVE FORM
cut	**kiri-masu**	**ki-ru**	**ki-rareru**	**kirare-nai**
sit down	**suwari-masu**	**suwa-ru**	**suwa-rareru**	**suwa-rare-nai**
roll up	**makuri-masu**	**maku-ru**	**maku-rareru**	**maku-rare-nai**
not speak/ be silent	**damari-masu**	**dama-ru**	**dama-rareru**	**dama-rare-nai**
do/play*	**shi-masu**	**su-ru**	**nasa-rareru**	**nasa-rere-nai**
come*	**ki-masu**	**ku-ru**	**ko-rareru**	**ko-rare-nai**

* Irregular

4. The suffix phrase **naku-naru/naku-nari-masu**

The suffix phrase **naku-naru/narimasu** means "not . . . anymore" and is used in the following kinds of constructions:

a) Verb: STEM VERB + **naku-naru/narimasu**.

> **(Watakushi wa) Miruku ga nome-naku-narimashita.** (intransitive)
> I could not drink milk anymore.

> **(Kodomo ga) Miruku o noma-naku narimashita.** (transitive)
> The child does not drink milk anymore.

> **Kanjya-san wa tsūin o shinaku narimashita.**
> The patient does not visit the hospital anymore.

> **Nemure-naku-naru to omoimasu.**
> I think I cannot sleep anymore.

b) **i**-ADJECTIVE + **nakunaru**. The adjective stem drops the **-i** ending and adds **-ku** before adding **-naku-naru/narimasu**.

> **Onaka ga itaku-nakunari-mashita.**
> My stomach could not hurt anymore.

> **Asemo ga kayuku-nakunaru to omoimasu.**
> I think that heat rash is not itchy/doesn't itch anymore.

> **Kusuri o non de, karada ga daruku nakunari-mashita ka.**
> From taking medicine, could your body not be tired anymore?

c) **Na**-ADJECTIVE OR NOUN + **nakunaru**. The **na**-adjective or noun is followed by **dewa** and then **naku-naru/narimasu**. To make this informal, add **jyā naku-naru/narimasu**.

> **Aka-chan wa seijyō hattatsu dewa naku-naru yō desu.**
> It seems that the baby is not developing normally anymore (*lit.*, The baby seems not to have normal development anymore).

> **Kanjya-san wa mō gengo-shōgai dewa nakunari-mashita.**
> The patient no longer has a speech impediment anymore.

> **Aka-chan wa shizuka jyā nakunarimasu.**
> The baby cannot be quiet anymore.

5. The suffix phrase **-ba yokkata**

We studied the suffix **-ba** in Lessons 17 and 28. The expression **-ba yokkata** states the speaker's regret and literally means "I wish; it would have been good if . . ." It consists of a conditional clause with **-ba** (if) and **yokkata** (was good).

> **Tsuberukurin-kensa o sureba yokkata noni (shimasen deshita).**
> I wish you had had the tuberculosis test (but you didn't it) (*lit.*, You should have had the tuberculosis test, but you didn't do it).

> **Shokumotsu arerugī no kusuri o nome-ba yokatta noni (nomimasen deshita).**
> I wish you had taken medicine for the allergy (but you didn't take it).

> **Shussei shōmei-sho o mireba yokatta.**
> I wish I had seen the birth certificate (but I didn't see it).

6. The pattern NOUN + **-go**

The pattern NOUN plus the suffix **-go** indicates a past event and is often translated as "since" or "after."

> **Ima shussei-go ni-shū-kan desu.**
> Now, it's (been) two weeks since the birth (*lit.*, Now, it's two weeks after childbirth).

> **Ima shussan-go san-ka-getsu desu.**
> Three months have passed since the delivery now.

> **Kensa-go-ni kanchō o shimasu.**
> After the examination, I will give an enema.

> **Shoku-go ni kusuri o nonde kudasai.**
> Please take medicine after meals.

Useful Expressions (CD 29-3)

Listen to the CD and repeat the sentences.

1. **Kigen ga warui desu ne.** You are in a bad mood, aren't you?
2. **Hikitsuke o okoshite imasu.** He has had convulsions.
3. **Ishiki ga arimasen.** She is unconscious.
4. **Shirome o muite imasu.** Her eyes are rolled back.
5. **Porio wakuchin wa sunde imasu ka.** Has he had a polio vaccine?
6. **Omutsu-kabure ga hidoi yō desu.** He seems to have bad diaper rash.
7. **Akai butsu-butsu ga karada-jyū ni dekite imasu.** She has red spots all over her body.
8. **Tsuberukurin-hannō wa insei deshita.** The tuberculin reaction was negative.
9. **Tamago o taberu to jinmashin ga demasu ka.** Do you get hives when you eat eggs?
10. **Dassui shōjyō o okoshite imasu node, suibun ga hitsuyō desu.** He needs liquid because he is dehydrated.

Key Sentences (CD 29-4)

Listen to the CD and repeat the sentences.

1. **Hikitsuke shi (ta ato de), shirome ni narimashita.** You had convulsions, and (then) your eyes rolled back.
2. **Seki ga dehajime-mashita ka.** Have you begun to cough?
3. **Aka-chan ga nemurete-inai yō desu.** It seems that the baby is not able to sleep.
4. **Nemure-naku-naru to omoimasu.** I think you cannot sleep any more.
5. **Arerugī no kusuri o nome-ba yokatta noni (nomimasen deshita).** I wish you had taken medicine for the allergy (but you didn't take it).

Additional Words

tataku/tatakimasu beat	**guttari** weak/listless
keru/kerimasu kick	**kigen ga warui** fussy/irritable
nageru/nagemasu throw	**kigen ga ii** good mood
obieru/obiemasu frighten	**naki-jyakuru** sob
kowagaru/kowagarimasu scare	**suibun-hokyū** hydration
hattatsu development	**shussei-mae** prenatal
ai-jyō love feeling	**shussei-ji** at birth
kūfuku hungry	**seichō** growth

gazō photo image

taijyū-zōka-furyō insufficient weight gain

netsu-sei keiren febrile seizure

tamago egg

chūi-kekkan tadōsei-shōgai attention deficit hyperactivity disorder (ADHD)

nyūji-totsuzen-shi-shōkōgun sudden infant death syndrome (SIDS)

Language Notes

1. The expression **zei-zei** is an onomatopoeia that imitates a sick breathing sound.

> **Tashika-ni, zei-zei itte iru yō desu.**   I can definitely hear a wheezing sound.
> **Mune ga zei-zei shite imasu.**   Your chest is making a wheezing sound.

A healthy lung or breathing sound is usually expressed by saying:

> **Mune no oto wa kirei desu.**   The sound of your breathing is clear.

2. **Aān** means "a wide-open mouth." **Aān** is considered an onomatopoeia that imitates the sound a human makes, and when healthcare professionals ask a child to open his or her mouth, this is the expression they use. When asking an adult, to use **aān** would be impolite. Instead, you should say, **Kuchi o ōkiku akete kudasai.** "Please open your mouth wide."

> **Aān, nodo ga harete akaku natte iru yō desu ne.**
> Say, "Aaah." Your throat looks red and inflamed.
> **Nodo ga itai yō desu ne. Aān shite (kudasai).**
> It looks like you have a sore throat. (Please) open your mouth wide and say, "Aaah."

The expression **bē**, accompanied by the gesture of showing the tongue (**shita**), is used by healthcare professionals to ask a child to show his or her tongue. For adults, the expression is **Shita o dashie kudasai.** "Show me your tongue."

> **Shita o misete (kudasai).**   Please show me your tongue.
> **Bē shite.**   Show me your tongue.

The expression **nobi-nobi** means "stretch (the body)." "Open and close your eyes" is **pachi-kuri**, and "open and close your hands" is **gū-pā**. For stretch your arm or neck, the verb is **nobasu** (stretch).

Karada o nobi-nobi shite kudasai.	Please stretch your body.
Me o pachi-kuri shite kudasai.	Please open and close your eyes.
Te o gū-pā shite kudasai.	Please open and close your hand.
Ude o nobashite kudasai.	Please stretch your arms.
Kubi o mawashite kudasai.	Please turn your neck.

3.   There are many onomatopoetic expressions for children in Japanese.

ogyā-ogyā to naku	to mewl (for babies)
meso-meso to naku	to whimper with sadness
wan-wan to naku	to howl with pain
ēen-ēn to naku	to cry
yochi-yochi to aruku	to toddle
niko-niko to warau	to smile and laugh
chū-chū to nomu/sū	to suck (for babies)
goku-goku to nomu	to gulp
hai-hai suru	to crawl (for babies)
guzu-guzu suru	to do something slowly and hesitantly
chan to suru	to meet a certain standard
choro-choro suru.	to move with quick movement
gero-gero suru	to vomit, throw up
taion ga poka-poka (to) suru	body temperature feels pleasant (for babies)
hada ga gasa-gasa	dry skin
hada ga fuwa-fuwa	soft skin
hada ga sube-sube	smooth skin
onaka ga peko-peko	to be hungry
onaka ga pī	has diarrhea (*lit.*, stomach has diarrhea)

4.   For a negative test result, use **insei**. For a positive test result, use **yōsei**. A pseudo-positive or false positive is **giji yōsei**.

Tsuberukurin-hannō no kekka wa insei deshita.
The result of tuberculosis reaction was negative.

Tamago-arerugī kensa no kekka wa yōsei deshita.
The result of the egg allergy test was positive.

Shokumotu-arerugī kensa no kekka wa giji-yōsei desu.
The result of food allergy test was a false positive.

5.   There are many kinds of allergies:

shoku-motsu-arerugī	food allergy
kusuri-arerugī	drug allergy

tamago-arerugī	egg allergy
pīnattsu-arerugī	peanuts allergy
gyū-nyū-arerugī	milk allergy
kokumotsu-arerugī	grain allergy

Language Roots

The word **ryō** (良) means "good, pleasing, benign." It is also pronounced **yo(i)**.

ryō-sei shuyō	benign tumor
ryō-shin	good conscience
kigen ga yo(i)	good mood
yoi hōhō	good method

The word **aku** (悪) has a range of meanings on the order of "bad, evil, false, wrong." It is also pronounced **waru(i)**.

aku-sei shuyō	malignant tumor
aku-sei hinketsu	pernicious anemia
kigen ga waru(i)	fussy/cranky/fretful
ashi ga warui desu ka.	Do you have a bad leg/foot?
anata wa aku-nin dewa arimasen.	You are not bad man.

Culture Notes

MMR: M=Mumps (**otafuku kaze**), M=Measles (**hashika**), and R=Rubella (**fūshin**)

Mumps (**ryūkō-sei jikasen-en**) is the so-called **otafuku kaze**. **Otafuku** means "woman who has an ugly swollen face." The name **otafuku** refers to the fact that when people catch the mumps, their faces become horribly swollen.

Measles (**ma-shin**) is the so-called **hashika**. Literally, **hashika** is a plant whose name means "grain beard" and that has firm, tiny needles. When people touched the needle, they would get a red welt similar to measles.

Rubella (**fū-shin**), or German measles, is the so-called **mikka-bashika**. The symptoms of measles (**hashika**) last for about ten days, while rubella (**fū-shin**) has symptoms for about three days, like mild measles. For this reason, rubella is called **mikka bashika** (three-day measles).

It is said that the reason for catching a cold (**kaze**) is that one has gotten "wicked wind," and **fū-shin** means "catching a wind-virus, or wind-measles."

Comprehension

Answer the following questions.

1. Which of the following does NOT belong with the others?
   a. **Omutsu-kabure**   b. **Nōha**
   c. **Asemo**   d. **Hada-are**

2. Which of the following could be used to express a baby crying?
   a. **Meso-meso**   b. **Ogyā-ogyā**
   c. **Yochi-yochi**   d. **Ēn-ēn**

3. Which of the following best completes the sentence below?
   Guttari (   ), dassui-shōjyō ni narimashita.
   (You became weak, and this was followed by dehydration.)
   a. **ga**   b. **wa**
   c. **ni**   d. **shi**

4. Your patient has complained of a sore throat, and you wish to examine it. Which of the following means "Open wide" or "Open your mouth wide"?
   a. **Aā to kuchi o akete kudasai.**
   b. **Bē to shita o misete kudasai.**
   c. **Guru-guru to me o mawashite kudasai.**
   d. **Gohon-gohon to seki o shite kudasai.**

Select the appropriate meaning from the list below.

5. **Omutsu kabure shi [ta ato de], kasabuta ni narimashita.**   (   )
6. **Mizu-bukure ga dehajime-mashita ka.**   (   )
7. **Aka-chan wa oto ga kikoete inai yō desu.**   (   )
8. **Nemure-naku-naru to omoimasu.**   (   )
9. **Arerugī no kusuri o nome-ba yokatta noni.**   (   )

a. It seems that the baby is not able to hear the sound.
b. Have you started to have blisters?
c. I think I cannot sleep any more.
d. I wish you had medicine for allergies.
e. He had diaper rash, and (then) it turned into scabs.

Practice

Respond to the following in Japanese using the cues that have been provided.

1. Using onomatopoetic expressions to ask a child to do something.
    (Healthcare professional)   (Onomatopoetic expression)
    1. **Kuchi o akete kusasai.**   _____
    2. **Shita o misete kudasai.**   _____
    3. **Karada o nobashite kudasai.**   _____
    4. **Me o aketari, tojitari shite kudasai.** _____
    5. **Te o hiraitari, tojitari shite kudasai.** _____

2. Examining the patient and stating your opinion.
    (Patient's condition)   (Healthcare professional)
    1. **Aka-chan wa nemure-masen.**   _____
    2. **Aka-chan wa kigen ga warui(n) desu.** _____
    3. **Aka-chan wa omutsu kabure desu.**   _____
    4. **Aka-chan wa Porio wakuchin o shite imasen.** _____
    5. **Aka-chan wa tamago arerugī desu.**   _____

3. Conveying the results of the examination.
    (Patient)   (Healthcare professional)
    1. **Mune no oto wa dō-desu ka.**   _____
                                               (It's a clear sound.)
    2. **Mune no oto wa dō-desu ka.**   _____
                                               (I can hear a wheezing sound.)
    3. **Atopī-kensa no kekka wa dō-deshita ka.** _____
                                               (You are positive.)
    4. **Arerugii-kensa no kekka wa dō-deshita ka.** _____
                                               (You are pseudo positive.)
    5. **Tsuberukurin hannō no kekka wa dō-deshita ka.** _____
                                               (You are negative.)

4. Dialogue comprehension. Based on the dialogue, answer the following questions.
    1. **Kodomo wa itsu hatsu-netsu shimashita ka.** _____
    2. **Kodomo wa don-na mune no oto ga shimasu ka.** _____
    3. **Kodomo no nodo wa don-na shōjyō desu ka.** _____
    4. **Kodomo no byōki wa nan-dato omoimasu ka.** _____
    5. **Kodomo wa mazu don-na kensa o shimasu ka.** _____
    6. **Kao no akai hasshin wa itsu kara dete imasu ka.** _____

5. Free response questions.

(Questions)   (Healthcare professional)

1. **Suibun-hokyū wa jyūbun desu ka.**   _____
2. **Kyō wa kigen ga warui(n) desu ka, ii(n) desu ka.**_____
3. **Shoku-motsu arerugī ga arimasu ka.**   _____
4. **Kyojyaku-taishitsu desu ka.**   _____
5. **Gengo-shōgai ga arimasu ka.**   _____

Exercises

1. Say the following words in Japanese.   _____
   A. Developmental disorders   _____
   B. Infantile asthma   _____
   C. Muscular dystrophy   _____
   D. Cerebral palsy   _____
   E. Rolled-back eye   _____

2. Say the following expressions in Japanese.
   A. I would like to re-examine you to make   _____
      sure whether it is the atopic dermatitis or not.
   B. Has your nose begun to run?   _____
   C. It seems that the baby is not able to drink.   _____
   D. You had constipation, and (so) you need to   _____
      get an enema.
   E. I prescribed allergy medicine (in advance).   _____

3. How do you ask your patients the following questions in Japanese?
   A. You are in bad mood, aren't you?   _____
   B. Did she get an MMR vaccine?   _____
   C. Do you get eruptions when you eat eggs?   _____
   D. Does he seem to have bad diaper rash?   _____
   E. Do you have prickly heat all over the body?   _____

LESSON **30** **Dentistry**
(Shi-ka)

Basic Vocabulary (CD 30-1)

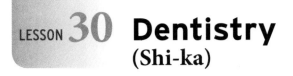

Listen to the CD and repeat the vocabulary.

1.	bite/chew	**kamu/kamimasu**	噛む/噛みます
2.	(dental) brushing	**hamigaki**	歯磨き
3.	cavity	**mushi-ba**	虫歯
4.	wisdom tooth	**oya-shirazu**	親知らず
5.	back tooth	**oku-ba**	奥歯
6.	front tooth	**mae-ba**	前歯
7.	gums	**ha-guki**	歯茎
8.	pyorrhea	**shishū-byō**	歯周病
9.	tartar	**shi-seki**	歯石
10.	plaque	**shi-kō**	歯垢
11.	denture	**ire-ba**	入れ歯
12.	false tooth	**sashi-ba**	差し歯
13.	extract teeth	**basshi**	抜歯
14.	sensitive	**shimiru**	沁みる
15.	nerve	**shinkei**	神経
16.	braces/teeth aligned	**kyōsei**	矯正
17.	baby tooth	**nyū-shi**	乳歯
18.	permanent tooth	**eikyū-shi**	永久歯
19.	buck tooth	**deppa**	出っ歯
20.	fluoride	**fusso**	フッ素
21.	crown	**kuraun-kan**	クラウン冠
22.	filling	**tsume-mono**	詰め物
23.	bad breath	**kōshū**	口臭
24.	gum infection	**haguki-no-enshō**	歯茎の炎症
25.	bleeding gums	**haguki-kara-no-shukketsu**	歯茎からの出血
26.	crooked tooth	**warui-ha-narabi**	悪い歯並び
27.	bad bite/malocclusion	**fusei-kōgō**	不正交合
28.	orthodontics	**shika-kyōsei**	歯科矯正
29.	dental hygienist	**shika-eisei-shi**	歯科衛生士
30.	dental technician	**shika-gikō-shi**	歯科技工士

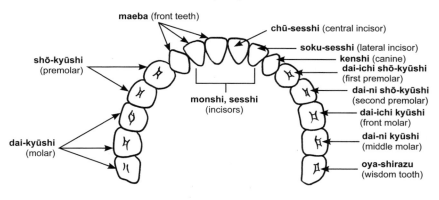

Ha (Teeth)

maeba (front teeth)

chū-sesshi (central incisor)

soku-sesshi (lateral incisor)

kenshi (canine)

dai-ichi shō-kyūshi (first premolar)

shō-kyūshi (premolar)

dai-ni shō-kyūshi (second premolar)

monshi, sesshi (incisors)

dai-ichi kyūshi (front molar)

dai-ni kyūshi (middle molar)

dai-kyūshi (molar)

oya-shirazu (wisdom tooth)

Dialogue (CD 30-2)

Listen to the CD and repeat the dialogue.

At the Dentist's Office

Dr. Lee (female dentist): **Kyō wa dō nasare mashita ka.**
Are you concerned about anything today?

Mr. Suzuki: **Hidari gawa no okuba ga sen-shū kara itakute tamarimasen.**
I've had an unbearable toothache in the upper back of my mouth since last week.

Dr. Lee: **Sō desu ka. Kuchi o akete kudasai. Tashika-ni, ue no okuba no haguki mo enshō o okoshite harete imasu ne.**
I see. Please open your mouth. Indeed, I can see your upper gum is also inflamed and swollen.

Rentogen o totte, shirabete mimashō ka.
Shall we take an X-ray and check it out?

Dewa, kono rentogen-yō purotekutā o tsukemasu. Ichi-ni fun de sugu(ni) owarimasu.
So, I'm putting a lead X-ray apron on you. It's will take just one or two minutes and be done in no time.

Mr. Suzuki: **Hai, (wakarimashita.) Onegai shimasu.**
Yes, I understand. Please go ahead.

Dr. Lee: **Rentogen kensa no kekka o mite kudasai.**
Please look at the X-ray result.

**Rentogen (kensa) de(mo) mirare-masu yōni, kanari ōkina mushi-
ba ni natte imasu ne.**
As you can see from the X-ray (result), it has become quite a big
cavity.

Kore wa basshi suru hitsyō ga arimasu.
The tooth needs to be removed.

Mr. Suzuki: **Kono ha wa dōshite mo nokose-masen ka.**
Is there any way I can keep the tooth?

Dr. Lee: **Sudeni kanari waruku natte imasu node, nokosu-nowa hotondo
muzukashii to omoimasu.**
It's already very bad, so I think that keeping the tooth is not possible.

Mr. Suzuki: **Aā so desu ka. Nokose-masen ka. Dewa, nuite kudasai.**
Really, is that so? It can't be saved? Then please extract it.

Dr. Lee: **Basshi-go no enshō o osaeru tame(ni) kōsei-zai to, itami o osaeru
tame(ni) chintsū-zai o shohō shimasu.**
I will prescribe an antibiotic to reduce the inflammation and a pain-
killer for your pain after the extraction.

**Sorekara, basshi-go wa sukunaku-tomo mikka-kan wa yoku ugai
o tsuzukete kudasai ne.**
And then, please (continue to) gargle for at least three days after the
extraction.

Grammar

1. ### The verb suffix **-kute** and the construction **te**-FORM + **tamaranai**

The verb suffix **-kute** and the construction **te**-FORM plus **tamaranai** both
emphasize the inability to cope with a situation and can be translated as "extreme, extremely; unbearable, unbearably; cannot cope with." **Tamaranai**
can be replaced by **shikataga nai**, but **tamaranai** is much more emotive than
shikataga nai.

Haguki ga shimite tamaranai.
I have extremely sensitive gums. (*lit.*, My gums are extremely sensitive).

Ha ga itakute itakute tamarimasen.   I cannot cope with this toothache.
Amai-mono ga tabetakute tamarimasen. I want badly to eat sweets.

2. The direct and indirect passive

We studied the passive forms in Lessons 18, 25, 27, and 29. Japanese has passive expressions for indicating actions or events that are not under control of the person or persons affected by them. The passive form -**rareru** is also an honorific. The object of the verb using -**rareru** is marked by the object particle **o**.

> **Shika-i wa mushi-ba o naoserareta.**
> The dentist can treat cavities. (polite)

> **Senseiwa rentogen kensa de fusei-kōgō o miraremashita.**
> The doctor can see a malocclusion from the X-rays. (polite)

Among Japanese passive forms, there are two types, the direct passive and indirect passive. The direct passive is used when the person or thing affected by an event or someone's action is the direct recipient of that action and is the grammatical subject marked by **wa**. With the indirect passive, the person or thing that is the grammatical subject is not the direct recipient of someone's action.

> **Ha wa shika-i ni yotte, chiryō saremashita.** (direct passive)
> The tooth was treated by a dentist.

> **Oya-shirazu wa shika-i ni nukarareta.** (direct passive)
> The wisdom tooth was removed by a dentist.

> **Uketsuke wa kanjya ni takusan shitsumon o sarareta.** (indirect passive)
> The receptionist was asked many questions by the patient.

> **Shika-eisei-shi wa kanjya ni shikō o torase-rareta.** (indirect passive)
> The dental hygienist was asked to remove the plaque by the patient.

The passive formed with -**rareru** also expresses possibility, and the object of the action is marked by the particle **ga**.

> **Rentogen kensa de fusei-kōgō ga miraremashita.**
> Malocclusion could be seen from the X-ray (result).

3. The conjunction yō(ni)

We studied the conjunction **yō(ni)** (be like, similar to) in Lesson 17, and in Lesson 27 we studied the construction STEM VERB plus **yōni suru** (make sure). There is another usage of **yō(ni)**. Used with non-past verbs, **yō(ni)** also expresses a potential action or result and can be translated as "so that."

Mushiba ni naranai yō(ni) ha o migaite kudasai.
Please brush your teeth so that you can prevent cavities.

Mushiba ni naranai yō(ni) fusso o nurimasu ka.
Do you like to use fluoride so that you can prevent cavities?

Shinkei ga shiminai yō(ni) ha o chiryō shimasu.
I will treat your teeth so that your nerve will not be sensitive.

4. The adverb **kanari**

The adverb **kanari** indicates that the degree of something is extremely high, though lower than **tottemo** (very), **sugoku** (awfully), or **hontōni** (really). **Kanari** can be translated as "quite, considerably, fairly."

Kono chiryō wa kanari itakatta desu.
This treatment is quite painful.

Kanari ōkina mushiba ni natte imasu ne.
It has become a fairly big cavity, hasn't it?

Shika-eisei-shi wa shikō o toru tame ni kanari jikan o kakemashita.
The dental hygienist spent a considerable time cleaning the tartar.

5. The adverb **dōshite-mo**

The adverb **dōshite-mo** expresses the strong will to achieve something and translates as "at any cost; by any means; by whatever means: whatever it takes; no matter what."

Haguki no enshō o dōshite-mo osaetai desu.
I would like to control my gum inflammation at any cost.

Dōshite-mo eikyū-shi wa nokoshitai desu.
No matter what, I would like to keep my permanent tooth.

Ha wa dōshite-mo nokose masen ka.
Won't you save the tooth at any cost?

6. The adverb **sukunaku-tomo**

The adverb **sukunaku-tomo** is used with a noun or number and translates as "at least." It takes the particle **wa**.

Basshi-go wa sukunaku-tomo itsuka-kan wa yoku ugai o tsuzukete kudasai.
After the tooth is extracted, please (continue to) try gargle for at least five days.

Basshi-go wa sukunaku-tomo ichi-ji-kan wa kuruma no unten o shinai de kudasai.
After the extraction, please do not drive a car for at least one hour.

Sukunak-tomo eikyū-shi wa nokoshimashō.
Let's at least keep the permanent teeth.

Useful Expressions (CD 30-3)

Listen to the CD and repeat the sentences.

1. **Mushiba wa ippon mo arimasen.** You don't have any cavities.
2. **Dōmo migi-ue-no oya-shirazu ga mushiba no yō desu.** I think you have a cavity on your upper right wisdom tooth.
3. **Tsumetai mono ga ha ni shimi-masu ka.** Are you sensitive to cold foods?
4. **Hidari-shita no oyashirazu ga itami-masu ka.** Does your lower left wisdom tooth hurt?
5. **Haguki-kara shukketsu o shite imasu.** Your gums are bleeding.
6. **Kodomo no ha ni fusso o nurimasu ka.** Do you need to apply a fluoride treatment on the child's tooth?
7. **Shiseki ga takusan arimasu.** You have a lot of tartar.
8. **Musume-san wa kyōsei ga hitsuyō mitai desu.** Your daughter may need to have braces/orthodontic treatment.
9. **Itai toki wa migi-te o agete kudasai.** Pleases raise your hand when you feel pain.
10. **Dono ha ga itami-masu ka.** In which tooth do you have pain?

Key Sentences (CD 30-4)

Listen to the CD and repeat the sentences.

1. **Oku-ba ga itakute itakute tamarimasen.** I cannot cope with the pain in my back tooth.
2. **Shika-gikō-shi wa kanjya ni ireba o tsukurase-rareta.** The dental technician was asked by the patient to make dentures.
3. **Shikō ga tsukanai yō(ni) ha o migaite kudasai.** Please brush your teeth so that you can prevent plaque.
4. **Dōshite-mo mae-ba wa nokoshitai(n) desu ka.** No matter what, would you like to keep the front tooth?
5. **Basshi-go wa sukunaku-tomo mikka-kan wa yoku ugai o tsuzukete kudasai.** After the extraction, please (continue to) try to gargle for at least three days.

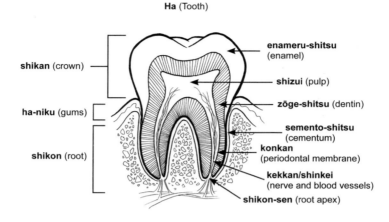

Ha (Tooth)

shikan (crown)

enameru-shitsu (enamel)

shizui (pulp)

zōge-shitsu (dentin)

ha-niku (gums)

semento-shitsu (cementum)

konkan (periodontal membrane)

shikon (root)

kekkan/shinkei (nerve and blood vessels)

shikon-sen (root apex)

Additional Words

nuku/nukimasu extract/pull out/remove

kezuru/kezurimasu grind

tsumeru/tsumemasu fill

kabuseru/kabusemasu cover

konkan chiryō root canal

migaku/migakimasu brushing

osaeru/osaemasu gain control/hold

nokosu/nokoshimasu save/remain

toru/torimasu take off

haeru/haemasu grow up

fusegu/fusekimasu prevent

nemuru/nemurimasu sleep

mu-kankaku numb

ippan-shika general dentistry

shinbi-shika cosmetic dentistry

kōkū-geka-i dental surgeon

yobō prevention

shishū-byō-chiryō periodontal treatment

kichin-to precisely

hagishiri gnash

shikon root

enameru-shitsu enamel

ha-burashi toothbrush

ha-migaki-ko toothpaste

furosu floss

shinsatsu-dai dentist's chair

ugai-gusuri mouthwash (expectorant)

doriru drill

kōkū senjyō-ki water pick

buriji bridge

inpuranto dental implant

mausu-pīsu night guard

tabe-kasu food particles

kyōsei-shika-i orthodontist

Language Notes

1. The following are some of the cavity-related expressions frequently used by dentists. All the grammar and vocabulary in the expressions has been studied.

   1. **Mushi-ba wa yoku itami masu ka.**
      Does this cavity often cause pain?

2. **Mushi-ba darake desu yo.**
   You have a lot of decayed teeth.

3. **Dō-mo mushi-ba no yō desu.**
   I think you probably have a decayed tooth.

4. **Mushi-ba wa ippon mo arimasen yo.**
   You don't have any cavities at all.

5. **Mushi-ba o nukimashō ka.**
   Shall we pull out your decayed tooth?

6. **Kono ha ga mushi-ba ni natte imasu yo.**
   This tooth is decayed.

7. **Amai-mono o taberu-to mushi-ba ni narimasu yo.**
   If you eat sweets, it will cause your teeth to decay.

8. **Hamigaki o shinai node, mushi-ba ni natta to omoimasu.**
   I think your tooth decayed because you neglected to brush. (*lit.*, You did not brush your teeth, so I think your tooth decayed.)

9. **Ha o kichin-to migake-ba, mushi-ba o fusegemasu.**
   If you brush well, you can prevent cavities.

10. **Tsumetai-mono ga ha ni shimimasu ka.**
    Are your teeth sensitive to cold?

2. There are several special expressions for teeth problems. As usual, to make a question using the expression, add **ka** at the end of sentence.

Ha ga zukin-zukin shimasu.	The tooth has a sharp pain.
Ha ga shimi-masu.	The tooth is sensitive.
Ha ga itami-masu.	The tooth is painful.
Ha ga gura-gura shimasu.	The tooth is loose.
Ha ga gaku-gaku shimasu.	The tooth is wobbly.
Ha ga gaku-gaku shimasu ka.	Is the tooth wobbly?

3. The following are some directions a dentist may give to a patient.

Kuchi o akete kudasai.	Please open your mouth.
Kuchi o motto ōkiku akete kudasai.	Please open your mouth wide.
Kuchi o tojite kudasai.	Please close your mouth.
Kan-de kudasai.	Please bite down.
Mōichi-do kande kudasai.	Please bite one more time.
Shita o agete kudasai.	Please lift your tongue up.
Shita o dashite kudasai.	Please move your tongue forward.
Sukoshi, matte kudasai.	Please wait a moment.

Ugai o shite kudasai.	Please rinse your mouth.
Hai, owari-mashia.	That's the end.

4.   Anesthesia-related expressions:

Masui-chūsha o shimasu.	I will give you an anesthetic injection.
Kyoku-bu masui o shimasu.	I will give you a local anesthetic.

Masui-go(ni) sukoshi shibire masu.
You will have a little numbness after the anesthesia.

Masui no toki(ni), chikuri to shimasu.
You may feel a slight prick when you have injection.

Language Roots

The word **shi** (歯) means "tooth." It is also pronounced **ha/ba**.

eikyū-shi	permanent tooth
shi-kō	plaque
mushi-ba	cavity

The word **sei/shō** (正) conveys the meaning of "correct, exact."

kyō-sei	braces/teeth aligned
sei-jyō	normal
sei-shiki	official, formal
shō-jiki	honesty

Culture Notes

Origin of the term for **oya-shirazu** (wisdom tooth)

There are two interpretations for the origin of the name for wisdom teeth, **oya-shirazu**. The literal meaning of **oya** is "parents," and of **shirazu (shiranai)** is "unknown." One interpretation is that the wisdom teeth come out when a parent (**oya**) is not showing interest in children's teeth. The other is that when the children's wisdom teeth begin to grow, the parents were usually deceased.

June 4th is Cavities Prevention Day (**Mushi-ba Yobō-bi**)

In 1928, the Japanese government established Cavities Prevention Day. Japanese enjoy playing on words and sound, and the name of the day is a pun. The number 6, for the sixth month, is **Mu(ttsu)** and the number 4 is **shi**. Therefore, June 4th is pronounced **Mu-shi-(ba)**, making it the obvious choice for **Mushi-ba Yobō-**

bi. After 1958, Cavities Prevention Day was extended to the Cavities Prevention Week (**Mushiba Yobō Shūkan**).

Comprehension

Answer the following questions.

1. Which of the following word does NOT belong with the others?
   a. **Tsume-mono**   b. **Ha-guki**
   c. **Ire-ba**   d. **Sashi-ba**

2. Which of the following could be used to say "sensitive teeth"?
   a. **Kami-masu**   b. **Itami-masu**
   c. **Shimi-masu**   d. **Shini-masu**

3. Which of the following best completes the sentence below?
   Basshi-go sukunaku-tomo ni-ji-kan (   ) kuruma o unten shinai de kudasai.
   (After the extraction, please do not drive a car for at least two hours.)
   a. **ga**   b. **wa**
   c. **ni**   d. **de**

4. A patient has complained about his teeth and you're examining him. Which of the following expressions is NOT related to tooth problems?
   a. **Ha ga gura-gura shimasu.**   b. **Ha ga zukin-zukin shimasu.**
   c. **Ha ga gasa-gasa shimasu.**   d. **Ha ga gaku-gaku shimasu.**

Select the appropriate meaning from list below.

5. **Shikō ga tsukanai yōni ha o migaite kudasai.**   (   )
6. **Dōshite-mo oyashirazu wa nokoshitai desu ka.**   (   )
7. **Oku-ba ga itakute itakute tamarimasen.**   (   )
8. **Shika-gikō-shi wa kanjya ni ire-ba o tsukurasa-rareta.**   (   )
9. **Ha no chiryō-go wa, sukunaku tomo futsu-kan wa yoku**   (   )
   ugai o tsuzukete kudasai.

a. Please brush your teeth so that you can prevent plaque.
b. I cannot cope with my back tooth pain.
c. The dentures were made for the patient by the dental technician.
d. No matter what, would you like to keep the wisdom tooth?
e. After treating the teeth, please continue to (try to) gargle for at least two days.

Practice

Respond to the following in Japanese using the cues that have been provided.

1. How do you state the following situations?
   (Patient)   (Healthcare professional)
   1. No cavities   _____
   2. The back tooth has a cavity.   _____
   3. Sensitive to cold   _____
   4. Gum bleeding   _____
   5. Need fluoride treatment.   _____

2. Give the patient the following directions.
   (Patient's situation)   (Healthcare professional)
   1. Need to rinse.   _____
   2. Need to give a sign when there is pain. _____
   3. Need to open mouth.   _____
   4. Need to lift tongue up.   _____
   5. Need to wait a moment.   _____

3. How do you ask about the patient's pains and problems?
   (Patient's problems)   (Healthcare professional)
   1. The tooth is sensitive.   _____
   2. The tooth is painful.   _____
   3. The tooth has a sharp pain.   _____
   4. The tooth is wobbly.   _____
   5. The tooth is loose.   _____

4. Dialogue comprehension. Based on the dialogue, answer the following questions.
   1. **Suzuki-san wa dono ha ga itai(n) desu ka.**   _____
   2. **Rentogen kensa no kekka wa dō deshita ka.**   _____
   3. **Ha no basshi ga hitsuyō desu ka.**   _____
   4. **Suzuki-san wa ha o nokoshitai desu ka.**   _____
   5. **Don-na kusuri ga shohō saremashita ka.**   _____
   6. **Suzuki-san wa basshi-go, nani o tsuzuke**   _____
      nakereba narimasen ka.

5. Free response questions.
   (Questions)   (Healthcare professional)
   1. **Ha no teiki-kenshin o shite imasu ka.**   _____
   2. **Hamigaki o ichi-nichi(ni) nan-kai shimasu ka.** _____

3. **Mushi-ba ga arimasu ka.**   _____

4. **Ire-ba ya sashi-ba o shite imasu ka.**   _____

5. **Haguki kara shukketsu ga arimasu ka.**   _____

Exercise

1. How to say the following words in Japanese.
    A. Gums   _____
    B. Tartar   _____
    C. Plaque   _____
    D. Denture   _____
    E. Permanent tooth   _____

2. Translate the following in Japanese.
    A. I cannot cope with my wisdom tooth pain.
    B. The dental technician made a false tooth for the patient.
    C. Please brush your teeth so that you can prevent bad breath.
    D. No matter what, would you like to keep the baby tooth?
    E. After the extraction, please continue to gargle for at least a week.

3. How do you ask patients the following questions in Japanese?
    A. Does this cavity often cause pain?
    B. Do you need to apply a fluoride treatment on child's tooth?
    C. Do you have pain in your lower left wisdom tooth?
    D. Are you sensitive to cold foods?
    E. In which tooth do you have pain?

4. Answer the following questions in Japanese.

    Q: **Amai-mono o taberuto mushi-ba ni shimi-masu ka.**
    A: _____
    (Yes, but if you brush well, you can prevent cavities.)

    Q: **Sensei, mushi-ba ga arimasu ka.**
    B: _____
    (Yes, you have a lot of decayed teeth.)

    Q: **Dono ha ga mushi-ba desu ka.**
    C: _____
    (This back tooth is decayed.)

Basic Medical Terms
(English-Japanese)

I. Facilities, Departments, and Specialists

adult medicine **seijin-byō-ka** 成人病科

allergy **arerugī-ka** アレルギー科

allergy specialist **arerugī senmon-i** アレルギー専門医

anesthesiologist **masui-ka-i** 麻酔科医

anesthetist **masui-shi** 麻酔士

attendant **tsukisoi-nin** 付添人

attending doctor **tantō-i(shi)** 担当医(師)

bonesetter **sekkotsu-i** 接骨医

brain surgeon **nō-ge-ka-i** 脳外科医

brain surgery **nō-ge-ka** 脳外科

cardiac surgery **shinzō ge-ka** 心臓外科

cardiologist **shinzō-byō senmon-i** 心臓病専門医

cardiovascular **jyun-kanki-ka** 循環器科

children's doctor **shōni-ka-i** 小児科医

children's hospital **kodomo-byōin** 子供病院

city hospital **shiritsu-byōin** 市立病院

clinic **shinryō-jyo/ i-in** 診療所・医院

clinical laboratory technician **rinshō-kensa-gishi** 臨床検査技師

community hospital **shimin-byōin** 市民病院

cosmetic surgery **biyō-seikei-ge-ka** 美容整形外科

counselor **kaunserā** カウンセラー

custodian, janitor **seisō-in** 清掃員

dental hygienist **shika-eisei-shi** 歯科衛生士

dental surgeon **kōkū-ge-ka-i** 口腔外科医

dental technician **shika-gikō-shi** 歯科技工士

dentist **shika-i-shi** 歯科医師

dentistry **shi-ka** 歯科

dermatologist **hifu-ka-i** 皮膚科医

dermatology **hifu-ka** 皮膚科

dispensary **ikyoku** 医局

doctor **i-shi/i-sha/ sensei** 医師・医者・先生

doctor's office **i-in** 医院

ear, nose and throat (ENT) **jibi-inkō-ka** 耳鼻咽喉科

ENT doctor **jibi-inkō-ka-i** 耳鼻咽喉科医

emergency doctor **kinkyū-i** 緊急医

emergency hospital **kinkyū-byōin** 緊急病院

emergency medical assistance team (EMAT) **kinkyū-iryō-chīmu** 緊急医療チーム

eye doctor **gan-ka-i** 眼科医

family care department **ippan-shinryō-ka** 一般診療科

family doctor **shu-ji-i** 主治医

field hospital **yasen-byōin** 野戦病院

gastroenterologist **i-chō-ka senmon-i** 胃腸科専門医

gastroenterology **shōkaki-ka, ichō-ka** 消化器科、胃腸科

general dentistry **ippan shi-ka** 一般歯科

general hospital **sogō-byōin** 総合病院

general practioner **ippan kaigyō-i** 一般開業医

general surgeon **ippan ge-ka-i** 一般外科医

genetics **iden-gaku** 遺伝学

geriatrics **rōjin i-gaku** 老人医学

gynecologist **fujin-ka-i** 婦人科医

gynecology **fujin-ka** 婦人科

head (chief) doctor **i-in-chō** 医院長

head (chief) nurse **kango-shi-chō** 看護師長

health center **hoken-jyo** 保健所

health insurance doctor **kenkō hoken-i** 健康保険医

healthcare worker **kaigo-shi** 介護士

heart specialist **shinzō senmon-i** 心臓専門医

heart surgeon **shinzō ge-ka-i** 心臓外科医

heart surgery **shinzō ge-ka** 心臓外科

hematologist **ketsu-eki senmon-i** 血液専門医

herb specialist (doctor) **kanpō-i** 漢方医

hospital nurse **byōin-kango-shi** 病院看護師

information **an-nai gakari** 案内係り

intern **intān** インターン

internal medicine **nai-ka** 内科

internist **nai-ka-i** 内科医

maternity clinic **sanka-i-in** 産科医院

medical doctor **i-shi/i-sha** 医師/医者

mental hospital **seishin-ka byō-in** 精神科病院

medical practitioner **kaigyō-i** 開業医

medical radiographer **shinryō-hōsha-sen gishi** 診療 放射線技師

medical social worker **iryō sōsharu-wākā** 医療ソーシャル ワーカー

midwife **jyosan-shi** 助産師

neurological surgery **shinkei ge-ka** 神経外科

neurologist **shinkei-ka-i** 神経科医

neurology **shinkei-ka** 神経科

neurosurgeon **nō shinkei ge-ka-i** 脳神経外科医

neurosurgery **nō shinkei-ka** 脳神経科

non-profit hospital **jizen-byōin** 慈善病院

nurse **kango-shi** 看護師

nurse's aid **kango-jyoshu** 看護助手

nursing home **kaigo-shisetsu/rōjin-fuku-shi-shi-setsu** 介護施設・老人福祉施設

obstetrician **san-ka-i** 産科医

obstetrics **san-ka** 産科

obstetrics and gynecology **san-fujin-ka** 産婦人科

office worker **jimu-in** 事務員

operating room nurse **shujyutsu-shitsu tantō-kango-shi** 手術室担当看護師

ophthalmologist **gan-ka-i** 眼科医

ophthalmology **gan-ka** 眼科

optician **megane-ya (-san)** 眼鏡屋(さん)

orderly **yōmu-in** 用務員

orthodontist **kyōsei shi-ka-i** 矯正歯科医

orthopedics **seikei ge-ka** 整形外科

orthopedic surgeon **seikei ge-ka-i** 整形外科医

orthopedic surgery **seikei ge-ka** 整形外科

osteopath **sekkotsu-i** 接骨医

otolaryngologist **jibi-inkō-ka-i** 耳鼻咽喉科医

otolaryngology **jibi-inkō-ka** 耳鼻咽喉科

pathology **byōri-gaku** 病理学

pediatrician **shōni-ka-i** 小児科医

pediatrics **shōni-ka** 小児科

plastic surgery **seikei ge-ka** 成形外科

pneumology **kokyūki-ka** 呼吸器科

pharmacist **yakuzai-shi** 薬剤師

pharmacy **yakkyoku** 薬局

primary care doctor **shuji-i** 主治医

private hospital **shiritsu-byōin** 私立院

private nurse **tsukisoi-kango-shi** 付添看護師

proctologist **kōmon-ka-i** 肛門科医

psychiatrist **seishin-ka-i** 精神科医

psychiatry **seishin-ka** 精神科

psychosomatic medicine **seishin-i-gaku** 精神医学

physician **i-shi, i-sha** 医師・医者

pulmonary disease specialist **kokyūki senmon-i** 呼吸器専門医

pulmonology **kokyūki-ka** 呼吸器科

radiologist **hōshasen-ka-i** 放射線科医

radiology department **hōshasen-ka** 放射線科

receptionist **uketsuke-gakari** 受付係り

school doctor **kō-i** 校医

school infirmary **hoken-shitsu** 保健室

school nurse **yōgo-kyōyu** 養護教諭

security officer/ guard **keibi-in** 警備員

specialist **senmon-i** 専門医

specialized hospital **senmon-byōin** 専門病院

student nurse **kango-gakusei** 看護学生

surgeon **ge-ka-i** 外科医

surgery **ge-ka** 外科

teaching hospital **daigaku-fuzoku-byōin** 大学付属病院

thoracic surgery **kyōbu ge-ka** 胸部外科

translator **tsūyaku** 通訳

urologist **hinyōki-ka-i** 泌尿器科医

urology **hinyōki-ka** 泌尿器科

II. Body Parts, Internal Organs, and Related Terms

abdomen **ka-fukubu** 下腹部

abdominal muscles **fukkin** 腹筋

Achilles tendon **akiresu-ken** アキレス腱

adrenal glands **fuku-jin** 副腎

ankle **ashi-kubi** 足首

ankle bone **kurubushi** 踝

anus **kōmon** 肛門

aorta **dai-dōmyaku** 大動脈

appendix **chūsui** 虫垂

arch (of foot) **tsuchi-fumazu** 土踏まず

arm **ude** 腕

armpit **waki-no-shita** 脇の下

artery **dōmyaku** 動脈

atrium **shinbō** 心房

ascending colon **jōkō-dai-chō** 上行大腸

auricle **gai-ji** 外耳

baby tooth **nyū-shi** 乳歯

back **senaka** 背中

back of the hand **te-no-kō** 手の甲

back of the head **kōtō-bu** 後頭部

backbone **sebone** 背骨

back tooth **oku-ba** 奥歯

barefoot **hadashi** 裸足

belly **hara/onaka** 腹・お腹

belly button **heso** へそ

big toe **ashi-no-oya-yubi** 足の親指

bladder **bōkō** 膀胱

blood **chi, ketsu-eki** 血・血液

blood plasma **kesshō** 血しょう

blood platelet **kesshō-ban** 血小板

blood vessel **kekkan** 血管

body **karada** 体

bone **hone** 骨

bone marrow **kotsu-zui** 骨髄

bottom/ buttocks **(o) shiri** お尻

bowel **chō** 腸

brain **nō** 脳

breast **mune/kyōbu/ chibusa** 胸・胸部・乳房

breastbone **kyō-kotsu** 胸骨

bronchus **ki-kan-shi** 気管支

calf **fukurahagi** ふくらはぎ

capillaries **mōsai-kekkan** 毛細血管

carotid artery **keidōmyaku** 頚動脈

cartilage **nan-kotsu** 軟骨

cecum **mō-chō** 盲腸

cell **saibō** 細胞

cervical spine **kei-tsui** 頚椎

cervix **shikyū-kei** 子宮頸

cervix of the uterus **shikyū-kō** 子宮口

cheek **hoho** ほお

cheek bone **hoho-bone** 頬骨

chest **mune** 胸・胸部

chin **ago-no-saki** あごの先

collarbone **sa-kotsu** 鎖骨

colon **kecchō** 結腸

cornea **kakumaku** 角膜

crotch **mata** 股

descending colon **kakō-dai-chō** 下行大腸

diaphragm **ōkakumaku** 横隔膜

digestive system **shōkaki-kei** 消化器系

digestive tract **chō-kan** 腸管

dimple **ekubo** えくぼ

duodenum **jyunishi-chō** 十二指腸

ear **mimi** 耳

eardrum **komaku** 鼓膜

earlobe **mimi-tabu** 耳たぶ

elbow **hiji** ひじ

enamel **enameru-shitsu** エナメル質

endocrine gland **nai-bunpitsu-sen** 内分泌線

esophagus **shokudō** 食道

eye **me** 目

eyeball **gan-kyū** 眼球

eyebrow **mayu-ge** 眉毛

eyelash **matsu-ge** まつげ

eyelid **mabuta** まぶた

face **kao** 顔

fat **shibō** 脂肪

femoral artery **daitai-dōmyaku** 大腿動脈

femoral vein **daitai-jyōmyaku** 大腿静脈

finger **yubi** 指

fingertip **yubi-saki** 指先

fist **kobushi** こぶし

flank **wakibara** 脇腹

foot **ashi** 足

forearm **zen-wan** 前腕

forefinger **hitosashi-yubi** 人差し指

forehead **hitai** 額

freckle **sobakasu** そばかす

front tooth **mae-ba** 前歯

gallbladder **tannō** 胆嚢

genital organ **sei-ki** 性器

genitalia **seishoku-ki** 生殖器

glabella **miken** 眉間

glands **nai-bunpitsu-sen** 内分泌腺

glans **kitō** 亀頭

gums **haguki** 歯茎

hair **kami** 髪

hand **te** 手

head **atama** 頭

heart **shinzō** 心臓

heel **kakato** かかと

hip **koshi** 腰

hymen **shojyo-maku** 処女膜

index finger **hito-sashi-yubi** 人差し指

intestine **chō** 腸

jaw **ao** あご

jejunum **kū-chō** 腔腸

joint **kansetsu** 関節

joint cavity **kansetsu-kō** 関節腔

kidney **suizō** 膵臓

knee **hiza** ひざ

large bowel **dai-chō** 大腸

latissimus dorsi muscle **(kō) hai-kin** (広) 背筋

leg **ashi** 足

lens **suishōtai** 水晶体

ligament **jintai** 靭帯

lip **kuchi-biru** 唇

little finger/pinky **ko-yubi** 小指

liver **kanzō** 肝臓

lower abdomen **ka-fukubu** 下腹部

lower back/hips **koshi** 腰

lower body **ka-han-shin** 下半身

lumbar spine **yō-tsui** 腰椎

lung **hai** 肺

lymph **rinpa-eki** リンパ液

lymph node **rinpa-setsu** リンパ節

lymphatic gland **rinpa-sen** リンパ腺

main vein (vena cava) **dai-jyōmyaku** 大静脈

mammary gland **nyū-sen** 乳腺

marrow **kotsu-zui** 骨髄

middle finger **naka-yubi** 中指

mole **hokuro** ほくろ

mouth **kuchi** 口

mucous membrane **nen-maku** 粘膜

mucus **nen-eki** 粘液

muscle **kin-niku** 筋肉

mustache **kuchi-hige** 口ひげ

nail **tsume** 爪

nasal cavity **bikō/nana no ana** 鼻腔・鼻の穴

navel **heso** へそ

neck **kubi** 首

nerve **shinkei** 神経

nipple **chi-kubi/nyū-tō** 乳首・乳頭

nose **hana** 鼻

organs **kikan/zōki** 器官・臓器

ovary **ran-sō** 卵巣

oviduct **ran-kan** 卵管

ovum **ran-shi** 卵子

palm **te-no-hira** 手のひら

pancreas **sui-zō** すい臓

pelvis **kotsu-ban** 骨盤

penis **penisu/dankon** ペニス・男根

peripheral nervous system **masshō-shinkei** 末梢神経

peritoneum **fuku-maku** 腹膜

permanent tooth **eikyū-shi** 永久歯

pit of the stomach **mizo-ochi** みぞおち

placenta **taiban** 胎盤

plantar arch **tsuchi-fumazu** 土踏まず

pleura **roku-maku** 肋膜

prostate gland **zenritsu-sen** 前立腺

pubic bone **chikotsu** 恥骨

pupil **hitomi** 瞳

rectum **choku-chō** 直腸

retina **mō-maku** 網膜

rib **rokkotsu** 肋骨

rib cage **kyō-kaku** 胸郭

ring finger **kusuri-yubi** 薬指

root (of tooth) **shi-kon** 歯根

sciatic nerve **zakotsu-shinkei** 坐骨神経

sex organ **seishoku-ki** 生殖器

shin **sune** すね

shoulder **kata** 肩

shoulder blade **kenkō-kotsu** 肩甲骨

sigmoid colon **esu-jyō-kkechō** S状結腸

skeletal muscle **kokkaku-kin** 骨格筋

skin **hifu/ hada** 皮膚・肌

skull **zugai-kotsu** 頭蓋骨

small bowel **shō-chō** 小腸

sole **ashi-no-ura** 足の裏

spinal cord **sekizui** 脊髄

spine **sebone** 背骨

spleen **hizō** 脾臓

stomach **i** 胃

temple **kome-kami** こめかみ

tendon **ken** 腱

testicles **kōgan** 睾丸

thigh **momo** もも

thighbone **daitai-kotsu** 大腿骨

thoracic spine **kyō-tsui** 胸椎

throat **nodo** のど

thumb **oya-yubi** 親指

thyroid gland **kōjyō-sen** 甲状腺

tip of tongue **shita-saki** 舌先

toe **tsuma-saki** つま先

toenail **ashi-no-tsume** 足の爪

tongue **shita** 舌

tonsil **hentō-sen** 扁桃腺

tooth **ha** 歯

transverse colon **ōkō-dai-chō** 横行大腸

trunk **dō** 胴

tummy **onaka** お腹

umbillical cord **heso-no-o** へその緒

underarm hair **waki-ge** わき毛

upper arm **jyō-an** 上腕

upper back **senaka** 背中

upper body **jyō-han-shin** 上半身

urethra **nyō-dō** 尿道

urinary bladder **bōkō** 膀胱

uterus **shikyū** 子宮

uvula **kōgai-sui/ nodo-chinko** 口蓋垂・のどちんこ

vagina **chitsu** 膣

vein **jyō-myaku** 静脈

ventricle **shin-shitsu** 心室

vocal cords **seitai** 声帯

waist **koshi** 腰

wisdom tooth **oya-shirazu** 親しらず

womb **shikyū** 子宮

wrinkle **shiwa** しわ

wrist **te-kubi** 手首

III. Diseases, Disorders, and Symptoms

abdominal pain **fuku-tsū** 腹痛

abnormal **ijyō** 異常

abnormal bleeding **fusei-shukketsu** 不正出血

abrasion **suri-kizu** すり傷

ache **itami** 痛み

acid stomach **isan-kata** 胃酸過多

acidosis **sanketsu-byō** 酸欠病

acne **nikibi** にきび

acute myocardial infarction **kyūsei shinkin-kōsoku** 急性心筋梗塞

acute pericarditis **kyūsei-shin-maku-en** 急性心膜炎

addiction **izon-shō** 依存症

adult disease **seijin-byō** 成人病

aftereffect **kōi-shō** 後遺症

aging process **rōka genshō** 老化現象

AIDS **e-i-zu** エイズ

alcoholism **arukōru izon-shō** アルコール依存症

allergic constitution **arerugī tai-shitsu** アレルギー体質

allergic disease **arerugī shikkan** アレルギー疾患

allergic rhinitis **arerugī-ei bi-en** アレルギー性鼻炎

allergy **arerugī** アレルギー

allergy to pollen **kafun-shō** 花粉症

alopecia **datsu-mō-shō** 脱毛症

alopecia areata **enkei-datsu-mō-shō** 円形脱毛症

alveolar pyorrhea **shisō-nōrō** 歯槽のう漏

Alzheimer's areata **arutsuhaimā-byō** アルツハイマー病

amnesia **kioku-sōshitsu** 記憶喪失

anal fistula **jirō** 痔ろう

anemia **hin-ketsu** 貧血

angina pectoris **kyōshin-shō** 狭心症

anorexia **kyoshoku-shō** 拒食症

anthropophobia **taijin kyōfu-shō** 対人恐怖症

anxiety **fuan** 不安

anxiety attack **fuan-hossa** 不安発作

apastia **kyoshoku-shō** 拒食症

apnea **mu-kokyū** 無呼吸

aphthous atomatitis **afuta-sei kōnai-en** アフタ性口内炎

apoplexy **nō-socchū** 脳卒中

appendicitis **mōchō-en/chūsui-en** 盲腸炎・虫垂炎

arrythmia **fusei-myaku** 不整脈

arsenic poisoning **hiso-chūdoku** 砒素中毒

arteriosclerosis **dōmyaku-kōka-shō** 動脈硬化症

arthritis **kansetsu-en** 関節炎

asthma **zen-soku** 喘息

astigmatism **ran-shi** 乱視

attention deficit hyperactivity disorder **chūi-kekkan tadōsei-shōgai** 注意欠陥多動性障害

athlete's foot **mizu-mushi** 水虫

atopic dermatitis **atopī-sei hifu-en** アトピー性皮膚炎

attack **hossa** 発作

auditory hallucination **genchō** 幻聴

autism **jihei-shō** 自閉症

autointoxication **jika-chū-doku** 自家中毒

autonomic imbalance **jiritsu shinkei-shichō-shō** 自律神経失調症

back pain **senaka-no-itami/ haibu-tsū** 背中の痛み・背部痛

bacteria **saikin** 細菌

bad bite **fusei-kōgo** 不正咬合

bad breath **kōshū** 口臭

baldness **datsu-mō-shō** 脱毛症

bed sore **tokozure** 床ずれ

bed wetting **onesho/ya-nyō-shō** お寝小・夜尿症

belching **geppu** げっぷ

(benign) prostate hypertrophy **(ryosei)zen-ritsu-sen hidai** (良性)前立腺肥大

beriberi **kakke** かっけ

bipolar disorder **sō-utsu-byō** 躁鬱病

birth defect **senten-sei ijyō** 先天性異常

birthmark **bohan** 母斑

bite wound **kami-kizu** 噛み傷

bladder cancer **bōkō-gan** 膀胱癌

bladder inflammation **bōkō-en** 膀胱炎

bladder stone **bōkō kesseki** 膀胱結石

bleary eye **kasumi** かすみ

bleeding **shukketsu** 出血

bleeding gums **haguki-kara-no-shukketsu** 歯茎からの出血

blepharitis **ganken-en** 眼瞼炎

blindness **shitsumei** 失明

blister **sui-hō/mizu-bukure/hi-bukure** 水泡・水ぶくれ・火ぶくれ

bloodshot **jyū-ketsu** 充血

bloody phlegm **kettan** 血痰

bloody stools **ketsu-ben** 血便

bloody urine **ketsu-nyō** 血尿

blurred vision **boyakeru** ぼやける

body odor **tai-shū** 体臭

boil **deki-mono** できもの

bone marrow transplantation **kotsuzui-ishoku** 骨髄移植

bowlegged **ō-kyaku** O脚

brain death **nō-shi** 脳死

brain stroke **nō-sochū** 脳卒中

brain tumor **nō-shiyō** 脳腫瘍

breast cancer **nyū-gan** 乳癌

broken bone **kossetsu** 骨折

broken tooth **ha ga oreru** 歯が折れる

bronchial asthma **kikanshi-zensoku** 気管支喘息

bronchitis **kikanshi-en** 気管支炎

bruise **uchimi/daboku-shō/ aza** 打ち身・打撲傷・痣

bubonic plague **sen-pesuto** 腺ペスト

bulimia **kashoku-shō** 過食症

bump **kobu** こぶ

burn **yakedo** やけど

buzzing in the ear **mimi-nari** 耳鳴り

caesarian section **teiō-sekkai** 帝王切開

calcipenia **karushūmu ketsubō-shō** カルシュウム欠乏症

callus **tako** たこ

cancer **gan** 癌

cancer-causing substance **hatsu-gan-sei-bushitsu** 発ガン性物質

cancer of the esophagus **shokudō-gan** 食道癌

cancer of the pancreas **suizō-gan** すい臓ガン

cancer of the rectum **choku-chō-gan** 直腸ガ

candidiasis **kanjida-shō** カンジダ症

carbon monoxide poisoning **issanka-chū-doku** 一酸化中毒

carbuncle **menchō** 面疔

carcinogen **hatsu-gan-sei-bushitsu** 発ガン性物質

cardiac asthma **shinzō-zensoku** 心臓喘息

cardiac failure **shin-fuzen** 心不全

cardiomyopathy **shin-kin-shō** 心筋症

caries **kariesu** カリエス

car sickness **kuruma-yoi** 車酔い

cataract **hakunai-shō** 白内障

catarrh **kataru** カタル

catatonia **kinchō-byō** 緊張病

cavity **mushi-ba** 虫歯

cerebral anemia **nō-hinketsu** 脳貧血

cerebral apoplexy **nō-socchū** 脳卒中

cerebral death **nō-shi** 脳死

cerebral hemorrhage **nō-shukketsu** 脳出血

cerebral infarction **nō-kōsoku** 脳梗塞

cerebral palsy **nō-sei-mahi** 脳性麻痺

cerebral thrombosis **nō-kkesen** 脳血栓

cerebral tumor **nō-shuyō** 脳腫瘍

cervix cancer **shikyū-kei-gan** 子宮頸癌

cesarean section/ C-section **teiō-sekkai** 帝王切開

change of voice **koe-gawari** 声変わり

chap, chapped skin **aka-gire** あかぎれ

character disorder **ijyō-jinkaku** 異常人格

chest pain **kyo-tsū/mune-no-itami** 胸痛・胸の痛み

chicken pox **suitō/mizu-bōso** 水痘・水ぼうそう

children's dysentery **ekiri** 疫痢

chill **samuke/okan** 寒気・悪寒

chilblain **shimo-yake** 霜焼け

cholelithiasis **tanseki** 胆石

cholera **korera** コレラ

cholesterol **koresuterōru** コレステロール

chronic disease **mansei-byō/ji-byō** 慢性病・持病

chronic fatigue syndrome **mansei-hirō shōkō-gun** 慢性疲労症候群

chronic hepatitis **mansei kan-en** 慢性肝炎

chronic nephritis **mansei jin-en** 慢性腎炎

chronic pain **mansei-tsū** 慢性痛

chronic pancreatitis **mansei sui-en** 慢性膵炎

circulatory disease **jyunkanki-kei shikkan** 循環器系疾患

cirrhosis **kankō-hen** 肝硬変

clogged arteries **dōmyaku kkesen** 動脈血栓

cognitive disease **ninchi-shō** 認知症

cold **kaze** かぜ

coldness **hie-shō** 冷え性

colitis **daichō-en/ kechō-en** 大腸炎・結腸炎

collagen disease **kōgen-byō** こうげん病

colon cancer **dai-chō-gan** 大腸ガン

color blindness **shiki-mō** 色盲

coma **konsui** 昏睡

comminuted fracture **funsui-kkosetsu** 粉砕骨折

complications **gappei-shō** 合併症

concussion **nō-shintō** 脳しんとう

compound fracture **fukuzatsu-kkosetsu** 複雑骨折

congestion **jyū-ketsu/ukketsu** 充血・うっ血

conjunctivitis **ketsumaku-en** 結膜炎

constipation **benpi** 便秘

consumption **hai-kekaku** 肺結核

contagious disease **densen-byō** 伝染病

contractions **jin-tsū** 陣痛

contusion **daboku-shō** 打撲傷

convulsion **hikitsuke** 引きつけ

corn **uo-no-me** 魚の目

corneal infection **kakumaku-kansen-shō** 角膜感染症

corneal xerosis **kakumaku-kansō-shō** 角膜乾燥症

coronary artery disease **kan-dōmyaku-shukkan** 冠動脈疾患

cough **seki** 咳

crack **hibi(-ware)** 輝(割れ)

cracked tooth **ha ga kakeru** 歯が欠ける

cramps **keiren/ashi-no-tsuri** 痙攣・足の攣り

crooked tooth **warui-ha-narabi** 悪い歯並び

cross-eyed **nai-sha-shi/yabu-nirami** 内斜視・やぶにらみ

cross-reaction **kōsa-hannō** 交差反応

cure **kaifuku** 回復

cuts **kiri-kizu** 切り傷

cyanosis **chianōze** チアノーゼ

cystitis (of bladder) **bōkō-en** 膀胱炎

dandruff **fuke** フケ

deafness **nan-chō** 難聴

death **shibō** 死亡

decayed tooth **mushi-ba** 虫歯

decreasing function **kinō-teika** 機能低下

dehydration **dassui-shōjyō** 脱水症状

delusion **mōsō** 妄想

delivery **bunben** 分娩

dementia **chihō** 痴ほう

depression **utsu-byō** うつ病

depressed condition **utsu-jyōtai** うつ状態

dermatitis **hifu-en** 皮膚炎

developmental disorder **hattatsu-shōgai** 発達障害

diabetes **tōnyō-byō** 糖尿病

diaper rash **omutsu-kabure** おむつかぶれ

diarrhea **geri** 下痢

die of old age **rōsui-shi** 老衰死

difficult delivery **nan-zan** 難産

dim vision **kasumu** かすむ

diphtheria **jifuteria** ジフテリア

discharge **ori-mono/bunpitsu-butsu** おりもの・分泌物

discharge from the ear **mimi-dare** 耳垂れ

discharge from the eyes **me-yani** 目やに

discomfort **fukai (kan)** 不快感

disease **byōki** 病気

dilated cardiomyopathy **kakuchō-gata shinkin-shō** 拡張型心筋症

dislocation **dakkyū** 脱臼

distortion **yugami** 歪み

dizziness **memai** めまい

dizzy spells **memai no jyumon** めまいの呪文

double vision **fuku-shi** 複視

Down's syndrome **daun-shō** ダウン症

drug addiction **mayaku-chūdoku** 麻薬中毒

drug allergy **kusuri-aregurī** 薬アレルギー

drug eruptions **yaku-shin** 薬疹

drug rash **yaku-shin** 薬疹

dry eyes **gan-kansō** 眼乾燥

dry skin **kansō-hada** 乾燥肌

dull ache **don-tsū** 鈍痛

duodenitis **jyūnishi-chō-en** 十二指腸炎

duodenitis ulcer **jyūnishi-chō-kaiyō** 十二指腸潰瘍

dysentery **sekiri** 赤痢

dysfunction **kinō-shōgai** 機能障害

dyslexia **shitsu-doku-shō** 失読症

dysmenorrhoea **seiri-fujyun** 生理不順

dyspnea **kokyū-kon-nan** 呼吸困難

ear infection **mimi-kansen-shō** 耳感染症

ear rash **mimi-kabure** 耳かぶれ

earache **mimi-no-itami** 耳の痛み

early cancer **sōki-gan** 早期ガン

earwax **mimi-aka** 耳垢

easy fatigability **kyojyaku-taishitsu** 虚弱体質

eczema **shissin** 湿疹

embolism **sokusen-shō** 塞栓症

emotional disorder **kanjyō-shōgai** 感情障害

emphysema **hai-kishu** 肺気腫

encephalitis **nō-en** 脳炎

encephalomalacia **nōnanka-shō** 脳軟化症

endometrial cancer **shikyūtai-gan** 子宮体癌

endometriosis **shikyū-nai-maku-shō** 子宮内膜症

endemic disease **fūdo-byō** 風土病

enlarged heart **shinzō-hidai** 心臓肥大

enlarged prostate gland **zenritsusen-hidai** 前立腺肥大

enlarged tonsils **hentōsen-hidai** 扁桃腺肥大

enteritis **chō-en** 腸炎

enuresis **ya-nyō-shō** 夜尿症

epidemic conjunctivities **ryūkō-sei ketsumaku-en** 流行性結膜炎

epidemic hepatitis **ryūkō-sei kan-en** 流行性肝炎

epidemic keratoconjunctivitis **ryūkō-sei kaku-ketsu-maku-en** 流行性角結膜炎

epilepsy **tenkan** 癲癇

eruptions **fukide-mono** 吹き出物

erysipelas **tan-doku** 丹毒

erythema **shimi** シミ

exanthema subitum **toppatsu-sei hasshin** 突発性発疹

excessive bleeding **shukketsu taryō** 出血多量

exhaustion **hirō** 疲労

extrauterine pregnancy **shikyū-gai-ninshin** 子宮外妊娠

eyestrain **gansei hirō** 眼精疲労

facial furuncle **menchō** 面疔

facial neuralgia **ganmen shinkei-tsū** 顔面神経痛

faint **kizetsu/nō-hinketsu** 気絶・脳貧血

fainting spell **shisshin/kizetsu** 失神・気絶

false nearsightedness **kasei-kin-shi** 仮性近視

farsightedness **en-shi** 遠視

fat **shibō/himan** 脂肪・肥満

fatigue **kentai-kan/hirō** 倦怠感/疲労

fear of people **taijin-kyōfu-shō** 対人恐怖症

febrile seizure **netsu-sei keiren** 熱性痙攣

fever **netsu** 熱

fibroid tumors **shikyū-kinshu** 子宮筋腫

fit **hossa** 発作

flat foot **henpei-soku** 扁平足

floaters **hibun-shō** 飛蚊症

flu **infuruenza** インフルエンザ

food poisoning **shoku-chūdoku** 食中毒

fracture **kossetsu** 骨折

frequent urination **hin-nyō** 頻尿

frigidity **fukan-shō** 不感症

frostbite **tōshō** 凍傷

frozen shoulder **gojyū-kata** 五十肩

fundus bleeding **gantei-shukketsu** 眼底出血

functional disorder **kinō-shōgai** 機能障害

gallstone **tanseki** 胆石

gas poisoning **gasu-chūdoku** ガス中毒

gastric catarrh **i-kataru** 胃カタル

gastric ulcer **i-kaiyō** 胃潰瘍

gastritis **i-en** 胃炎

gastrointestional disease **i-chō-byō** 胃腸病

gastroptosis **i-kasui** 胃下垂

gastrospasm **i-keiren** 胃けいれん

genital herpes **seiki herupesu** 性器ヘルペス

genital infectious disease **sei-kansen-shō** 性感染症

geriatrics disease **rōjin byō** 老人病

germ (bacillus) **byōgen-kin** 病原菌

German measles **fūshin/mikka-bashika** 風疹・三日麻疹

giddiness/light-headedness **tachi-kurami** 立眩み

gingivitis **shiniku-en** 歯肉炎

glandular fever **hakkekyū zōka-shō** 白血球増加症

glaucoma **ryokunai-shō** 緑内障

glycosuria **tō-nyō** 糖尿

gonorrhea **rin-byo** 淋病

gout **tsūfū** 痛風

Graves' disease **basedō-byō** バセドウ病

graze **suri-kizi/ kasuri-kizu** すり傷・かすり傷

green-stick fracture **wakagi kossetsu** 若木骨折

grind teeth **ha-gishiri** 歯ぎしり

growing pain **seichō-tsū** 成長痛

growl (stomach or bowel) **onaka-ga-naru** お腹が鳴る

gum infection **haguki-no- enshō** 歯茎の炎症

hair fall **nuke-ge** 抜け毛

hair loss **datsu-mō** 脱毛

hallucination **genkaku** 幻覚

hallux valgus **gaihan-boshi** 外反母趾

hangnail **sakamuke** さかむけ

Hansen's disease **rai-byō** らい病

hard of hearing **nanchō** 難聴

hard to breathe **iki-gurushii** 息苦しい

harelip **kōshinretsu/ mitsu-kuchi** 口唇裂・三つ口

hay fever **kafun-shō** 花粉症

head and neck cancer **tōkei-bu-gan** 頭頸部癌

head cold **hana-kaze** 鼻風邪

headache **zutsū** 頭痛

hearing impairment **chōkaku-shōgai** 聴覚障害

heart attack **shinzō-hossa** 心臓発作

heartburn **mune-yake** 胸焼け

heart failure **shin-fuzen** 心不全

heart transplant **shjnzō-ishoku** 心臓移植

heat rash **asemo** あせも

heat stroke **nissha-byō/nessha-byō** 日射病・熱射病

heaviness of the head **zujyū-kan** 頭重感

hemiplegia **hanshin-fuzui** 半身不随

hemophilia **ketsuyū-byō** 血友病

hemoptysis **kakketsu** 喀血

hemorrhage **shukketsu** 出血

hemorrhoids **ji** 痔

hepatitis **kan-en** 肝炎

hereditary disease **iden-sei-shikkan** 遺伝性疾患

hernia **herunia** ヘルニア

herniated disc **tsui-kanban-herunia** 椎間板ヘルニア

herpes **herupesu** ヘルペス

hiccup **shakkuri** しゃっくり

high blood pressure **kō-ketsu-atsu** 高血圧

hives **jinma-shin** 蕁麻疹

hoarse voice **shiwagare-goe** しわがれ声

Hong Kong flu **honkon-kaze** ホンコン風邪

hopelessness **zetsubō-kan** 絶望感

human vegetable **shokubutsu ningen** 植物人間

humming in the ear **mimi-nari** 耳鳴り

hydronephrosis **suijin-shō** 水腎症

hyperacidity **i-san-kata** 胃酸過多

hypermetropia **en-shi** 遠視

hyperphagia **kashoku-shō** 過食症

hypertension **kō-ketsuatsu-shō** 高血圧症

hypertrophic cardiomyopathy **hidai-gata shinkin-shō** 肥大型心筋症

hypertrophy of the heart **shinzō-hidai** 心臓肥大

hypobulia **shoku-yoku-gentai** 食欲減退

hypotension **tei-ketsua-tsu** 低血圧

hysteria **hisuterī** ヒステリー

idiosyncrasy **tokui-taishitsu** 特異体質

illness/disease **byōki** 病気

illusion **genkaku** 幻覚

impaired hearing **nan-chō** 難聴

impaired vision **shiryoku shōgai** 視力障害

impetigo **nōka-shin** 膿痂疹

impetigo contagiosa **tobihi/densen-sei nōka-shin** とびひ・伝染性膿痂疹

impotence **bokki fuzen/funō** 勃起不全/不能

indigestion **shōka-furyō** 消化不良

infantile asthma **shōni-zensoku** 小児喘息

infantile paralysis **shōni-mahi** 小児麻痺

infection of the bladder **bōkō-en** 膀胱炎

infectious disease **densen-byō** 伝染病

infectious hepatitis **ryūkōsei kan-en** 流行性肝炎

infertile **funin-shō** 不妊症

inflammation **enshō** 炎症

inflammation of external ear **gai-ji-en** 外耳炎

inflammation of inner ear **nai-ji-en** 内耳炎

inflammation of middle ear **chū-ji-en** 中耳炎

inflammation of urethra **nyōdō-en** 尿道炎

influenza **infuruenza** インフルエンザ

injury **kega** けが

insanity **seishin-ijyō** 精神異常

insect bites **mushi-sasare** 虫さされ

insomnia **fumin-shō** 不眠症

insufficient weight gain **taijyū-zōka-furyō** 体重増加不良

intercostal neuralgia **rokkan-shinkei-tsū** 肋間神経痛

internal bleeding **nai-shukketsu** 内出血

internal bruises **naibu-daboku-shō** 内部打撲傷

internal cramps **fukubu keiren** 腹部けいれん

intestinal catarrh **chō-kataru** 腸カタル

intestinal obstruction **chō-heisoku** 腸閉塞

intestinal TB **chō-kekkaku** 腸結核

intestinal volvulus **chō-nenten** 腸捻転

irregular pulse **fusei-myaku** 不整脈

itch **kayumi** かゆみ

Japanese encephalitis **nihon-nō-en** 日本脳炎

jaundice **ōdan** 黄疸

jock itch **hassin** 発疹

joint pain **kansetsu-tsū** 関節痛

juvenile diabetes **jyaku-nen-sei tōnyō-byō** 若年性糖尿病

keloid **keroido** ケロイド

kidney inflammation **jin-en** 腎炎

kidney stones **jinzō kesseki** 腎臓結石

Koplik spot **kopurikku-han** コプリック斑

labor pains **jintsū** 陣痛

laceration **resshō/haretsu-shō** 裂傷・破裂傷

lack of sleep **suimin-busoku** 睡眠不足

languid **darui** 怠い

laryngitis **kōto-en** 喉頭炎

learning disabilities **gakushū-shōgai** 学習障害

leg cramps **komura-gaeri** こむら返り

leprosy **rai-byō** らい病

lethargic **datsuryoku-kan** 脱力感

leukemia **hakketsu-byō** 白血病

lie heavy on one's stomach **motareru** もたれる

lifestyle disease **sekatsu shūkan-byō** 生活習慣病

light-headedness **ishiki-mōrō-jyōtai** 意識もうろう状態

liver cancer **kanzō-gan** 肝臓ガン

liver cirrhosis **kankō-hen** 肝硬変

liver disease **kanzō-byō** 肝臓病

loose bowels **geri** 下痢

loose stools **geri** 下痢

lose eyesight **shitsu-mei** 失明

loss of appetite **shoku-yoku-fushin** 食欲不振

loss of blood **shukketsu-taryō** 出血多量

loss of consciousness **ishiki-fumei** 意識不明

lost vision **shitsumei** 失明

low abdominal pain **kafukubu-tsū** 下腹部痛

low blood pressure **tei-ketsu-atsu** 低血圧

lower back pain **yōtsū** 腰痛

lumbago **yōtsū** 腰痛

lumbar disc herniation **tsuikanban- herunia** 椎間板ヘルニア

lump **shikori** しこり

lung abscess **hai-nōyō** 肺膿瘍

lung cancer **hai-gan** 肺ガン

lung hemorrhage **kakketsu** 喀血

lung TB **hai-kekkaku** 肺結核

lying **uso** 嘘

Lyme disease **raimu-byō** ライム病

malaria **mararia** マラリア

malformation **kikei** 奇形

malignant **aku-sei** 悪性

malignant tumor **aku-sei-shiyō** 悪性腫瘍

malnutrition **eiyō-shichō** 栄養失調

malocclusion **fusei-kōgō** 不正交合

mania **sō-byō** 躁病

manic depression **sō-utsu-byō** 躁鬱病

mastitis **nyū-sen-en** 乳腺炎

measles **hashika** はしか

medical poisoning **yakubutsu-chūdoku** 薬物中毒

membrance rupture **hasui** 破水

Meniere's disease **menierushi-byō** メニエル氏病

meningitis **nōmaku-en/ kotsuzui-en** 脳膜炎・骨髄炎

menopausal symptoms **kōnenki-shōgai** 更年期障害

menopause **hei-kei** 閉経

menstrual cramps **seiri-tsū** 生理痛

menstrual irregulaity **seiri-fujyun** 生理不順

menstrual pain **seiri-tsū** 生理痛

mental disease **seishin byō** 精神病

mental disorder **seishin shōgai** 精神障害

mental illness **seishin-byō** 精神病

mental irritation **ira-ira** イライラ

mental retardation **seishin-haku-jyaku** 精神薄弱

mercy killing **anraku-shi** 安楽死

metabolic disorder **taisha-ijyo** 代謝異常

metabolism **shinchin-taisha** 新陳代謝

migraine **hen-zutsū** 偏頭痛

miscarriage **ryū-zan** 流産

mononucleosis, mono **densen-sei-tankaku** 伝染性単核

morning sickness **tsuwari** つわり

motion sickness **nori-mono-yoi** 乗り物酔い

mountain sickness **kōzan-byō** 高山病

mucous discharge from eyes **me-yani** 目やに

mucous stool **nen-eki-ben** 粘液便

mucus **nen-eki** 粘液

multi-fracture **tahatsu-kossetsu** 多発骨折

multiple sclerosis **tahatsu-sei-kōka-shō** 多発性硬化症

munps **otafuku-kaze** おたふく風邪

muscle pain **kin-niku-tsū** 筋肉痛

muscle strain **kin-zashō** 筋挫傷

muscular dystrophy **kin-jisutorofī** 筋ジストロフィー

myalgia **kin-niku-tsū** 筋肉痛

myelitis **kotsuzui-en** 骨髄炎

myocardial infarction **shinkin-kōsoku** 心筋梗塞

myoma **kinshu** 筋腫

myoma of the uterus **shikyū-kinshu** 子宮筋腫

myopic **kin-shi** 近視

mysophobia **fuketsu-kyōfu-shō** 不潔恐怖症

nasal discharge **hana-kuso** 鼻くそ

nasal inflammation **bi-en** 鼻炎

nasal voice **hana-goe** 鼻声

nausea **hakike** 吐き気

nearsightedness **kin-shi** 近視

negative **insei** 陰性

nephritis **jin-en** 腎炎

nephrolith **jinzō kesseki** 腎臓結石

nephrosis **nefurōze** ネフローゼ

nervous **shinkei-shitsu** 神経質

nervous breakdown **shinkei-suijyaku** 神経衰弱

nervous prostration **shinkei-suijyaku** 神経衰弱

nervous stomach **shinkei-sei i-en** 神経性胃炎

nettle rash **jinma-shin** 蕁麻疹

neuralgia **shinkei-tsū** 神経痛

neuritis **shinkei-en** 神経炎

neurosis **shinkei-shō** 神経症

neurotic disease **shinkei-shō** 神経症

night blindness **tori-me** 鳥目

night eating syndrome **yashoku-shōkō-gun** 夜食症候群

night sweat **ne-ase** 寝汗

nonulcer dyspepsia **shinkei-sei-i-en** 神経性胃炎

normal **heijyō/seijyō** 平常・正常

normal temperature **hei-netsu** 平熱

nosebleed **hana-ji** 鼻血

numbness **shibire** しびれ

obese **himan** 肥満

obese child **himan-ji** 肥満児

obesity **himan-shō** 肥満症

obsessive-compulsive disorder **kyōhaku-shinkei-shō** 強迫神経症

old complaint **ji-byō** 持病

organ transplantation **zōki-ishoku** 臓器移植

osteomyelitis **kotsuzui-en** 骨髄炎

osteoporosis **kotsu-soshō-shō** 骨粗しょう症

otitis externa **gai-ji-en** 外耳炎

otitis media **chu-ji-en** 中耳炎

out of breath **iki-gire** 息切れ

ovarian cancer **ransō-gan** 卵巣癌

ovarian tumor **ransō-shuyō** 卵巣腫瘍

overeating **tabe-sugi** 食べ過ぎ

overweight **himan** 肥満

overweight child **himan-ji** 肥満児

overwork **karō** 過労

oxygen deficiency **sanso ketsubō-shō** 酸素欠乏症

pain **itami** 痛み

painless **mutsū** 無痛

palpitation **dōki** 動悸

palsy **chū-bū** 中風

pancreatic cancer **suizō-gan** すい臓ガン

pancreatitis **suizō-en** すい臓炎

paralysis **mahi** 麻痺

paranoia **henshitsu-kyō** 偏執狂

parasite **kisei-chū** 寄生虫

Parkinson's disease **Pākinson-byō** パーキンソン病

parotiditis **jika-sen-en** 耳下腺炎

pelvic inflammatory disease **kotsuban-nai-enshō** 骨盤内炎症

pelvis **kotsuzui-en** 骨髄炎

period pains **seiri-tsū** 生理痛

periodontal disease **shishū-byō** 歯周病

peritonitis **fukumaku-en** 腹膜炎

pernicious anemia **akusei-hinketsu** 悪性貧血

personality disorder **jinkaku-shōgai** 人格障害

perspire while sleeping **ne-ase** 寝汗

pertussis **hyaku-nichi-zeki** 百日咳

pest **pesuto/koku-shi-byō** 黒死病

pharyngitis **intō-en** 咽頭炎

phimosis **hōkei** 包茎

phlegm **tan** たん

phlebitis **jyōmyaku-en** 静脈炎

phobia **kyōfu-shō** 恐怖症

piles **ji** 痔

pimple **nikibi** にきび

pityriasis **hikō-shin/ hatake** 粃糠疹・はたけ

plague **eki-byō** 疫病

plaque **shikō** 歯垢

pleurisy **kyōmaku-en** 胸膜炎

pleurodynia **kyōmaku-tsū** 胸膜痛

plugged nose **hana-zumari** 鼻づまり

pneumonia **hai-en** 肺炎

pneumonic plague **hai pesuto** 肺ペスト

poisoning **chūdoku** 中毒

polio **shōni-mahi/ porio** 小児麻痺

pollakiuria **hin-nyō** 頻尿

pollinosis **kafun-shō** 花粉症

poor health condition **taichō-furyō** 体調不良

poor physical condition **kyojyaku-taihishitsu** 虚弱体質

positive **yōsei** 陽性

post-traumatic stress disorder **shin-teki gaishō-go sutoresu-shōgai** 心的外傷後ストレス障害

Pott's fracture **potto-kossetsu** ポット骨折

powerlessness **muryoku-kan** 無力感

pregnant **ninshin** 妊娠

premature ejaculation **sōrō** 早漏

premature rupture **sōki-hasui** 早期破水

premenstrual syndrome **gekkei-zen shōkō-gun (PMS)** 月経前症候群

presbyopia **rōgan** 老眼

prickly heat **asemo** あせも

progressive muscular atrophy **shinkō-sei kin-ishuku-shō** 進行性筋萎縮症

prostate hypertrophy **zenritsu-sen-hidai** 前立腺肥大

pseudo myopia **kasei-kin-shi** 仮性近視

pseudo positive **giji-yōsei** 疑似陽性

psoriasis **kansen** 乾癬

psychasthenia **seishin-suijyaku** 精神衰弱

psychosis **seishin-byō** 精神病

psychosomatic disorder **shinshin-shō** 心身症

puffy **mukumi** 浮腫み

pulled muscle **niku-banare** 肉離れ

pulmonary cancer **hai-gan** 肺癌

pulmonary tuberculosis **hai kekkaku** 肺結核

purulent **kanō** 化膿

pus **umi** うみ

pyelitis **jin-u-en** 腎盂炎

pyorrhea alveolaris **shisō-nōrō** 歯槽のう漏

rabies **kyōken-byō** 狂犬病

rash **hasshin/kabure** 発疹・かぶれ

razor cut **sori-kizu** そり傷

reaction **hannō** 反応

recover **kaifuku-(suru)** 回復（する）

recurrence **saihatsu-(suru)** 再発（する）

renal insufficiency **jin-fuzen** 腎不全

renal stone **jinzō kesseki** 腎臓結石

residual hearing **zan-chō** 残聴

respiratory failure **kokyū-fuzen** 呼吸不全

respiratory illness **kokyū-ki shikkan** 呼吸器疾患

rest **ansei** 安静

restrictive cardiomyopahty **kōsoku-gata shinkin-shō** 拘束型心筋症

retinal detachment **mōmaku-hakuri** 網膜剥離

retinitis **mōmaku-en** 網膜炎

rheumatic fever **ryūmachi-netsu** リュウマチ熱

rheumatism **ryūmachi** リュウマチ

rheumatoid arthritis **ryūmachi-sei kansetsu-en** リュウマチ性関節炎

rhinitis **bi-en** 鼻炎

rickets **kuru-byō** くる病

ringing in the ear **mimi-nari** 耳鳴り

ringworm **ta-mushi** たむし

rolled-back eye **shiro-me** 白目

rough skin **hada-are** 肌荒れ

roundworm **kaichū** 回虫

rubella **fūshin** 風疹

runny ear **mimi-dare** 耳垂れ

runny nose **hana-mizu** 鼻水

sarcoma **nikushu** 肉腫

satisfaction **manzoku-kan** 満足感

scab **kasabuta** かさぶた

scar **kizu-ato** 傷跡

scarlet fever/scarlatina **shōkō-netsu** 猩紅熱

schizophrenia **sōgō-shichō-shō** 総合失調症

sciatica **zakotsu-shinkei-tsū** 坐骨神経痛

scrape **suri-muku** すりむく

scratches **hikkaki-kizu** 引っかき傷

scurvy **kaiketsu-bō** 壊血病

seasickness **funa-yoi** 船酔い

secondary disease **yobyō** 余病

seizure **tenkan** 癲癇

self-mutilation **jishō-kōi** 自傷行為

senile dementia **rōjin-sei chihō-shō** 老人性痴呆症

senility **rōka-genshō** 老化現象

sepsis, septicemia **hai-kketsu-shō** 敗血症

serious illness **jyū-shō** 重症

serious injury **jyū-shō** 重傷

serum hepatitis **kessei-kan-en** 血清肝炎

sexual desire **sei-yoku** 性欲

sexual frigidity **sei-kō fukan-shō** 性交不感症

sexually transmitted disease **sei-kōi-kansen-shō** 性行為感染症

shaking **furue** 震え

shock **sochū/shokku-shō** 卒中・ショック症

shoe sores **kutsu-zure** 靴ずれ

short breath **iki-gire** 息切れ

shortsighted **kin-shi** 近視

side effects **fukusayō** 副作用

sign of aging **rōka-genshō** 老化現象

simple fracture **tanjyun-kossetsu** 単純骨折

sinusitis **chikunō-shō** 蓄膿症

skin cancer **hifu-gan** 皮膚癌

skin disease **hifu-byō** 皮膚病

sleep disorder **suimin-shōgai** 睡眠傷害

sleepwalking **muyū-byō** 夢遊病

slight fever **bi-netsu** 微熱

slight injury **kei-shō** 軽傷

slipped disk **tsuikanban-herunia** 椎間板ヘルニア

smallpox **tennen-tō** 天然痘

sneeze **kushami** くしゃみ

snore **ibiki** いびき

sob **naki-jyakuru** 泣きじゃくる

softening of the brain **nō-nanka-shō** 脳軟化症

sore **itami** 痛み

sore throat **nodo-no-itami/ intō-en** 喉の痛み・咽頭炎

speech impediment **gengo-shōgai** 言語障害

spew **hedo** ヘド

spit **tsuba/haku** 唾・吐く

sprain **nenza** 捻挫

sprained finger **tsuki-yubi** 突き指

sputum **tan** たん

squint **sha-shi** 斜視

stammering symptom **kitsuon-shō** 吃音症

sterility **funin-shō** 不妊症

sterilization **funin-shujyutsu** 不妊手術

stiff neck **kubi no kori** 首の凝り

stiff shoulder **kata-kori** 肩こり

stillbirth **shi-zan** 死産

stomachache **fuku-tsū/hara-ita** 腹痛・はら痛

stomach cancer **i-gan** 胃ガン

stomach cramps **i-keiren** 胃けいれん

stomach ulcer **i-kaiyō** 胃潰瘍

stomatitis **kōnai-en** 口内炎

strained back **gikkuri-goshi** ぎっくり腰

strep throat **yōren-kin-kansen-shō** 溶連筋感染症

stress **sutoresu** ストレス

stridor **zenmei** 喘鳴

stroke **nō-socchū** 脳卒中

stuttering **kitsuon-shō/ domori** 吃音症・どもり

stuffed nose **hana-zumari** 鼻ずまり

sty **mono-morai** ものもらい

subaracnoidal hemorrhage **kumo-makka-shukketsu** くも膜下出血

subjective symptom **jikaku-shōjyō** 自覚症状

sudden heart attack **shinzō-hossa** 心臓発作

sudden infant death syndrome **nyūyōji kyūshi shōkōgun** 乳幼児急死症候群

suffering **kurushii** 苦しい

suffocate **kokyū-kon-nan** 呼吸困難

suicide **jisatsu** 自殺

summer heat fatigue **natsu-bate** 夏バテ

sunburn **hi-yake** 日焼け

sunstroke **nissha-byō** 日射病

suppuration **kanō** 化膿

suspended animation **kashi-jyōtai** 仮死状態

sweat **ase** 汗

swell **mukumi** むくみ

swelling **hare-mono** 腫れ物

swollen tonsils **hentōsen-hidai** 扁桃腺肥大

symptom **shōjyō** 症状

syncope **shisshin** 失神

syndrome **shōkō-gun** 症候群

syphilis **bai-doku** 梅毒

tartar **shiseki** 歯石

tear (from eye) **namida** 涙

temper **kanshaku** かんしゃく

temporary near-sightedness **kasei-kinshi** 仮性近視

tendonitis **kenshō-en** 腱鞘炎

terminal cancer **makki-gan** 末期ガン

tetanus **hashōfū** 破傷風

thrombosis **kessen-shō** 血栓症

thyroiditis **kōjyōsen-en** 甲状腺炎

tinnitus **mimi-nari** 耳鳴り

tipped uterus **shikyū-kōkutsu** 子宮後屈

tiredness **horō** 疲労

tonsillitis **hentōsen-en** 扁桃腺炎

tooth extraction **basshi** 抜歯

toothache **ha-ita** 歯痛

torn ligament **jintai-danzetsu** 靭帯断絶

torn muscle **niku-banare** 肉離れ

toxemia of pregnancy **ninshin-chūdoku-shō** 妊娠中毒症

trachoma **torahōmu** トラホーム

tremor **kin-niku shūshuku** 筋肉収縮

trichiasis **sakasa-matsuge** さかさまつげ

tuberculosis **kekkaku** 結核

tumor **shuyō** 腫瘍

twitch **hiki-tsuru** 引きつる

typhoid fever **chō-chifusu** 腸チフス

typhus **hasshin-chifusu** 発疹チフス

ulcer **kaiyō** 潰瘍

unconscious **mu-ishiki** 無意識

unbalanced nutrition **eiyō-shicchō** 栄養失調

underarm odor **waki-ga** わきが

uremia **nyō-doku-shō** 尿毒症

ureteral stone **nyō-kan-kesseki** 尿管結石

urethral stone **nyōdō-kesseki** 尿道結石

urethritis **nyōdō-en** 尿道炎

urinary incontinence **nyō-shikkin** 尿失禁

urinary problem **hainyō-shōgai** 排尿障害

urinary sediment test **nyō-chinsa-kensa** 尿沈渣検査

urinary tract stone **nyōro-kesseki** 尿路結石

urination **hai-nyō** 排尿

urticaria **jinma-shin** 蕁麻疹

uterine cancer **shikyū-gan** 子宮癌

uterine fibroids **shikyū-kinshu** 子宮筋腫

uterine myoma **shikyū-kinshu** 子宮筋腫

vagina infections **chitsu-en** 膣炎

vaginal discharge **orimono** 下り物

vaginal itching **chitsu no kayumi** 膣の痒み

vaginitis **chitsu-en** 膣炎

valvular disease of the heart **shinzō-ben-maku-shō** 心臓弁膜症

varicella **sui-tō/mizu-bōsō** 水痘/水疱瘡

varix **jyō-myaku-ryū** 静脈瘤

vascular bruit **kekkan-zatsuon** 血管雑音

vasectomy **paipu-katto** パイプカット

venereal disease (V.D.) **sei-byō** 性病

viral disease **uirusu-sei-shikkan** ウイルス性疾患

viral pneumonia **uirusu-sei-hai-en** ウイルス性肺炎

vitamin deficiency **bitamin-ketsubō-shō** ビタミン欠乏症

vocal polyp **seitai-porīpu** 声帯ポリープ

volvulus **chō-nenten** 腸捻転

vomit **haku/modosu** 吐く・もどす

vomiting **ōto** 嘔吐

wall-eyed **gai-sha-shi** 外斜視

wart **ibo** いぼ

washed-out feeling **kentai-kan** 倦怠感

watery eye **urunda-me** 潤んだ目

watery nose **hana-mizu** 鼻水

weak constitution **kyojyaku-taishitsu** 虚弱体質

weakness **datsu-ryoku-kan** 脱力感

wheal **bō-shin** 膨疹

wheezing **zenmei** 喘鳴

whiplash (injury) **muchi-uchi-shō** むち打ち症

whitlow (felon) **hyōsō** ひょうそう

whooping cough **hyakunichi-zeki** 百日咳

withdrawal symptoms **kindan-shōjyō** 禁断症状

wild fancy **mōsō** 妄想

women's disease **fujin-byō** 婦人病

worry **shinpai** 心配

wound **kizu** 傷

wryneck (torticollis) **shakei** 斜頸

yellow fever **ōnetsu-byō** 黄熱病

IV. Medicines

analgesic **chin-tsū-zai** 鎮痛剤

anesthetic **masui-zai** 麻酔剤

anti-acid tablet **shōka-zai** 消化剤

antibiotic **kōsei-bushitsu** 抗生物質

anticancer drug **kōgan-zai** 抗ガン剤

antidepressant drug **kō-utsu-yaku** 抗うつ薬

antidiabetic drug **tōnyō-byō-yaku** 糖尿病薬

antidiarrheal **geri-dome** 下痢止め

antidote **gedoku-zai** 解毒剤

antihistamine **kō-hisutamin-zai** 抗ヒスタミン剤

antihypertensive drug **kō-atsu-zai** 抗圧剤

anti-itch cream **kayumi-dome** かゆみ止め

antipyretic **genetsu-zai** 解熱剤

antiseptic **shōdoku-yakui** 消毒薬

antiseptic solution **shōdoku-eki** 消毒液

aspirin **asupirn** アスピリン

ataractic **seishin-antei-zai** 精神安定剤

ataraxic **seishin-antei-zai** 精神安定剤

azidothymidine (AZT) **ajidochimijin** アジドチミジン

bronchodilator **kikanshi-kakuchō-zai** 気管支拡張剤

calcium **karushūmu** カルシューム

capsule **kapuseru-zai** カプセル剤

carcinostatic **sei-gan-zai** 制ガン剤

cardiotonic **kyōshin-zai** 強心剤

chemicals **kagaku-yakuhin** 化学薬品

Chinese herbal medicine **kanpō-yaku** 漢方薬

cold compress **rei-shippu** 冷湿布

cold medicine **kaze-gusuri** 風邪薬

compress **shippu-yaku** 湿布薬

condom **kondōmu** コンドーム

contraceptive **hinin-yaku** 避妊薬

cough drop **seki-dome-doroppu** 咳止めドロップ

cough medicine **seki-dome/ chingai-yaku** 咳止め/鎮咳薬

cough syrup **sekidome-shiroppu** 咳止めシロップ

crack **ma-yaku** 麻薬

decoction **senji-gusuri** 煎じ薬

diabetes remedy **tōnyō-byō-yaku** 糖尿病薬

digestant **shōka-zai** 消化剤

digestive **shōka-zai** 消化剤

disinfectant **sakkin-zai** 殺菌剤

diuretic **ri-nyō-zai** 利尿剤

DPT shot **sanshu-kongō-sesshu** 三種混合接種

DPT vaccine **sanshu-kongō-wakuchin** 三種混合ワクチン

drug **kusuri/ma-yaku** 薬・麻薬

drug fact **yūkō-seibun** 有効成分

drug store **yakkyoku** 薬局

enema **kanchō** 浣腸

expectorant **kyotan-yaku** 去痰薬

external application medicine **nuri-gusuri** 塗り薬

eyedrops **me-gusuri** めぐすり

fertility drug **hairan-yūhatsu-zai** 排卵誘発剤

floss **furosu** フロス

fluoride **fusso** フッ素

gargle **ugai-gusuri** うがい薬

genetic drug **generikku-iyakuhin/kō-hatsu-iyakuhin** ジェネリック医薬品・後発医薬品

granulated **karyū** 顆粒

hematinic **zōketsu-zai** 増血剤

hematopoietic drugs **ketsueki-seizai** 血液製剤

herb medicine **kanpō-yaku** 漢方薬

hormone active drugs **horumon-zai** ホルモン剤

hot compress **on-shippu** 温湿布

household medicine **jyōbi-yaku** 常備薬

hydrogen peroxide **okishifuru** オキシフル

hypnotic **suimin-yaku** 睡眠薬

inhaler **kyūnyū-yaku** 吸入薬

insulin **insurin** インスリン

intestinal medicine **ichō-yaku** 胃腸薬

intravenous drip infusion **tenteki** 点滴

intravenous fluid **tenteki** 点滴

iodine tincture **yōdo-chinki** ヨードチンキ

itch lotion **kayumi-dome** かゆみ止め

I. V. **tenteki** 点滴

labor-inducing drugs **jintsū-sokushin-zai** 陣痛促進剤

laxative **ge-zai** 下剤

lip salve **kuchibiru-yō-nankō** 唇用軟膏

liquid **ekitai** 液体

liquid mdicine **mizu-gusuri** 水薬

local anesthetic **kyokusho-masui-yaku** 局所麻酔薬

lotion **rōshon** ローション

LSD (lysergic acid diethylamide) **eru-esu-dī** エルエスディ

MMR vaccine **emu-emu-āru wakuchin** エム・エム・アール・ワクチン

marijuana **marifana** マリファナ

medical herb **yakusō** 薬草

medicine **kusuri** 薬

medicine for external application **nuri-gusuri** 塗り薬

medicine for fever **genetsu-zai** 解熱剤

medicine to relieve itching **kayumi-dome** かゆみ止め

mouthwash **ugai-gusuri** うがい薬

multiple vitamin **sōgō-bitamin-zai** 総合ビタミン剤

narcotic drug **mayaku** 麻薬

narcotic addict **mayaku jyōshū-sha** 麻薬常習者

non-prescription drugs **mu-shohō-yaku** 無処方薬

nonpyrazolone **hi-pirin-kei** 非ピリン系

novocaine **nobokein** ノボケイン

ointment **nankō** 軟膏

oral contraceptive **keikō-hinin-yaku** 経口避妊薬

orally dispensed drug **kōkūyō-yaku** 口腔用薬

oral medicine **nomi-gusuri/ naifuku-yaku** 飲み薬・内服薬

over-the-counter drugs **shihanyō-iyakuhin** 市販用医薬品

ovulation inducing drug **hairan-yūhatsu-zai** 排卵誘発剤

oxytocics **jintsū-sokushin-zai** 陣痛促進剤

pain killer **itami-dome/ chintsū-zai** 痛み止め・鎮痛剤

pain reliever **itami-dome** 痛み止め

panacea **ban-nō-yaku** 万能薬

pessary **pessarī** ペッサリー

pesticide **sacchū-zai** 殺虫剤

pharmacy **yakkyoku** 薬局

pill **piru (keikō-hinin-yaku)** ピル（経口避妊薬）

placebo **gi-yaku** 偽薬

poison **doku** 毒

polio vaccine **porio wakuchin** ポリオ ワクチン

pot **marifana** マリファナ

powder **kona-gusuri/ funmatsu-zai** 粉薬・粉末剤

preparation drug **chōgō-zai** 調合剤

prescription **shohō-sen** 処方箋

preventative **bōfu-zai** 防腐剤

preventive medicine **yobō-yaku** 予防薬

psychotropic drug **kō-seishin-yaku** 向精神薬

pyrazolone **pirin-kei** ピリン系

remedy against poison **gedoku-zai** 解毒剤

restorative **kyōsō-zai** 強壮剤

sedative **chinsei-zai** 鎮静剤

serum **kessei** 血清

shot **chūsha** 注射

sleeping pill **suimin-dōnyū-zai** 睡眠導入剤

spermicide **satsu-seishi-yaku** 殺精子薬

stimulants **kōfun-zai** 興奮剤

stomach medicine **i-gusuri** 胃薬

suppository **za-yaku** 座薬

syrup **shiroppu** シロップ

tablet **jyō-zai** 錠剤

tranquilizer **seishin-antei-zai** 精神安定剤

tuberculin **tsuberukurin** ツベルクリン

vaccine **wakuchin** ワクチン

vaseline **waserin** ワセリン

vitamin pill **bitamin-zai** ビタミン剤

worm capsule **mushi-kudashi** 虫下し

wonder drugs **tokkō-yaku** 特効薬

V. Other Medical and Related Terms

abdominoplasty **fukubu-seikei** 腹部整形

abortion **jinkō-chūzetsu** 人工中絶

absolute rest **zettai-ansei** 絶対安静

absorbent cotton **dasshimen** 脱脂綿

accident **jiko** 事故

accident insurance **shōgai-hoken** 傷害保険

action of the bowels **bentsū** 便通

acupressure **shiatsu** 指圧

acupuncture **hari/shinkyū** 針・針灸

acute **kyūsei** 急性

adhesive (tape) **bansōkō** 絆創膏

admission to a hospital **nyūin** 入院

after bed **shūshin-go** 就寝後

afterbirth **san-go** 産後

after every meals **mai-shoku-go** 毎食後

after meals **shoku-go** 食後

aging process **kaire** 加齢

alcohol **arukōru/(o) sake** アルコール・お酒

allergic tendency **arerugī no keikō** アレルギーの傾向

ambulance **kyūkyū-sha** 救急車

amniocentesis **yōsui-kensa** 羊水検査

amputate **setsudan** 切断

anesthesia **masui** 麻酔

anaesthesia apparatus **masui-sōchi** 麻酔装置

annual checkup **teiki-kenshin** 定期検診

appearance/lōks **yōsu** 様子

appetite **shoku-yoku** 食欲

artificial insemination **jinkō-jyusei** 人工授精

artificial kidney machine **jinkō-tōseiki-ki** 人工透析機

artificial respiration **jinkō-kokyū** 人工呼吸

artificial teeth **ire-ba/gi-shi** 入れ歯・義歯

aspiration **kyū-in** 吸引

aspirator **kyūin-ki** 吸引機

baby **aka-chan** 赤ちゃん

baby bottle **honyū-bin** ほ乳びん

baby lotion **bebī-rōshon** ベビー・ローション

baby oil **bebī-oiru** ベビー・オイル

baby powder **bebī-paudā** ベビー・パウダー

baby soap **bebī-sekken** ベビー石鹸

baggage **nimotsu** 荷物

balloon sinuplasty **barūn kaku-chō-jyutsu** バルーン拡張術

bandage **bansōkō/hōtai** 絆創膏・包帯

Band-Aid **bando-eido** バンドエイド

basal body temperature **kiso-taion** 基礎体温

basin **senmen-ki** 洗面器

BCG vaccine **bī shī jī** ビーシージー

bedpan **ben-ki** 便器

bedridden **neta-kiri** 寝たきり

bed urinal **ben-ki** 便器

before bed **shūshin-mae** 就寝前

before every meals **mai-shoku-zen** 毎食前

before meals **shoku-zen** 食前

benign **ryōsei** 良性

between meals **shokkan** 食間

bifocal lenses **nijyū-shōten-renzu** 二重焦点レンズ

bifocal glasses **en-kin-ryōyō-megane** 遠近両用メガネ

bile **tan-jyū** 胆汁

birth certificate **shussei-shōmei-sho** 出生証明書

birth control **hinin** 避妊

blind person **shiryoku-shōgai-sha** 視力障害者

blinking **ma-bataki** 瞬き

bloated **hara-no-hari** 腹の張り

blockage **heisoku** 閉塞

blood **ketsu-eki** 血液

blood donation **ken-ketsu** 献血

blood pressure **ketsu-atsu** 血圧

blood pressure gauge **ketsuatsu-kei** 血圧計

blood sugar **kettō** 血糖

blood sugar level test **kettōchi-kensa** 血糖値検査

blood test **ketsu-eki-kensa** 血液検査

blood transfusion **yu-ketsu** 輸血

blood type **ketsu-eki-gata** 血液型

body shape **taikei** 体形

body waste **rōhai-butsu** 老廃物

boiled water **nettō** 熱湯

bottle feeding **jinkō-eiyō** 人工栄養

bowel movements **ben-tsū** 便通

braces **kyōsei** 矯正

braille **ten-ji** 点字

brain waves **nō-ha** 脳波

breast augmentation **hōkyō-shujyutsu** 豊胸手術

breast feeding **bonyū-eiyō** 母乳栄養

breast milk **bonyū** 母乳

breast self-examination **nyū-gan jiko-kenshin** 乳癌自己検診

breath **iki** 息

breathing capacity **haikatsu-ryō** 肺活量

breech presentation **saka-go** 逆子

bronchoscopy **kikanshi-kyō-kensa** 気管支鏡検査

bulletin **yōdai-sho** 容態書

caesarean section **teiō-sekkai** 帝王切開

caloric test **ondo-ganshin kensa** 温度眼振検査

calorie **karorī** カロリー

cancel **torikeshi** 取り消し

cancer causer **hatsu-gan-bushitsu** 発ガン物質

cap/hat **bōshi** 帽子

car accident **kōtsū-jiko** 交通事故

carbohydrate **tansui-kabutsu** 炭水化物

carbon dioxide **nisanka-tanso** 二酸化炭素

carbon monoxide **issanka-tanso** 一酸化炭素

carcinogen **hatsu-gan-bushutsu** 発ガン物質

cardiac massage **shizō-masāji** 心臓マッサージ

carrier **hokin-sha** 保菌者

cast **gibusu** ギブス

caterpillar **ke-mushi** 毛虫

cause **genin** 原因

cause of a disease **byōki-no-genin** 病気の原因

centigrade **sesshi** 摂氏

change of voice **koe-gawari** 声変わり

change to positive **yō-ten** 陽転

checkup **kenkō-shindan** 健康診断

chemotheraphy **kagaku-ryohō** 化学療法

child/children **ko/kodomo** 子・子供

child abuse **yōji-gyakutai** 幼児虐待

childbirth **shussan** 出産

cholesterol **koresuterōru** コレステロール

cholesterol test **koresuterōru kensa** コレステロール検査

chronic **mansei** 慢性

cigarette/tobacco **tabako** 煙草

clean **seiketsu** 清潔

client **kanjya** 患者

clinical chart **karute** カルテ

clinical history **byō-reki** 病歴

clinical test **rinshō-tesuto** 臨床テスト

clinical thermometer **taion-kei** 体温計

closed ward **heisa-byōtō** 閉鎖病棟

clothes **fuku** 服

cold **tsumetai/samui** 冷たい・寒い

collecting a blood sample **sai-ketsu** 採血

colon & rectal surgery **kecchō/choku-chō shijyutsu** 結腸・直腸手術

commute to the hospital **tsū-in** 通院

company employee **kaisha-in** 会社員

complaining **fuhei/monku** 不平・文句

complete medical checkup **ningen-dokku** 人間ドック

complete recovery **kanchi/zenkai** 完治・全快

complexion **kao-iro** 顔色

complications **yobyō** 余病

concern **ki-ni-naru** 気になる

condition **chōshi/guai/ yōtai** 調子・具合・様態

condition of a patient **byōjyō** 病状

confirmation **kakunin** 確認

congenital **senten-sei** 先天性

constitution **tai-shitsu** 体質

consultation **sōdan** 相談

consulting room **shinryō-shitsu** 診療室

contagious **densen-sei** 伝染性

contraceptive device **hinin-gu** 避妊具

contract **sesshoku** 接触

contact lense **kontakuto-renzu** コンタクト・レンズ

convalescence **byō-go** 病後

convenience **tsugō** 都合

corrected vision **kyōsei-shiryoku** 矯正視力

corrective lenses **kyōsei-renzu** 矯正レンズ

corset **korusetto** コルセット

cosmetic surgery **seikei-shujyutsu** 整形手術

cosmetics **keshō-hin** 化粧品

cosmetic dentistry **shinbi-shi-ka** 審美歯科

cotton ball **men** 綿

cotton swabs **men-bō** 綿棒

critical condition **kitoku** 危篤

crown **kuraun-kan** クラウン冠

crutches **matsuba-zue** 松葉杖

crying (of infant) at night **yo-naki** 夜泣き

CT scan **dansō-satsuei** 断層撮影

cute **kawaii** かわいい

cystoscopy **bōkō-kyō-kensa** 膀胱鏡検査

danger **kiken** 危険

days of hospital treatment **nyūin-nissū** 入院日数

decompression chamber **genatsu-shitsu** 減圧室

defecation **hai-ben** 排便

delivery room **bunben-shitsu** 分娩室

delivery unit **bunben-dai** 分娩台

delicate **kyojyaku-taishitsu** 虚弱体質

dental brushing **ha-migaki** 歯磨き

dental floss **ito-yōji** 糸楊子

dental implant **inpuranto** インプラント

dentist's chair **shika-chiryō-isu** 歯科治療椅子

denture **ire-ba** 入れ歯

diagnosis **shindan** 診断

dialysis **tōseki** 透析

die of illness **byō-shi** 病死

diet **daietto** ダイエット

dietary cure **shokuji-ryōhō** 食事療法

diet regimen **shokuji-ryōhō** 食事療法

diet therapy **shokuji-ryōhō** 食事療法

difficulty hearing high pitched sound **kō-on-sei nan-chō** 高音性難聴

difficulty hearing low pitched **tei-on-sei nan-chō** 低音性難聴

directions **shiyō-hōhō** 使用方法

discharge (from hospital) **tai-in** 退院

discomfort **fukai-kan** 不快感

discomfort index **fukai-shisū** 不快指数

disposable diapers **tsukai-sute kami-omutsu** 使い捨て紙おむつ

doctor's fee **chiryō-hi/ chiryō-dai** 治療費・治療代

doctor's note **shindan-sho** 診断書

dosage **yōryō** 用量

dose **yōryō** 用量

doubt/suspect **utagai** 疑い

due date **shussan-yotei-bi** 出産予定日

draw blood **sai-ketsu** 採血

dream **yume** 夢

during one's illness **byō-chū** 病中

drug abuse **yaku-butsu ranyō** 薬物乱用

early birth **sō-zan** 早産

early detection **sōki-hakken** 早期発見

early pregnancy **ninshin-shoki** 妊娠初期

early stage **shoki** 初期

earpick **mimi-kaki** 耳かき

eat out **gai-shoku** 外食

effectiveness **kōka/yūkō-sei** 効果・有効性

ejaculate **sha-sei** 射精

elastic bandages **shinshuku-no-hōtai** 伸縮の包帯

elderly persons **(o) toshiyoi/ rōjin** お年寄り・老人

electrocardiogram **shin-den-zu** 心電図

electroencephalogram **nō-ha** 脳波

eliminate **kaishō** 解消

emaciate **suijyaku** 衰弱

emergency **kinkyū** 緊急

emergency patient **kyū-kan** 急患

emergency room **ōkyū-shochi-shitsu** 応急処置室

endocrine **nai-bunpitsu** 内分泌

endoscope **naishi-kyō** 内視鏡

endoscopy **naishi-kyō kensa** 内視鏡検査

enough/plenty **jūbun** 十分

environment **kankyō** 環境

epidemic **ryūkō-sei** 流行性

euthanasia **anraku-shi** 安楽死

examination **kensa/shinsatsu** 検査・診察

examination fee **kensa-dai/hiyō** 検査代・費用

examination of feces/stool **ken-ben** 検便

examination of urine **ken-nyō** 検尿

examination room **shinsatsu-shitsu** 診察室

examination table **shinsatsu-dai** 診察台

excessive bleeding **shukketsu taryō** 出血多量

exercise **undō** 運動

exocrine **gai-bunpitsu** 外分泌

expiration date **yūkō-kigen** 有効期限

extract teeth **basshi** 抜歯

eye chart **shiryoku kensa-hyo** 視力検査表

eye ground examination **gantei-kensa** 眼底検査

eyeglasses **megane** めがね

eyesight **shi-ryoku** 視力

eyesight test **shi-ryoku kensa** 視力検査

Fahrenheit **kashi** 華氏

fales teeth **sashi-ba/gishi** 差し歯・義歯

family planning **kazoku-keikaku** 家族計画

fart **onara/he** おらな・へ

fasting **zesshoku** 絶食

fat **shibō** しぼう

fatal dose **chishi-ryō** 致死量

feel oppressed in the chest **muna-kurushii** 胸苦しい

feeling **kibun** 気分

fetal heart sound **shin-on** 心音

fetal movement **taidō** 胎動

fetus **taiji** 胎児

fill out **kinyū** 記入

filling **tsume-mono** 詰め物

fine wrinkles **kojiwa** 小じわ

first aid **ōkyū-shochi** 応急処置

first aid kit **kyūkyū-bako** 緊急箱

first aid treatment **ōkyū-shochi** 応急処置

first childbirth **uizan** 初産

first period **shochō** 初潮

first visit **shoshin** 初診

flea **nomi** 蚤

fluid **suibun** 水分

focus **byōsō** 病巣

food allergy **shokumotsu-arerugī** 食物アレルギー

food particles **tabe-kasu** 食べかす

food value **eiyōka** 栄養価

freckles **sobakasu** そばかす

free consulation **muryō sōdan** 無料相談

free examination **muryō kenshin** 無料検診

funduscopy **gantei-kensa** 眼底検査

gargle **ugai** 嗽

gas **gasu** ガス

gastric camera **i-kamera** 胃カメラ

gastric juice **i-eki** 胃液

gastrocamera **i-kamera** 胃カメラ

gauze **gāze** ガーゼ

gene **iden-shi** 遺伝子

gene splicing **iden-shi-kumikae** 遺伝子組み替え

genetic engineering **iden-shi-kōgaku** 遺伝子工学

gnash **hagishiri** 歯軋り

going out **gaishutsu** 外出

grape suger **budō-tō** ブドウ糖

grind teeth **hagishiri** 歯ぎしり

group medical examination **shūdan kenshin** 集団検診

growth **seichō** 成長

habitual offender **jyōshū-sha** 常習者

hangover **futsuka-yoi** 二日酔い

hangnail **saka-muke** さかむけ

HDL cholesterol **zendama koresuterōru** 善玉コレステロール

health education **kenkō kyōiku** 健康教育

health hazard **yūgai shokuhin** 有害食品

healthy **kenkō** 健康

hearing aid **hochō-ki** 補聴器

hearing aid test **hochō-ki tekigō-kensa** 補聴器適合検査

hearing test **chō-ryoku-kensa** 聴力検査

heartbeat **shinpaku/shinzō-no-kodō** 心拍・心臓の鼓動

heart massage **shinzō-masāji** 心臓マッサージ

heart transplantation **shinzō-ishoku** 心臓移植

hemophiliac **ketsuyū-byō kanjya** 血友病患者

heredity **iden** 遺伝

high fat diet **kō-shibō-shoku** 高脂肪食

high fiber diet **kō-seni-shoku** 高繊維食

high temperature **kō-netsu** 高熱

history of illness **byō-reki** 病歴

homeostasis **karada no baransu** 体のバランス/ホメオスタシス

hormone therapy **horumon-ryōhō** ホルモン療法

hospital charges **nyūin-ryō** 入院料

hospitalization **nyūin** 入院

hospital room **byō-shitsu** 病室

hospital ward **byō-tō** 病棟

hot **atsui** 熱い

hot water **oyu** お湯

hot-water bottle **yu-tanpo** 湯たんぽ

house call **ōshin** 往診

housewife **shufu** 主婦

human rights **jinken** 人権

human vegetable **shokubutsu ningen** 植物人間

hungry **kū-fuku** 空腹

hydration **suibun-hokyū** 水分補給

hypodermic needle **chūsha-bari** 注射針

hypodermic injection **hika-chūsha** 皮下注射

ice bag **hyōnō** 氷のう

ice pack **hyōnō/aisu-pakku** 氷のう/アイス・パック

ICU **shūchū-chiryō-shitsu** 集中治療室

ID card **mibun-shōmei-sho** 身分証明書

idiosyncrasy **tokui-taishitsu** 特異体質

in vitro fertilization **taigai jyusei** 体外受精

initial medical examination **shoshin** 初診

immunity **meneki** 免疫

immunization **yobō-sesshu** 予防接種

improvement **kaizen** 改善

improvement of constitution **taishitsu-kaizen** 体質改善

imunotheraphy **meneki-ryōhō** 免疫療法

inadequate intake **sesshu-busoku** 摂取不足

incubation period **senpuku-ki** 潜伏期

incubator **hoiku-ki** 保育器

infant **nyūyō-ji** 乳幼児

infant mortality **nyūyō-ji shibō-ritsu** 乳幼児死亡率

infection **kansen** 感染

infectious **densen-sei** 伝染性

infertile **funin** 不妊

influence **eikyō** 影響

infusion **tenteki** 点滴

inhalater **kyū-nyū-ki** 吸入器

initial visit **shoshin** 初診

injection **chūsha** 注射

injection syringe **chūsha-ki** 注射器

injured person **fushō-sha** 負傷者

inoculation **sesshu** 接種

inpatient **nyū-in-kanjya** 入院患者

insecticide **sacchū-zai** 殺虫剤

instruction **shiji** 指示

instruction for use **setsumei-sho** 説明書

intake **sesshu** 摂取

intensive care **shūchū-kango** 集中看護

intensive care unit (ICU) **shūchū-chiryō-shitsu** 集中治療室

internal examination **nai-shin** 内診

intraocular pressure test **gan-atsu-kensa** 眼圧検査

intravenous injection **jyōmyaku chūsha** 静脈注射

isolation ward **kakuri-byōto** 隔離病棟

IV drip **tenteki** 点滴

lack/insufficient **fusoku** 不足

lack of exercises **undō-busoku** 運動不足

labyrinth **meiro** 迷路

lack of sleep **suimin-busoku** 睡眠不足

lactation **jyu-nyū** 授乳

lactation period **jyu-nyū-ki** 授乳期

laparoscopy **shikyū-naishi-kyō** 子宮内視鏡

large quantity **tairyō** 大量

lasik **rēshiku-shujyutsu** レーシック手術

last month of pregnancy **rin-getsu** 臨月

late child-bearing **kōrei-shussan** 高齢出産

LDL cholesterol **akudama koresuterōru** 悪玉コレステロール

left **hidari** 左

legal communicable disease **hōtei-densen-byō** 法定伝染病

lethal dose **chishi-ryō** 致死量

letter **moji** 文字

lie on your back **aomuke** 仰向け

lie on your stomach **utsubuse** うつ伏せ

life expectancy **heikin-jyumyō** 平均寿命

life span **jyumyō** 寿命

lifestyle **seikatsu yōshiki** 生活様式

life support system **seimei-iji-sōchi** 生命維持装置

liquid food **ryūdō-shoku** 流動食

lotion **rōshon** ローション

louse **shirami** シラミ

lung capacity **hai-katsu-ryō** 肺活量

lymph **rinpa-eki** リンパ液

lymphatic gland **rinpa-sen** リンパ腺

lymphocyte **rinpa-kyū** リンパ球

lymph node **rinpa setsu** リンパ節

magnetic resonance imaging (MRI) **jiki-kyōmei-eizō-hō** 磁気共鳴映像法

malformation **kikei** 奇形

malfunction **kinō-shōgai** 機能障害

malocclusion **fusei-kōgō** 不正咬合

malpractice **iryō-misu** 医療ミス

mammogram **chibusa satsuei** 乳房撮影

mammography **chibusa satsuei-hō** 乳房撮影法

massage **masāji** マッサージ

meals/steamed rice **gohan** ご飯

measurement **sokutei** 測定

medical chart **karute** カルテ

medical checkup **kenshin** 検診

medical cost/fees **iryō-hi** 医療費

medical examination **shin-satsu** 診察

medical expenses **iryō-hi** 医療費

medical history **byō-reki** 病歴

medical science **i-gaku** 医学

medical thermometer **taion-kei** 体温計

memories **kioku** 記憶

menstrual cycle **gekkei shūki** 月経周期

mental cruelty **seishin-teki gyakutai** 精神的虐待

mental disorder **seishin shōgai** 精神障害

mental health **seishin-teki kenkō** 精神的健康

mental hygiene **seishin-eisei** 精神衛生

mental test **shinri-kensa** 心理検査

Mercurochrome **makyuro** マーキュロ

metastasis **ten-i** 転移

middle-aged spread **chūnen-butori** 中年太り

middle of urination **chūkan-nyō** 中間尿

mind **kokoro** 心

miscarriage **ryū-zan** 流産

mobile blood unit **saiketsu-sha** 採血車

mole **hokuro** ほくろ

money **okane** お金

mood **kigen** 機嫌

mortality rate **shibō-ritsu** 死亡率

mother **haha-oya** 母親

mouse **nezumi** ねずみ

mouthwash **ugai** うがい

multipara **kesisan-pu** 経産婦

naked eye **ra-gan** 裸眼

name of a disease **byōmei** 病名

natural childbirth **shizen bunben** 自然分娩

neonatal intensive care unit (NICU) **shinsei-ji toku-tei shūchū chiryō-shitsu** 新生児特定集中治療室

nervousness **shinkei-shitsu** 神経質

new type **shin-gata** 新型

newborn baby **shinsei-ji** 新生児

night guard **mausu-pīsu** マウスピース

no visitors **menkai-shasetsu** 面会謝絶

nocuous substance **yūgai-bushitsu** 有害物質

noise **zatsu-on** 雑音

normal development **seijō-hattatsu** 正常発達

normal pulse **hei-myaku** 平脈

nose cosmetic surgery **hana no seikei-shujyutsu** 鼻の整形手術

nursing bottle **honyū-bin** ほ乳びん

nutrition **eiyō** 栄養

nutrition deficiency **eiyō-busoku** 栄養不足

nutritive value **eiyō-ka** 栄養価

nystagmus test **ganshin-kensa** 眼振検査

old people **otoshiyori** お年寄り

old type **kyū-gata** 旧型

open air **gai-ki** 外気

open ward **kaihō-byōtō** 開放病棟

operating room **shujyutsu-shitsu** 手術室

operating table **shujyutsu-dai** 手術台

operation **shujyutsu** 手術

ophthalmoscope **kengan-kyō** 検眼鏡

optical shop **megane-ya** 眼鏡屋

optometric **ken-gan** 検眼

ordinary temperature **hei-netsu** 平熱

organ **zōki/kikan** 臓器・器官

organ transplantation **zōki-ishoku** 臓器移植

origin of a disease **byōgen** 病原

orthodontics **shika-kyōsei** 歯科矯正

orthopnoea **kiza-kokyū** 起座呼吸

osteopathy **seikotsu-ryōhō** 整骨療法

outpatient **gairai-kanjya** 外来患者

overconsumption **kajyō-sesshu** 過剰摂取

overdose **taryō-sesshu** 多量摂取

overeat **bō-shoku** 暴食

overwork/overdo **muri** 無理

ovulation **hai-ran** 排卵

ovulation day **hai-ran yotei-bi** 排卵予定日

oxygen **sanso** 酸素

oxygen concentration **sanso-nōdo** 酸素濃度

oxygen mask **sanso-masuku** 酸素マスク

pad **gāze** ガーゼ

pain **itami** 痛み

pain of sickness **byōku** 病苦

painless **mutsū** 無痛

palpation **shoku-shin** 触診

pandemic **sekai-ryūkō** 世界流行

paranoid personality disorder **mōsō-sei jinkaku-shōgai** 妄想性人格障害

parasite **kisei-chū** 寄生虫

pathogen **byōgen-kin** 病原菌

patience **gaman** 我慢

patient **kanjya** 患者

pelvic examination **nai-shin** 内診

period **seiri/gekkei** 生理/月経

periodical check up **teiki-kenshin** 定期検診

periodically **shūki-teki** 周期的

periodontal treatment **shishū-byo-chiryō** 歯周病治療

permission **kyoka** 許可

perspiration **ase** 汗

petroleum jelly **waserin** ワセリン

pharmacotherapy **yakubutsu-ryōhō** 薬物療法

phimosis **hōkei** 包茎

photo image **gazō** 画像

physical balance **heikō-kankaku** 平衡感覚

physical constitution **taishitsu** 体質

physical examination **kenkō-shindan** 健康診断

physical position **tai-i** 体位

pillow **makura** 枕

platelet **kesshō-ban** 血小板

plaster **bansōkō** 絆創膏

pleural effusion **kyō-sui** 胸水

pleasant feeling **kai-kan** 快感

poison **doku** 毒

poison ivy **urushi** うるし

poisonous insect **doku-mushi** 毒虫

possibility **kanō-sei** 可能性

postmature infant **kajyuku-ji** 過熟児

postnatal **sei-go** 生後

postpartum **san-go** 産後

potty **omaru** おまる

pregnancy **ninshin** 妊娠

pregnancy test **ninshin-kensa** 妊娠検査

pregnant **ninpu** 妊婦

premature baby **mijyuku-ji** 未熟児

premature birth **sō-zan** 早産

preparation **junbi** 準備

prevention **yobō** 予防

preventive care **yobō-teki-kea** 予防的ケア

prickle **toge** とげ

primipara **shosan-pu** 初産婦

private room (LDRP room) **koshitsu** 個室

problem **mondai** 問題

procedure **tetsuzuki** 手続き

professional ethics **shokugyō-rinri** 職業倫理

progressive lenses **en-kin-ryōyō-renzu** 遠近両用レンズ

protection of human rights **jinken-yōgo** 人権擁護

protein **tanpaku** 蛋白

pulmonary function tests **hai-kinō kensa** 肺機能検査

pulse **myaku** 脈

pushing **ikimi** 息み

psychological examination **shinri-kensa** 心理検査

psychotherapy **seishin-ryōhō** 精神療法

Q-tip **menbō** 綿棒

quackery **ikasama-chiryō** いかさま治療

quacks **yabu-i-sha** やぶ医者

quarantine **ken-eki** 検疫

question **shitsumon** 質問

quick relief **sōki-kaifuku** 早期回復

radiotherapy **hōsha-sen ryōhō** 放射線療法

reception **uketsuke** 受付

recovery **kaifuku** 回復

recuperation **ryōyō** 療養

recurrence **sai-hatsu** 再発

rectal examination **choku-chō-shin** 直腸診

red blood cell **sekkekkyū** 赤血球

re-examination **sai-kensa** 再検査

reference ranges **kijun-chi** 基準値

referral **shōkai-jyō** 紹介状

referrer/referred person **shōkai-sha** 紹介者

reflex reaction **hansha hannō** 反射反応

refractive index test **kussetsu-ritsu-kensa** 屈折率検査

regular checkup **teiki-kenshin** 定期検診

regimen **sessei-keikaku** 摂生計画

registration window **uketsuke madoguchi** 受付窓口

rehabilitation **rehabiri-tēshon** リハビリテーション

rejection **kyozetsu-hannō** 拒絶反応

removal surgery **tekishitsu-shujyutsu** 摘出手術

remove **tekishitsu-(suru)** 摘出（する）

remove the stitches **basshi-(suru)** 抜糸(する)

renal function tests **jin-kinō-kensa** 腎機能検査

Rentgen examination **rentogen-kensa** レントゲン検査

respirator **jinkō-kokyū-ki** 人工呼吸器

rescue **kyūshitsu** 救出

research **kenkyū** 研究

rest **kyūyō/seiyō** 休養・静養

restrain **kyōsei** 強制

result **kekka** 結果

return to home **kitaku** 帰宅

RH negative **RH mainasu** ＲＨマイナス

rhythm method **ogino-shiki hinin-hō** オギノ式避妊法

right **migi** 右

ring **yubiwa** 指輪

risk **kiken-sei** 危険性

root canal **konkan-chiryō** 根管治療

rubber **kondōmu** コンドーム

rubbing alcohol **shōdoku-yō arukōru** 消毒用アルコール

rupture of the bag **hasui** 破水

safe **anzen** 安全

safety **anzen-sei** 安全性

saliva **daeki** 唾液

salivary glands **daeki-sen** 唾液腺

sample of feces **ken-ben** 検便

sampling urine **sai-nyō** 採尿

sanitary napkin **seiri-yō napukin** 生理用ナプキン

secretion **bunpitsu-butsu** 分泌物

sedation **chinsei-sayō** 鎮静作用

semen **sei-eki** 精液

senility **rōka** 老化

serum **kessei** 血清

sense of hearing **chōka-ku** 聴覚

sense of smell **shūka-ku** 臭覚

sense of touch **shokka-ku** 触覚

sex organs **seishoku-ki** 生殖器

sexual intercourse **sei-kō** 性交

shock therapy **shokku-ryōhō** ショック療法

shoes **kutsu** 靴

shot **chūsha** 注射

sick bay **byō-shitsu** 病室

sick person **byō-nin** 病人

sickbed **byōshō** 病床

sickroom **byō-shitsu** 病室

side effects **fukusayō** 副作用

sign of aging **rōka-genshō** 老化現象

sleep **suimin** 睡眠

slender type **yase-gata** 痩せ形

sling **sankaku-kin** 三角巾

sneeze **kushami** くしゃみ

snore **ibiki** いびき

socks **kutsu-shita** 靴下

sodium **en-bun** 塩分

soap **sekken** 石鹸

specimen **kentai** 検体

sphygmomanometer (blood pressure gauge) **ketsu-atsu-kei** 血圧計

spider **kumo** クモ

standard **hyōjyun** 標準

stay quiet **ansei** 安静

sterilization **sakkin** 殺菌

sterilization operation **funin-shujyutsu** 不妊手術

stethoscope **chōshin-ki** 聴診器

sticking plaster **bansōkō** 絆創膏

stillbirth **shi-zan** 死産

stool **dai-ben/unchi** 大便・うんち

stretcher **tanka** 担架

student (after secondary school) **gakusei** 学生

student (before college) **seito** 生徒

sugar **tō-bun** 糖分

sunbathing **nikkō-yoku** 日光浴

surgical knife **mesu** メス

surgical spirit **shōdoku-yō-arukōru** 消毒用アルコール

swabs **menbō** 綿棒

syndrome **shōkō-gun** 症候群

syringe **chūsha-ki** 注射器

taking medicine **fukuyō** 服用

tapping **dashin** 打診

tear duct **rui-sen** 涙腺

test-tube baby **shikenkan-beibī** 試験管ベービー

taste **mikaku/aji** 味覚・味

tea **(o) cha** （お）茶

temperature **taion** 体温

terminal **makki** 末期

test of visual power **shiryoku-kensa** 視力検査

test tube **shiken-kan** 試験管

therapy **ryōyō** 療養

thermometer **taion-kei** 体温計

thorn **toge** とげ

thyroid hormone **kōjyōsen-horumon** 甲状腺ホルモン

tick **dani** ダニ

tocodynamometer **bunben kanshi-sōchi** 分娩監視装置

tonsillectomy **hentōsen-tekijyo-shujyutsu** 扁桃腺摘除手術

tools **kigu** 器具

toothbrush **ha-burashi** 歯ブラシ

toothpaste **ha-migki-ko** 歯磨き粉

traction therapy **kenin-ryōhō** 牽引療法

transfer to a different hospital **ten-in** 転院

transfusion **yuketsu** 輸血

transplant **ishoku** 移植

treatment **chiryō** 治療

trousers **zubon** ズボン

tuberculin reaction **tsuberukurin-hannō** ツベルクリン反応

tuberculin test **tsuberukurin-kensa** ツベルクリン検査

tummy tuck **fukubu-shibō-kyūin** 腹部脂肪吸引

tweezers **ke-nuki/pinsetto** 毛抜き・ピンセット

twins **futago/sōsei-ji** 双子・双生児

tympanostomy **komaku-sekkai-jyutsu** 鼓膜切開術

type of blood **ketsueki-gata** 血液型

ultrasound **chō-onpa** 超音波

underarm hair **waki-ge** わき毛

underwear **shitagi** 下着

urine **nyō/shō-ben/oshikko** 尿・小便・おしっこ

urine test **nyō-kensa** 尿検査

vaccination **yobō-sesshu/shutō** 予防接種・種痘

vaccination scar **shutō no ato** 種痘の痕

vasectomy **paipu katto** パイプカット

vaseline **waserin** ワセリン

violation of human rights **jinken-shingai** 人権侵害

virus **bīrusu** ビールス

vision **shiryoku** 視力

vision correcting surgery **shiryoku-kyōsei-shujyutsu** 視力矯正手術

vision test **shiryoku-kensa** 視力検査

visiting hospital/ medical office **rai-in** 来院

visual correction **shiryoku-kyōsei** 視力矯正

visual field test **shiya-kensa** 視野検査

visually impaired person **shiryoku-shōgai-sha** 視力障害者

waiting room **machiai-shitsu** 待合室

ward **byōtō** 病棟

warning **chūi-jikō** 注意事項

weaning period **rinyū-ki** 離乳期

weight **taijyū** 体重

weight scale **taijyū-kei** 体重計

water **(o) mizu** (お)水

water pick **kōkū-senjyō-ki** 口腔洗浄機

wheel chair **kuruma-isu** 車椅子

wheeled stretcher **tanka** 担架

white blood cell **hakkekkyū** 白血球

woman who has first childbirth **shosan-pu** 初産婦

woman who has given birth **keisan-pu** 経産婦

wounded person **fushō-sha** 負傷者

wrong diagnosis **go-shin** 誤診

World Health Organization **sekai hoken kikō** 世界保健機構

X-rays **rentogen** レントゲン

young persons **seinen** 青年

VI. Medical Forms and Related Terms

address **jyūsho** 住所

address in Japan **nihon-no-jyūsho** 日本の住所

address of referrer **shōkai-sha-no-jyūsho** 紹介者の住所

adjustment **seisan** 精算

adult **sei-jin** 成人

age **nenrei/toshi** 年齢・年

aged persons **kōrei-sha** 高齢者

agent/substitute **dairi-nin** 代理人

assets **shisan** 資産

attending physician **tantō-i-shi** 担当医師

basic charge **kihon-ryōkin** 基本料金

bill/invoice **seikyū-sho** 請求書

billing information **seikyū-an-nai** 請求案内

birth date **sei-nen-ga-ppi** 生年月日

birthday **(o) tanjyō-bi** (お)誕生日

birthplace **shussei-chi** 出生地

blood type **ketsu-eki-gata** 血液型

business address **kinmu-saki** 勤務先

car insurance **jidōsha hoken** 自動車保険

cardiac pacemaker **pēsu meikā** ペース・メーカー

cellular phone number **keitai-denwa-bangō** 携帯電話番号

child support **kodomo-no-fuyō** 子供の扶養

city **shi** 市

closest relative **moyori-no-shinseki** 最寄りの親戚

comments **komento** コメント

contact information **renraku-saki** 連絡先

copayment **jiko-futan-kin** 自己負担金

copy of bill **seikyū-sho-no-utsushi** 請求書の写し

copy of payment **ryōshū-sho-no-utsushi** 領収書の写し

country of birth **shussei-chi** 出生地

country of origin **shusshin-chi** 出身地

county **gun** 郡

credit card **kurejitto kādo** クレジット・カード

credit card number **kurejitto kādo bangō** クレジット・カード番号

date of admission **nyūin-bi** 入院日

date of birth **sei-nen-ga-ppi** 生年月日

date of procedure **shochi-bi** 処置日

dental insurance **shika-hoken** 歯科保険

diagnosis **shindan** 診断

deductible **menseki-gaku** 免責額

dependant **haigū-sha** 配偶者

divorced **rikon** 離婚

document **shorui** 書類

due date **(shussan) yotei-bi** (出産)予定日

duplicate card **fukusha-kādo** 複写カード

effective date **yūkō-kijyutsu** 有効期日

emergency **kinkyū** 緊急

emergency contact **kinkyū-renraku-saki** 緊急連絡先

employer's address **kinmu-gaisha-no-jyūsho** 勤務会社の住所

employer's name **kinmu-gaisha-mei** 勤務会社名

employer's phone number **kinmu-gaisha-no-denwa-bangō** 勤務会社の電話番号

employment history **shoku-reki** 職歴

explanation **setsumei** 説明

expiration date **yūkō-kigen** 有効期限

family **kazoku** 家族

female **on-na/joshi/jyosei** 女・女子・女性

fill in (form) **kinyū** 記入

financial responsibility **shiharai sekinin-sha** 支払い責任者

financial screening **zaisei-shinsa** 財政審査

first name **mei** 名

friend's name **yūjn-no-namae** 友人の名前

friend's phone number **yūjin-no-denwa-bangō** 友人の電話番号

group **gurūpu** グループ

group insurance **dantai-hoken** 団体保険

group number **gurūpu bangō** グループ番号

group plan **gurūpu puran** グループ・プラン

health insurance **kenkō-hoken** 健康保険

health insurance company **kenkō hoken-gaisha** 健康保険会社

health insurance society **kenkō hoken kumiai** 健康保険組合

Health Maintenance Organization **hoken-iji-kikō** 保険維持機構

home phone number **jitaku-no-denwa-bangō** 自宅の電話番号

hospital name **byōin-no-namae** 病院の名前

hotel name **hoteru-no-namae** ホテルの名前

informed consent **dōi-sho** 同意書

insurance **hoken** 保険

insurance card **hoken-shō** 保険証

insurance company **hoken-gaisha** 保険会社

insurance information **hoken-ni-tsuite** 保険について

insurance number **hoken-bangō** 保険番号

insurance provider **hoken-teikyō-gaisha** 保険提供会社

insurance subscriber **hoken-kanyū-sha** 保険加入者

insured person **hi-hoken-sha** 被保険者

insured's relationship to patient **kanjya-to-hoken-kanyu-sha-no-kankei** 患者と保険加入者の関係

last name **sei** 姓

length of employment **kinzoku-nensū** 勤続年数

maiden name **kyū-sei** 旧姓

male **otoko/danshi/ dansei** 男・男子・男性

marital status **konin-reki** 婚姻歴

married **kikon** 既婚

maximum charge **seikyū-gendo-gaku** 請求限度額

medication **fukuyō-chū-no-kusuri** 服用中の薬

medical center **iryō-sentā** 医療センター

medical history **byōreki** 病歴

medical questionnaire **monshin-hyō** 問診表

Medicare **rōjin-iroyō-hoken** 老人医療保険

member **kai-in** 会員

member name **kai-in-mei** 会員名

middle name **midoru-neimu** ミドルネーム

minor **mi-seinen-sha** 未成年者

modify **shūsei** 修正

mother's maiden name **haha-oya-no-kyūsei** 母親の旧姓

name **namae/shi-mei** 名前・氏名

name, first **mei** 名

name, last **sei** 姓

name, middle **midoru-neimu** ミドルネーム

nationality **kokuseki** 国籍

neighbor **tonari-kinjyo** 隣近所

new patient **shoshin-sha** 初診者

next of kin **kinshin-sha** 近親者

number **bangō** 番号

occupation **shoku-gyo** 職業

origin (town or city) **shusshin-chi** 出身地

overseas travelers insurance **kaigai ryokō-sha ho-ken** 海外旅行者保険

passport number **pasupōto-bangō** パスポート番号

patient name **kanjya-mei** 患者名

patient information **kanjya-jyōho** 患者情報

payment **shiharai** 支払い

phone number **denwa-bangō** 電話番号

phone number in Japan **nihon-no-denwa-bangō** 日本の電話番号

plan (insurance) **puran (hoken)** プラン（保険）

policy **kiyaku** 規約

policy number **hoken-bangō** 保険番号

pregnant **ninshin-chū** 妊娠中

previous name **kyū-sei** 旧姓

primary care physician **shuji-i** 主治医

print **katsu-ji-de-kinyū** 活字で記入

provider (insurance) **teikyō-sha (hoken)** 提供者（保険）

reason **riyū** 理由

referral **shōkai-jyō** 紹介状

referrer **shōkai-sha** 紹介者

register **tōroku** 登録

registration **uketsuke** 受付

registration date **uketsuke-bi** 受付日

registration information **tōroku-jyōho** 登録情報

relationship to patient **kanjya-tono-kankei** 患者との関係

religion **shūkyo** 宗教

re-registration date **sai-uketsuke-bi** 再受付日

responsible person **sekinin-sha** 責任者

room number **heya-bangō** 部屋番号

savings **chochiku** 貯蓄

school **gakkō** 学校

sex **sei-betsu** 性別

separate **ribetsu** 離別

signature **shomei** 署名

single **dokushin** 独身

smoker **kitsuen-sha** 喫煙者

social security number **shakai-hoken-bangō** 社会保険番号

spouse **haigū-sha** 配偶者

subscriber **kanyū-sha** 加入者

subscriber number **kanyū-sha-bangō** 加入者番号

taking medicine **fukuyō-chu-no-kusuri** 服用中の薬

telephone number **denwa-bangō** 電話番号

total adjustment **saishū-seisan** 最終の精算

total income **zen-shūnyū** 全収入

travelers insurance **ryokō-sha hoken** 旅行者保険

visa number **sashō-bangō** 査証番号

visiter hours **menkai jikan** 面会時間

widow **mibō-jin** 未亡人

woman **fu-jin/jyosei/on-na** 婦人・女性・女

work place **shigoto-ba** 仕事場

year previously admitted **zenkai-nyūin-shita-toshi** 前回入院した年

ZIP code **yūbin-bangō** 郵便番号

## PART FIVE

Appendices

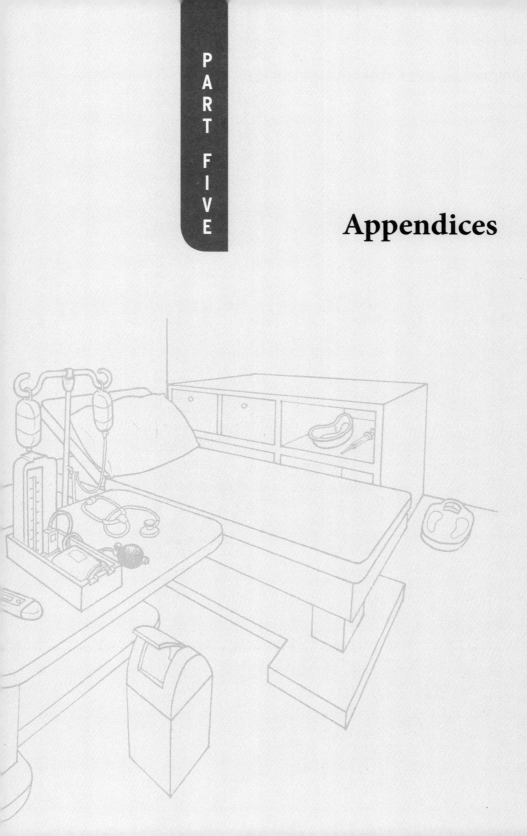

1. MEDICAL QUESTIONNAIRE (問診表)

All information given is strictly confidential. (秘密厳守)

Please fill out in English. (ローマ字で可能な限りご記入下さい)

PATIENT INFORMATION (患者情報)

Date_____/_____/_____ Soc.Sec #_____ Birthdate_____
今日の日付　　年　　月　　日 ソーシャル・セキュリティー番号　　誕生日

Name_____ _____ Sex: ___ Male ___ Female
名前　　　　Last Name 姓　　　　　　First Name 名　　　性別　　男　　　女

Hotel Name_____ Room Number_____
ホテルの名前　　　　　　　　　　　　　　　　　　　　　　　部屋番号

Address_____ Home Phone_____
住所　　番地　　　　　　　ストリート　　　　　　自宅電話番号

City_____ State_____ Zip_____ Cell Phone_____
市　　　　　　　　　州/県　　　　郵便番号　　　携帯電話番号

__ Minor (less than 18) Marital Status: __ Single ___Married __ Divorced __ Widowed __ Separated
未成年者(18歳以下)　結婚暦　　　独身　　既婚　　離婚　　　未亡人　　　離別

Employer_____ Business Phone_____
会社名　　　　　　　　　　　　　　　　　　　　　　会社の電話番号

Employer Address_____ Occupation_____
会社の住所　　　　　　　　　　　　　　　　　　　　職業

Fax_____ E-Mail_____ Nationality_____ Religion_____
ファックス　　　　メール　　　　　国籍　　　　　　　　宗教

Emergency Contact Person: Name_____ Phone number_____
緊急時の連絡先　　　　　　名前　　　　　　　　電話番号

Who should we thank for referring you, if any?_____
紹介者名(もし、何方かいらっしゃればご記入下さい)

PRIMARY INSURANCE (保険情報)

Insurance Company_____
保険会社名

Insurance Company Address_____
保険会社住所

Subscriber ID #_____ Group #_____
加入者番号　　　　　　　　　　　　　　　　　団体番号 (もしあれば)

Policy Holder's Name_____ Sex: __ Male __ Female
保険者名　　　　　Last Name 姓　　　　　First Name 名　　性別　　男　　　女

Relationship to Patient_____ Soc.Sec #_____ Birthdate_____
患者との関係　　　　　　　　　　ソーシャル・セキュリティー番号　　誕生日

Address_____ Home Phone_____
住所　　番地　　　　　　　ストリート　　　　　　自宅電話番号

City_____ State_____ Zip_____ Cell Phone_____
市　　　　　　　　　州/県　　　　郵便番号　　　携帯電話番号

Employer_____ Business Phone_____
会社名　　　　　　　　　　　　　　　　　　　　　　会社の電話番号

Employer Address_____ Occupation_____
会社の住所　　　　　　　　　　　　　　　　　　　　職業

ADDITIONAL INSURANCE（その他の保険情報）

Insurance Company _____
保険会社名

Insurance Company Address _____
保険会社住所

Subscriber ID # _____ Group # _____
加入者番号   団体番号（もしあれば）

Policy Holder's Name _____ _____ Sex: ___ Male ___ Female
保険者名   Last Name 姓   First Name 名   性別   男   女

Relationship to Patient _____ Soc.Sec # _____ Birthdate _____
患者との関係   ソーシャル・セキュリティー番号   誕生日

Address _____ Home Phone _____
住所   番地   ストリート   自宅電話番号

City _____ State_____ Zip_____ Cell Phone _____
市   州/県   郵便番号   携帯電話番号

Employer _____ Business Phone _____
会社名   会社の電話番号

Employer Address _____ Occupation _____
会社の住所   職業

REASON FOR VISIT（本日の受診の理由を教えてください）

Please state the reason for your visit, including your present health concerns, symptoms, and medications.

理由_____

症状_____

服用中の薬など_____

MEDICAL HISTORY（病歴について）

1. Are you currently under medical treatment? (Yes/No)
   現在、かかりつけの病気がありますか （はい/いいえ）

2. Have you ever had any serious illnesses or operations? (Yes/No)
   過去に重病や手術をしましたか （はい/いいえ）

   Have you had a blood transfusion? (Yes/No)
   過去に輸血をしましたか （はい/いいえ）

3. Are you taking any medications? (Yes/No)
   現在、服用中の薬がありますか （はい/いいえ）

4. Do you smoke? (Yes/No)
   タバコをすいますか （はい/いいえ）

5. Do you drink alcohol? (Yes/No)
   お酒を飲みますか （はい/いいえ）

6. Do you use cocaine or other drugs? (Yes/No)
   コカインや薬物を使用していますか （はい/いいえ）

7. Have you had any allergic reactions to the following（下記の薬でアレルギー反応がありましたか）
   Local anesthetics (e.g. Novocaine) (Yes/No)
   局所麻酔薬（ノボケインなど） （はい/いいえ）

   Penicillin or other Antibiotics (Yes/No)
   （ペニシリンや抗生物質など） （はい/いいえ）

   Sulfa Drugs (Yes/No)
   （サルファ剤：外傷などの治療薬） （はい/いいえ）

Barbiturates (Sleeping Pills)	(Yes/No)
(バルビツール酸塩：鎮痛剤・催眠剤用)	(はい/いいえ)
Other Sedatives	(Yes/No)
(鎮静剤)	(はい/いいえ)
Iodine	(Yes/No)
(ヨウ素)	(はい/いいえ)
Aspirin	(Yes/No)
(アスピリン)	(はい/いいえ)
Other	(Yes/No)
(その他の薬)	(はい/いいえ)

8. Women Only (女性への質問)

Do you have regular periods?	(Yes/No)
生理は順調ですか	(はい/いいえ)
Are you using birth control pills/patch/injection?	(Yes/No)
避妊薬を使用していますか	(はい/いいえ)
Are you pregnant now?	(Yes/No)
妊娠中ですか	(はい/いいえ)
Are you currently breastfeeding?	(Yes/No)
現在、授乳中ですか	(はい/いいえ)
Have you ever been pregnant?	(Yes/No)
妊娠をしたことがありますか	(はい/いいえ)
Number of pregnancies	_____回
妊娠回数は何回ですか	

HAVE YOU EVER HAD THE FOLLOWING? (過去に病気をしましたか)

	Yes/No		Yes/No
Anemia (low blood count) 貧血(低血圧)	(はい/いいえ)	Glaucoma 緑内障	(はい/いいえ)
Anorexia (no appetite) 拒食症(食欲不振)	(はい/いいえ)	Heart Disease 心疾患	(はい/いいえ)
Arthritis 関節リュウマチ	(はい/いいえ)	Heart Murmur 心雑音	(はい/いいえ)
Asthma 喘息	(はい/いいえ)	Hepatitis Type ___ 肝炎__型	(はい/いいえ)
Back Problems 腰痛	(はい/いいえ)	Hernia ヘルニア	(はい/いいえ)
Bleeding Tendency 出血しやすい	(はい/いいえ)	Herpes ヘルペス	(はい/いいえ)
Blood Disease 血液病	(はい/いいえ)	High Blood Pressure 高血圧	(はい/いいえ)
Cancer 癌	(はい/いいえ)	HIV/AIDS エイズ	(はい/いいえ)
Chemical Dependency (addiction to	(はい/いいえ)	Jaundice 黄疸	(はい/いいえ)
drugs) 薬物中毒		Kidney Disease 腎臓病	(はい/いいえ)
Chemotherapy 化学療法	(はい/いいえ)	Latex Sensitivity ラテックス・アレルギー	(はい/いいえ)
Chicken Pox 水痘	(はい/いいえ)	Liver Disease 肝臓病	(はい/いいえ)
Chronic Fatigue Syndrome 慢性疲労	(はい/いいえ)	Low Blood Pressure 低血圧	(はい/いいえ)
Circulatory Problems 循環器障害	(はい/いいえ)	Measles 麻疹	(はい/いいえ)
Congenital Heart Lesions 先天性心臓病	(はい/いいえ)	Migraine 偏頭痛	(はい/いいえ)
Cough – persistent or bloody 咳	(はい/いいえ)	Headaches 頭痛	
(持続性、又は血を含む)		Mitral Valve Prolapse 僧帽弁逸脱症	(はい/いいえ)
Diabetes 糖尿病	(はい/いいえ)	Mumps 流行性耳下腺炎	(はい/いいえ)
Emphysema 肺気腫	(はい/いいえ)	Multiple Sclerosis 多発性硬化症	(はい/いいえ)
Epilepsy 癲癇	(はい/いいえ)	Pacemaker ペースメーカー	(はい/いいえ)

	Yes/No		Yes/No
Pneumonia 肺炎	(はい/いいえ)	Skin Rash 発疹	(はい/いいえ)
Polio ポリオ	(はい/いいえ)	Stroke 脳卒中	(はい/いいえ)
Prostate Problem 前立腺障害	(はい/いいえ)	Thyroid Problems 甲状腺機能障害	(はい/いいえ)
Psychiatric Care 精神療養中	(はい/いいえ)	Tonsillitis 扁桃腺炎	(はい/いいえ)
Respiratory Disease 呼吸器疾患	(はい/いいえ)	Tuberculosis 結核	(はい/いいえ)
Rheumatic Fever リュウマチ熱	(はい/いいえ)	Ulcer 潰瘍	(はい/いいえ)
Scarlet Fever 猩紅熱	(はい/いいえ)	Venereal Disease 性病	(はい/いいえ)
Shortness of Breath 息切れ	(はい/いいえ)	Any Other Condition (Please describe) その他の症	
Sinus Trouble 蓄膿症	(はい/いいえ)	状があれば記入 _____	

FAMILY HISTORY（家族歴）

Please select any illnesses your immediate families have had.（家族の中で下記の病気になった方がいますか）

Cancer 癌   Diabetes 糖尿病   Hereditary diseases 遺伝子関連疾患

High blood pressure 高血圧   Kidney disease 腎臓病   Liver disease 肝臓病

Other (please write) その他の病歴があれば記入 _____

ASSIGNMENT AND RELEASE （権利の譲渡と放棄についての承諾書）

I hereby authorize payment directly to this medical provider of all insurance benefits otherwise payable to me for service rendered. I understand that I am financially responsible for all charges, whether or not paid by insurance, and for all services rendered for me or for my dependents.

私はここに保険会社が治療費・諸経費等を当医療機関に直接支払いすることを承諾します。又は、私に直接支払われる場合も承諾します。治療費・諸経費等の支払いは私に責任があることを理解し、もし保険が適用されない場合には私や家族の治療費・諸経費等は私が全額支払うことを承諾します。

I authorize the doctors and/or any provider or supplier of services in this office to release the information required to secure the payment of benefits. I authorize the use my signature on all insurance submissions.

保険適用に関して患者情報を関係機関に解除することを承諾します。この署名を全ての保険申請に使用することを承諾します。

Signature:_____ Date _____
署名   日付 Year年 Month月 Day日

If the patient is a minor (under 18 years of age), the responsible parent or guardian must sign above and fill in the information below.

もし患者が未成年者（１８歳以下）の場合は、親か保護者が上記に署名して、下記にも記入してください

Parent/Guardian Name (Print): _____ Patient Name: _____
親・保護者名   患者の名前

Relationship to Patient: Son; Daughter; Step Father; Step Mother; Grandchild; Legal Guardian; Other
患者との続柄   息子   娘   まま父   まま母   孫   後見人   その他

2. List of Grammar Covered in the Lessons

LESSON 1 (7 grammar points)

1. Noun + **desu** expresses "this is" or "it is."
2. Noun + **dewa arimasen** indicates a negative and translates as "this is not" or "it's not."
3. The particle **wa** indicates the topic of a sentence. **X wa Y desu** means "X is Y."
4. The particle **no** is used to indicate the affiliation of a person.
5. The question marker **ka** is added at the end of sentence.
6. The tag question marker **ne** is added at the end of sentence.
7. **Nan desu ka** means "What is it?"

LESSON 2 (9)

8. The particle **ga**: Noun/subject **ga arimasu** expresses "I have; there is."
9. The particle **wa** is used for all negative statements.
10. The particle **wa** is used in why-questions.
11. The verb **arimasu** means "I have; there is."
12. The negative form of **arimasu** is **arimasen**.
13. The particle **o** is an object marker used with transitive verbs.
14. The expression **onegai shimasu** expresses a request or favor
15. WH-words + **desu ka** express questions.
16. Noun or number + **gurai** indicates "about" or "approximately."

LESSON 3 (10)

17. The expression **ii desu ka** is asking a preference or choice.
18. The particle **ni** indicates a specific point in time, as with English *at*.
19. Place + the particle **ni** indicates "toward the place."
20. The article **de** indicates reasons, causes, and ways and means.
21. **Nan/nani + de** is used to ask about reason and means.
22. The usage of the verb **arimasu/imasu** for non-animate/animate subjects
23. The expressions **dō-desu ka** and **ikaga-desu ka** mean "how about?"
24. Verbs in the present and future tenses end with -**masu** and the past tense -**mashita**.
25. The expression **te kudasai** (**te**-form + **kudasai**) is used to make a request.
26. Noun **(o) shite+ imasu** expresses the present progressive tense (be doing).

LESSON 4 (9)

27. **Ko-so-a-do** words refer to location.
28. The particle **de** indicates a specific place.
29. The **te**-form + -**aru/-arimasu** expresses a condition that has resulted from an intentional action.
30. Japanese verb forms include the **masu** form and stem verb (dictionary form).
31. The stem verb past tense + **koto ga aru/arimasu** expresses experience, fact, and events in the past.
32. The stem verb present tense + **koto ga arimasu** express actions that occur occasionally.
33. The **te**-form + **oku/okimasu** is used for something done in advance
34. The interrogatives **dare** (who), **dore** (which), **doko** (where), **naze** (why), **itsu** (when), and **nan** (what)
35. The interjection **dewa** expresses "then."

LESSON 5 (6)

36. The **i**-adjectives modifying nouns
37. Adding **n** after the **i**-adjective conveys the speaker's feeling and emotion: (-**i(n) desu**).

38. The **i**-adjective + suffix **-kunai(n) desu** makes adjectives negative.
39. The particle **kara** indicates a starting point and means "from/since."
40. The particle **mo** can replace **wa** and **ga** and means "also" or "too."
41. The adverbs **bimyō-ni** (slightly), **sukoshi** (little) **chotto** (few), **hontō-ni** (really), **tottemo** (very)

Lesson 6 (11)

42. The verb suffix **-masen** indicates present tense negative form.
43. The verb suffix **-masen + deshita** indicates negative past tense.
44. The **te**-form + **imasu** expresses the present progressive (be doing).
45. The **te**-form + **imasen** expresses the negative progressive tense (not be doing).
46. The present negative **-masen + ka** is asking about a condition or inviting to action.
47. The **te**-form + **imasen ka** is used to ask about the present progress of an action.
48. To make an **i**-adjective into a noun, drop the suffix **-i** and replace it with **-mi**.
49. The expression **don-na** means "what kind of . . . ?"
50. The adverbs **ichiban** (most), **itsumo** (always), **tokidoki** (sometimes), **tamani** (once in a while), **yoku** (often), **tsuyoku** (strongly/hard), **yowaku** (weakly), and **tokuni** (especially/particularly)
51. The adverbs **zenzen** (not at all), **hotondo** (hardly), **amari** (not very much/often) are used only with negative sentences.
52. The adverb **hokani** expresses "Is there anything else?" when used with **arimasu ka**.

Lesson 7 (6)

53. The verb ending **mashō** is a volitional form that means "Let's."
54. The **te**-form + **imashita** expresses past progressive action.
55. The adverb **nani-ka** means "something else" or "anything else."
56. The expression **nani-ka** + **-te imasu ka** indicates a question about present progress.
57. The particle **to** is used to list noun in series and means "and."
58. Three uses of the conjunction **kara**: (noun + kara); (noun + **desu/da-kara**); (verb + **kara**)

Lesson 8 (7)

59. Connecting two sentences using **te**-form, which has the sense of "and"
60. The suffix **-ppoi** indicates some distinctive feature or characteristic.
61. The suffix **-gimi** means "feeling like."
62. The time expressions **saikin** (recently), **chikagoro** (nowadays), and **konogoro** (these days)
63. The conjunctions **soshite** (and), **sorekara** (and then), **shikashi** (but), and **demo** (but)
64. **Ko-so-a-do** words indicate general locations.
65. An interrogative followed by **ka** forms an adverb meaning "some."

Lesson 9 (7)

66. The suffix **-sō** added to the verb base means "it seems that."
67. The suffix **-yō(na)** expresses purpose/appearance/emphasis and means "appears, looks like."
68. The suffix **-ta nowa** indicates new and important information.
69. The expression **mitai desu** means "looks like."
70. The expression **kamo shiremasen** indicates possibility (might).
71. The adverb **nen-no-tame (ni)** means "making sure; just to be sure."
72. The verb ending **-mashō + ka** is used for making a suggestion (shall we).

Lesson 10 (6)

73. A noun followed by the particle **no** may modify another noun.

74. The expression **-te mo ii desu ka** means "may I? ; can I?"
75. The expression **hō ga ii** means "better to do (something)," and **nai hō ga ii** means "better not to do (something)."
76. The adverb **mushiro** expresses a suggestion and translates as "instead, rather, better."
77. The verb **te**-form + **iru/imasu** also express a present condition.
78. The sentence-final particle **yo** expresses the speaker's conviction, assertion, or suggestion.

LESSON 11 (6)
79. Place/body + **no atari/no tokoro** expresses the area around the place or body part
80. The **te**-form + **iru mitai** expresses an observation about a present condition and means "looks like, seems."
81. A noun or **na**-adjective + **dato omoimasu** means "I think that."
82. A verb or **i**-adjective + **to omoimasu** means "I think that."
83. The expression **shita koto ga arimasu ka** means "Have you ever?"
84. The expression **sore-dewa** means "in the case; well then."

LESSON 12 (8)
85. The adverb **mō** is used in an affirmative sentence and means "already."
86. The adverb **mada** expresses incomplete action in a negative sentence and means "yet."
87. The adverb **nani-yorimo** means "more than anything; above all; first of all."
88. Day/week/month/frequency + **no yōni** means "almost every (time)."
89. The suffix -**tari** . . . -**tari** expresses two actions at the same time.
90. The adverb **sugu (ni)** indicates immediate action and proximity.
91. The negative verb + **wake-ni(wa)-ikanai** means "cannot help; cannot help but do."
92. The expression **mazu saisho ni** means "first of all."

LESSON 13 (6)
93. Stem verb present tense + **tsumori** indicates plans or intentions for the future.
94. The stem verb + **deshō** means "probably," and stem verb + **nai-deshō** means "probably not."
95. The expression **mo sureba** . . . **narimasu** indicates an upper limit (as much as).
96. The stem verb + **hitsuyō ga arimasu** means "it's necessary to."
97. Verb + **ga** combines two sentences while expressing a contrast (but).
98. Verb + **ga** also is used for when the speaker trails off (but . . .).

LESSON 14 (9)
99. The polite expression **omochi-desu ka** means "Do you have?"
100. The adverb **nani-ka** means "something" in affirmative contexts and "anything" in questions.
101. **Nani-mo** . . . **masen** means "anything" in negative sentences.
102. Noun + **ni(wa)** places emphasis on a subject or topic.
103. The stem verb + **niwa** means "in order to; for the purpose of."
104. The interrogative pronoun **don-na** means "what kind of?"
105. The stem verb + **kamo** means "might."
106. Time + **goni** + verb base + **ni kite kudasai**; and time + **goni** + place + **ni kite kudasai** are used to request that an action be taken after a certain time.
107. The interrogative pronoun **dono-kurai** is used to ask "how long" or "how many."

LESSON 15 (7)
108. The verb base + -**kata** means "how to" or expresses a method.

109. Noun + **no hōhō** and stem verb + **hōhō** also mean "how to" and can be used to express a method.
110. The noun suffix **inai ni** means "within" or "less than" with respect to time.
111. The counters **ichi-nichi ni . . . kai** or **do** indicate how many time per day.
112. The counters **i-kkai ni** and **ichi-do ni** expresses quantity at one time for dosage.
113. The suffix **-ika** means "not more than; under" and is used with the negative for prohibition **naide**.
114. The expression X **ga** Y **ni kikimasu** states that X is effective/works well against Y.

Lesson 16 (8)
115. Place **ni** + subject **ga arawarete kimasu** expresses that someone or something has become visible.
116. The **i**-adjective + **-garu** means "to show signs of (a wish and desire)."
117. Verb + **-garu** means "to show signs of (a wish and desire)."
118. The expression **no mawari-de** indicates a surrounding area, neighborhood, or locality.
119. The expression **ni chigai arimasen** means"I think; there is no doubt that."
120. The **te**-form + **shimau** means "have done, have finished."
121. The noun **ni taishite** expresses a person's attitude or action toward something.
122. The adverbs **motto takusan** mean "even more, any more."

Lesson 17 (9)
123. The stem verb or **i**-adjective + **-yō (ni)** means "to be like/similar to."
124. The noun or **na**-adjective + **no yō-ni/na** means "like, similar."
125. The expression **ni natte inai ka tashikamete mimasu** means "I am trying to be sure whether it has became X or not."
126. Body part + **zentai-ni** means "the whole (body part)."
127. The **i**-adjective + **ku-naru** means "become, turn."
128. Changing the **i**-adjective to the **te**-form with **-kute**
129. The **te**-form + **iru no dewa naika(to) shinpai desu** means "I am worried about the risk of."
130. The adverbs **tashika-ni** (surely, certainly, definitely) and **toriaezu** (first of all; for the time being; anyway)
131. The conjunction **-ba** indicates that the preceding phrase expresses a conditional statement or if-statement.

Lesson 18 (9)
132. The stem verb plus the sentence-final particle **no** indicates a question.
133. The stem verb + particle **to** is used for when- and if-clauses.
134. The suffix **-rare-ru/-rare-masu** is used for the passive form.
135. The **i**-adjective + **ku-narimasu** expresses "become, turn."
136. The verb base + **-yasui** expresses the ease of an action; verb base + **-nikui(n)** expresses the difficulty of an action.
137. The **te**-form + the suffix **morau** expresses the notion of receiving some benefit from someone's action or getting someone to do something for your sake.
138. The expression **dō sureba ii(n) desu ka** means "What shall I do?"
139. **Nan + daka** (somehow): interrogatives plus **daka** express "some."
140. Changing the **i**-adjective to an adverb: **kuwashiku** (in detail) and **sugoku** (awfully, very, immensely)

Lesson 19 (10)
141. Sentences ending with **-te** express requests, instructions, and commands.
142. The expression **no guai wa ikaga desu ka** is a polite way to ask about a patient's condition.
143. The particle **yori** is a comparative marker.

144. The expression **ka oshiete kudasai** means "Could you tell me if/whether?"
145. The negative **te**-form of **i**-adjectives is **ku(wa)-nakute** and means "not X but Y."
146. The verb base + **sō ni narimasu** means "I feel like I am going to do (something)."
147. The negative **te**-form of nouns ends in **dewa naku(te)** (not X but Y).
148. The negative **i**-adjective of polite expression is **kuwa arimasen (deshita)**.
149. The expression **i**-adjective + **kuwa nai(n)-desu ka** means "Don't you have (something)?"
150. The suffixes **-nado** and **-ya** mean "and the like, et cetera, and so forth."

LESSON 20 (9)

151. Verb base + **taku-naru/narimasu** expresses the wish to begin an action.
152. The stem verb + **toki(ni)** means "when, at that time."
153. The verb base + **-seru/-saseru** means "to make or order someone to do something."
154. Subject **wa** + noun **no koto** is a noun phrase that can be used to explain or rephrase.
155. The stem verb + **noni** indicates the purpose of doing something or the process of doing it.
156. An interrogative followed by the suffix **-kurai** asks about approximate quantity, length, or extent.
157. Time + **teido de** indicates approximate time and translates as "about."
158. The negative form of **suru** is **sezu(ni)** and means "without (something)"; **shinai-de** is a synonym.
159. The adverb **narubeku** means "if possible, if you can."

LESSON 21 (10)

160. The **na**-adjective **genki** means "healthy."
161. The conjunction **node** indicates a reason or a cause
162. The **na**-adjective + **de** combines two statements and means "and."
163. The **na**-adjective + **da-kara** expresses a cause or reason.
164. Noun + **ni yoru-to** means "according to."
165. Adverbs with negative forms: **nani-mo** (nothing at all (for things)); **doko-mo** (nothing at all (place)); **mettani** (rarely, seldom); **kesshite** (never, by no means); **sappari** (not at all (informal)); **sukoshi-mo** (not a bit); **chitto-mo** (not a bit (informal))
166. The expression **itadake masu ka** is a more polite **kudasai**.
167. The expression **gozai masu ka** is a more polite **arimasu ka**.
168. Directions with respect to body part: **migi** (right), **hidari** (left); **ue** (up, above); **shita** (below, under); **naka** (inside); **soto** (outside); **man-naka** (center)
169. The expression noun + **no chōkō ga arimasu** means "show the signs of illness."

LESSON 22 (6)

170. The expression **yōto shita totan (ni)** means "at a moment that; just as."
171. The stem verb + **dake de(mo)** expresses the notion of just doing or doing just enough for something to happen.
172. The expression **dewa naika to omoimasu** means "I think that it's probably."
173. The past tense verb + **tokoro** expresses when someone has done something intentionally.
174. The suffix **-morau** expresses the notion of receiving some benefit from a person's action.
175. The verbs **ageru/agemasu** and **kureru/kuremasu** mean "give."

LESSON 23 (8)

176. Verb + **shi**; **i**-adjective + **shi** ; noun + **dashi**; **na**-adjective + **dashi** all indicate "and."
177. The quote marker **toiu** means "called, that says."
178. The expression **iwayuru** means "what is called; as it is called; the so-called; so to speak."
179. The adverb **osoraku (wa)** means "probably, likely, perhaps."

180. The verb **osoreru** means "worry, concern" and conveys seriousness.
181. Noun **no tame(ni)** or verb **tame(ni)** expresses purpose, benefit, reasons, cause.
182. The phrase **-tari . . . -tari** expresses a series of actions or states and translates as "and . . . and."
183. The phrase **koto ni naru/narimasu** means "It will be decided that; come about; be arranged that; turn out that."

Lesson 24 (7)

184. The adverb **totsuzen** (suddenly) + **na**-adjective is used for sudden action.
185. The **te**-form + **iraremasen** means "not able to do something."
186. The expression **tamaranai/tamarimasen** means "terrible, extreme, severe, unbearable."
187. The verb base + **nikui** means "difficult to do (something), and the verb base + **yasui** means "easy to do (something)."
188. The sentence-initial conjunction **sore-dewa** means "if that is the case."
189. The phrase **darō-to omoimasu** means "I think probably that."
190. The usage of **oi**; **ōku no**; **ōzei** (many)

Lesson 25 (9)

191. The verb base + **tara kaette** means "rather; on the contrary; more."
192. Adding the noun **mono** after a verb indicates things to do.
193. The compound verb **omoi-ataru** means "come to mind; recall; think of."
194. Adding **-rareru/-rare** to the **te**-form makes honorific expressions.
195. The verb base + **-reru/-remasu** expresses the possibility of doing something.
196. Counters are used to indicate singular or plural in Japanese.
197. The adverb **nan-toka** expresses the notion of doing anything to achieve a seemingly impossible outcome.
198. The verb **omowareru/omowaremasu** means "appear, seem, apparently."
199. The construction stem verb + **tame(ni)** and the conjunction **node**

Lesson 26 (8)

200. The expression **koko** + duration of time + **hodo** indicates a recent time period.
201. The verb base + **-renai/-remasen** expresses that something is impossible to do/can't be done.
202. The noun suffix-**gimi** can mean "look (like), appear"; noun suffix -**gachi** means "tend to, apt to, show a tendency to, etc."
203. The negative short form of the verb + **ni[wa] irarenai/iraremasen** means "I cannot stand going without (action)."
204. X **niwa** Y **ga hitsuyō/kakasenai/taisetsu desu** expresses the necessity, indispensability, or importance of doing something.
205. The verb **susumeru/susumemasu** means "recommend, encourage, advise."
206. The adverbs **tonikaku** (anyway), **yatara-ni** (unexpectedly, incredibly), **muyami-ni** (unreasonably, carelessly, unthinkingly).
207. The adverb **naruhodo** expresses agreement.

Lesson 27 (10)

208. The adverbs **ichiō** (just in case; tentatively; for the time being;) and **toriaezu** (first of all; for now; at once)
209. The word **tada** is used to change topics (however, but, nevertheless).
210. Noun/**na**-adjective + **dattari** and the **i**-adjective + **kattari** express "like A and B; sometimes A, sometimes B."

211. The suffix **-sa** makes a noun out of an adjective and expresses the current condition, degree, or quality.
212. The phrase **hazu nano ni** means "I expected . . . , but; I can say with confidence . . . , but."
213. A number plus the suffix **-bai** means "times, -fold, twice, double."
214. The transitive verb (**o mitsukeru/mitsukemasu**) and intransitive verb (**ga mitsukaru/mitsukarimasu**)
215. The expression **ima-no-tokoro** means "for now; for the moment; so far; for the time being."
216. The phrase **kanō na gakiri/dekiru kagiri** means "by every possible means; as often as possible, etc."
217. The stem verb plus **yōni suru** means "to make sure."

LESSON 28 (7)
218. The conjunction word **jitsu-wa** indicates a change of topic for a true story and can be used with the copula **nan(o) desu** or **da** to emphasize the actual fact.
219. The noun + **no mae** or dictionary form of the verb + **mae-ni** expresses an action or event that occurred earlier.
220. The conjunction **mata wa** means "or, either . . . or . . . ."
221. The idiom **mo nai(desu)shi . . . mo nai(desu)/arimasen** means "neither . . . nor . . . ."
222. The idiom **moshi . . . ga areba** indicates hypothetical and conditional action.
223. The interjection **masaka** means "never thought; don't tell me that; surely not; absolutely not."
224. The suffix **-tara** expresses conditional action or supposition and means "when, if."

LESSON 29 (6)
225. The conjunction suffix **-shi** means "and, what's more."
226. The compound verb **de-hajimeru** and verb base + **hajimeru** mean "begin to."
227. **Nemureru** (passive, but spontaneously possible: can sleep), **nemurenai** (cannot sleep)
228. The words **naku-naru/nakunari-masu** mean "not anymore."
229. The expression **ba yokkata** states the speaker's regret (I wish; it would have been good if).
230. Noun + the suffix **-go** indicates a past event and means "after, since."

LESSON 30 (6)
231. The te-form + **tamaranai** means "extremely, unbearably, cannot cope with."
232. The passive form **-rareru** expresses an honorific and is used with the object marker **o**.
233. The conjunction **yō(ni)** expresses potential action with non-past verbs (so that).
234. The adverb **kanari** means "considerably, fairly, quite."
235. The adverb **dō shite mo** means "by all means, at any cost, no matter what."
236. The adverb **sukunaku-tomo** means "at least."

3. List of Language Roots in the Lessons

LESSON 1
Byō (病) indicates illness and disease and is used both as a prefix and a suffix.
The suffix **-shi** (士) indicates a person who has extensive knowledge and learning experience or superior social standing.

LESSON 2
The suffix **-sha/-jya** (者) indicates a person, **-sha** (車) indicates a car, and **-sha** (社) indicates a company.
The word **ban** (番) means "number" in a series and is used as either a prefix or a suffix.

LESSON 3

The suffix **-in** (院) indicates an institution, especially a government office, school, hospital, or institute for higher learning.

The word **ki** (気) indicates feelings, mood, spirit, mind, and heart.

LESSON 4

The word **kan** (患) indicates illness, disease, and ailment.

The word **shin** (診) indicates diagnosis, checkup, examination, and seeing.

LESSON 5

The word **ke/ge** (毛) indicates hair. It is also pronounced **mō**.

The suffix **-tsū** (痛) indicate pain, soreness, and hurt. It is also pronounced **-itai**.

LESSON 6

Jyō (上) means "upper" and "above." It is also pronounced **ue/uwa**.

Naka (中) means "inside, middle, center." If **naka** is pronounced **chū**, the meaning become the duration.

The prefix **ka-** (下) means "lower, below, under." The same character is pronounced **shita** and **ge**.

LESSON 7

Kei (計) indicates measurement, meter, measuring device, or plan.

The suffix **-ki** (器) indicates a device, instrument, or container. A different word **-ki** (機) with the same pronunciation means "machine."

LESSON 8

Chi (血) means "blood" and may be used as both a prefix and a suffix. **Chi** is also pronounced **ji** or **ketsu**.

Eki (液) is used for liquids or fluids.

LESSON 9

The prefix **kō-** (高) means "high."

The prefix **tei-** (低) means "low."

LESSON 10

The negative prefix **fu-/bu-** (不) means irregularity and often translates as "un-, non-, dis-, *or* a-."

The suffix **-yō** (養) indicates support or treatment.

LESSON 11

The word **zō** (臓) indicates internal organs, intestines, and viscera.

The word **chō** (腸) is also used for internal organs and indicates guts, bowels, and intestines.

LESSON 12

The suffix **-hō** (法) indicates a principle or method.

Ken (検) indicates an examination, inspection, or investigation. A similar meaning of "examination" is conveyed by **ken** (験) and **sa** (査).

LESSON 13

The word **sei** (性) indicates nature, gender, sex, quality, and condition. There are four homophones for **sei** that all have different meanings: **sei** (生) "birth," **sei** (正) "truth," **sei** (制) "system," and **sei** (精) "energy."

The word **hatsu** (発) conveys the sense of "start, depart, emit."

LESSON 14

The suffix **-kusuri/-gusuri** (薬) refers to medicine. The character is also pronounced **yaku**.

The suffix **-zai** (剤) also refers to medicine or a tablet.

LESSON 15

The prefix **kō-** (抗) means "against," like the English prefix anti-.

The prefix **kyō-** (強) indicates strength or potency.

LESSON 16

The word **netsu** (熱) indicates fever and temperature.

The word **shi** (死) indicates death and decease.

LESSON 17

The suffix **-gan** (癌) indicates cancer of the internal organs.

The suffix **-en** (炎) indicates an inflammatory disease and corresponds to the suffix *-itis*.

LESSON 18

Shin (心) indicates the heart and corresponds to the prefix *cardio-*.

Shō (症) indicates illness and corresponds to the suffix *-sis*.

LESSON 19
The prefix **i-** (胃) indicates the stomach and corresponds to the prefix *gastro-*.
The suffix **-kei** (系) means "group, lineage, system."

Lesson 20
Jin (腎) refers to the kidneys and corresponds to the prefix *nephr-*.
Kyū (急) means "urgent, sudden, fast."

LESSON 21
The suffix **-kan** (感) indicates feeling and sense.
Dō (動) can be either a prefix or a suffix and indicates motion and movement.

LESSON 22
The word **kotsu** (骨) means "bone." It's also pronounced **hone**.
The word **niku** (肉) indicates flesh, body, meat.
The word **tsui** (椎) indicates the spine and vertebral column.

LESSON 23
The word **shi** (視) indicates vision, sight, and the visual.
The word **gan** (眼) means "eyeball" and in compounds indicates the eye.

LESSON 24
The word **ji** (耳) means "ear" and "hearing" and in compounds indicates these meanings. The same character is also pronounced **mimi**.
The word **bi** (鼻) means "nose" and indicates the nose in compounds. The same character is also pronounced **hana**.

LESSON 25
The word **shō** (焼) indicates burn. It is also pronounced **yake**.
The word **shō** (傷) indicates a wound, cut, scrape, or scratch. The same character is also pronounced **kizu**.

LESSON 26
The word **shin** (神) indicates spirit and psyche.
The word **nō** (脳) indicates brain and memory.

LESSON 27
The word **kyū** (宮) indicates a holy place and womb.
The word **ri** (理) indicates a principle, rule, and reason.

LESSON 28
The word **san/zan** (産) indicates produce, confinement, and childbirth.
The word **nyuu** (乳) indicates breasts and milk. It's also pronounced **chi**.

LESSON 29
The word **ryō** (良) means "good, pleasing, benigh." It is also pronounced **yo(i)**.
The word **aku** (悪) has a range of meanings on the order of "bad, evil, false, wrong." It is also pronounced **waru(i)**.

LESSON 30
The word **shi** (歯) means "tooth." It is also pronounced **ha/ba**.
The word **sei/shō** (正) conveys the meaning of "correct, exact."

4. List of Culture Notes in the Lessons

LESSON 1
The world and Japanese populations
The Japanese bow is called **ojigi**.
Statistics for Japanese nationals overseas
The most popular Japanese family names
The origin of **arigatō** (thank you)

LESSON 2
Countries with the Highest Life Expectancy at Birth for 2005–2010 and 2045–2050 (chart)
Lucky and unlucky numbers in Japanese culture

LESSON 3
Yaku-doshi (Japanese bad luck year)
Appointment system in Japan
The first day of the month

Morita therapy
The word **okashii** and understanding of the Japanese view of natural beauty

LESSON 27
Hot springs and healing illnesses
Health-related Japanese proverbs XIII

LESSON 28
Hospitalization for the delivery
Lamaze and Zen meditation

Circumcision (**hōhi-setsudan**) in Japanese society and culture

LESSON 29
MMR: M=Mumps (**otafuku kaze**), M=Measles (**hashika**), and R=Rubella (**fūshin**)

LESSON 30
Origin of the term for **oya-shirazu** (wisdom tooth)
June 4th is Cavities Prevention Day (**Mushi-ba Yobō-bi**)

5. List of Common Verbs

U-verbs

English	Transitive Intransitive	**Masu** form Verb base	Stem verb Dictionary form	**Te**-form	Negative form
allow	tr	**yurushi-masu**	yurusu	yurushi-te	yurusa-nai
beat	tr	**tataki-masu**	tataku	tata-ite	tataka-nai
bind	tr	**maki-masu**	maku	ma-ite	maka-nai
bite/chew	tr	**kami-masu**	kamu	ka-nde	kama-nai
brush	tr	**migaki-masu**	migaku	miga-ite	migaka-nai
buy	tr	**kai-masu**	kau	ka-tta	kawa-nai
catch/pull	tr/intr	**hiki-masu**	hiku	hi-ite	hika-nai
cool/cool off	tr	**hiyashi-masu**	hiyasu	hiyashi-te	hiyasa-nai
comb	tr	**tokashi-masu**	tokasu	tokashi-te	toka-nai
cross/put together	tr	**kumi-masu**	kumu	ku-nde	kama-nai
depress	intr	**ochimomi-masu**	ochikomu	ochiko-nde	ochikoma-nai
die	intr	**shini-masu**	shinu	shi-nde	shina-nai
drink	tr	**nomi-masu**	nomu	no-nde	noma-nai
effect	intr	**kiki-masu**	kiku	ki-ite	kika-nai
empty/be hungry	intr	**suki-masu**	suku	su-ite	suka-nai
erase	tr	**keshi-masu**	kesu	keshi-te	kesa-nai
exhale	tr	**haki-masu**	haku	ha-ite	haka-nai
extract	tr	**nuki-masu**	nuku	nu-ite	nuka-nai
fall down	intr	**korobi-masu**	korobu	koro-nde	koroba-nai
follow/obey	intr	**shitagai-masu**	shitagau	shitaga-tte	shitagawa-nai
go	intr	**iki-masu**	iku	i-tte	ika-nai
hit	tr	**uchi-masu**	utsu	u-tte	uta-nai
inhale/smoke	tr	**sui-masu**	suu	su-tte	suwa-nai

English	Transitive Intransitive	**Masu** form Verb base	Stem verb Dictionary form	**Te**-form	Negative form
include	tr	fukumi-masu	fukumu	fuku-nde	fukuma-nai
keep	tr	tamochi-masu	tamotsu	tamo-tte	tamota-nai
leave	tr	nokoshi-masu	nokosu	nokoshi-te	nokosa-nai
lend	tr	kasha-masu	kasu	kasha-te	kasa-nai
listen	tr	kiki-masu	kiku	ki-ite	kika-nai
live in (place)	tr	kurashi-masu	kurasu	kurashi-te	kurasa-nai
massage	tr	momi-masu	momu	mo-nde	moma-nai
miss/lack	tr	kakashi-masu	kakasu	kakashi-te	kakasa-nai
move	intr	ugoki-masu	ugoku	ugo-ite	ugoka-nai
open	tr	hiraki-masu	hiraku	hira-ite	hiraka-nai
pay	tr	harai-masu	harau	hara-tte	harawa-nai
peel off	tr	muki-masu	muku	mu-ite	muka-nai
pinch	tr	hasami-masu	hasamu	hasa-nde	hasama-nai
point out	tr	sashi-masu	sasu	sashi-te	sasa-nai
prescribe/send out	tr	dashi-masu	dasu	dashi-te	dasa-nai
prevent	tr/intr	fusegi-masu	fusegu	fuse-ide	fusega-nai
pull down	intr	hiki-masu	hiku	hi-ite	hika-nai
push down/strain	tr	ikimi-masu	ikimu	iki-nde	ikima-nai
reach/arrive	intr	todoki-masu	todoku	todo-ite	todoka-nai
read	tr	yomi-masu	yomu	yo-nde	yoma-nai
release	tr	nuki-masu	nuku	nu-ite	nuka-nai
rest/be absent	intr	yasumi-masu	yasumu	yasu-nde	yasuma-nai
say/tell	tr	ii-masu	iu	i-tte	iwa-nai
scrape	tr	surimuki-masu	surimuku	surimu-ite	surimuka-nai
scratch	tr	kaki-masu	kaku	ka-ite	kaka-nai
send out/pre-scribe	tr	dashi-masu	dasu	dashi-te	dasa-nai
shoot/hit	tr	uchi-masu	utsu	u-tte	uta-nai
smell/sniff	tr	kagi-masu	kagu	ka-ide	kaga-nai
speak	tr	hanashi-masu	hanasu	hanashi-te	hanasa-nai
sprain	tr	kujiki-masu	kujiku	kuji-ite	kujika-nai
stand up	intr	tachi-masu	tatsu	ta-tte	tata-nai
sting	tr	sashi-masu	sasu	sashi-te	sasa-nai
stitch	tr	nui-masu	nuu	nu-tte	nuwa-nai
stretch	tr	nobashi-masu	nobasu	nobashi-te	nobasa-nai

English	Transitive Intransitive	**Masu** form Verb base	Stem verb Dictionary form	**Te**-form	Negative form
stumble	intr	tsumazuki-masu	tsuma-zuku	tsumazui-te	tsumazaka-nai
swallow	tr	nomikomi-masu	nomiko-mu	nomiko-nde	nomikoma-nai
take off (accessories)	tr	hazushi-masu	hazusu	hazushi-te	hazusa-nai
take out/pull out	tr	toridashi-masu	toridasu	toridashi-te	toridasa-nai
tie	tr	musubi-masu	musubu	nusu-nde	musuba-nai
think	tr	omoi-masu	omou	omo-tte	omowa-nai
try	tr	tameshi-masu	tamesu	tameshi-te	tamesa-nai
throw up	tr	hakidashi-masu	hakidasu	hakidashi-te	hakidasa-nai
turn off	tr	keshi-masu	kesu	keshi-te	kesa-nai
undress/take off (clothes)	tr	nugi-masu	nugu	nu-ide	nuga-nai
unfasten/remove	tr	hazushi-masu	hazusu	hazushi-te	hazusa-nai
untie	tr	hodoki-masu	hodoku	hodo-ite	hodoka-nai
upset (mind)	intr	mukatsuki-masu	mukat-suku	mukatsui-te	mukatsuka-nai
use up	tr	tsukaikiri-masu	tsukaikiru	tsukaiki-tte	tsukaikira-nai
vibrate	intr	hibiki-masu	hibiku	hibi-ite	hibika-nai
vomit	tr	haki-masu	haku	ha-ite	haka-nai
wait	tr/intr	machi-masu	matsu	ma-tte	mata-nai
walk	intr	aruki-masu	aruku	aru-ite	aruka-nai
wash	tr	aria-masu	arau	ara-tte	arawa-nai
wear (shoes)	tr	haki-masu	haku	ha-ite	haka-nai
wipe	tr	fuki-masu	fuku	fu-ite	fuka-nai
worry	intr	nayami-masu	nayamu	naya-nde	nayama-nai
write	tr	kaki-masu	kaku	ka-ite	kaka-nai

Ru-verbs

English	Transitive Intransitive	**Masu** form Verb base	Stem verb Dictionary form	**Te**-form	Negative form
accumulate/build up	intr	tamari-masu	tamaru	tama-tte	tamara-nai
accumulate/save	tr	tame-masu	tameru	tame-te	tame-nai
anger/upset	intr	okori-masu	okoru	oko-tte	okora-nai
appear/be visible	intr	araware-masu	arawareru	awarare-te	araware-nai

English	Transitive Intransitive	**Masu** form Verb base	Stem verb Dictionary form	Te-form	Negative form
apply/paint	tr	nuri-masu	nuru	nu-tte	nura-nai
attach	tr	tsuke-masu	tsukeru	tsuke-te	tsuke-nai
avoid/restrain	tr	hikae-masu	hikaeru	hikae-te	hikae-nai
bandage/bind	tr	shibari-masu	shibaru	shiba-tte	shibara-nai
bandage/bind (can)	intr	shibare-masu	shibareru	shibare-te	shibare-nai
be silent/not speak	intr	damari-masu	damaru	dama-tte	damara-nai
become	intr	nari-masu	naru	na-tte	nare-nai
become angry/ upset	intr	okori-masu	okoru	oko-tte	okora-nai
become numb	intr	shibire-masu	shibireru	shibire-te	shibire-nai
begin/start	tr	hajime-masu	hajimeru	hajime-te	hajime-nai
begin/start	intr	hajimari-masu	hajimaru	hajima-tte	hajimara-nai
bend	tr	mage-masu	mageru	mage-te	mage-nai
bend	intr	magari-masu	magaru	maga-tte	magara-nai
bite off	tr	kuichigiri-masu	kuichigiru	kuichigi-tte	kuichigira-nai
block/close	intr	fusagari-masu	fusagaru	fusaga-tte	fusaga-nai
close up/fill	tr	fusagi-masu	fusageru	fusage-te	fusage-nai
break	tr	ore-masu	oreru	ore-te	ore-nai
break	intr	ori-masu	oru	o-tte	ora-nai
bump/collide	tr	butsuke-masu	butsukeru	butsuke-te	butsuke-nai
bump/collide	intr	butsukari-masu	butsukaru	butsuka-tte	butsukara-nai
change/substitute	tr	kae-masu	kaeru	kae-te	kae-nai
change/substitute	intr	kawari-masu	kawaru	kawa-tte	kawara nai
change (clothes)	tr	kigae-masu	kigaeru	kigae-te	kigae-nai
choke	tr	tsumari-masu	tsumaru	tsuma-tte	tsumara-nai
close (door/win-dow)	tr	shime-masu	shimeru	shime-te	shime-nai
close (door/win-dow)	intr	shimari-masu	shimaru	shima-tte	shimara-nai
close (eye/mouth)	tr	toji-masu	tojiru	toji-te	toji-nai
collapse/fall down	intr	taore-masu	taoreru	taore-te	taore-nai
come*	intr	ki-masu	kuru	ki-te	ko-nai
come out/show up/appear	intr	de-masu	deru	de-te	de-nai

English	Transitive Intransitive	**Masu** form Verb base	Stem verb Dictionary form	Te-form	Negative form
complete/finish	intr	owari-masu	owaru	owa-tte	owara-nai
continue	tr	tsuzuke-masu	tsuzukeru	tsuzuke-te	tsuzuke-nai
cost/take	intr	kakari-masu	kakaru	kaka-tte	kakara-nai
cover	tr	kabuse-masu	kabuseru	kabuse-te	kabura-nai
cure/recover/heal	intr	naori-masu	naoru	nao-tte	naora-nai
cut	tr	kiri-masu	kiru	ki-tte	kira-nai
decrease	tr	herashi-masu	herasu	herashi-te	herara nai
decrease	intr	heri-masu	heru	he-tte	herasa-nai
develop skin rash	intr	kabure-masu	kabureru	kabure-te	kabure-nai
dim	intr	boyake-masu	boyakeru	boyake-te	boyake-nai
disappear/die	intr	nakunari-masu	nakunaru	nakuna-tte	nakunara-nai
do/play*	tr	shi-masu	suru	shi-te	shi-nai
eat	tr	tabe-masu	taberu	tabe-te	tabe-nai
end/stop/quit	tr	yame-masu	yameru	yam-te	yame-nai
enter/break into	intr	hairi-masu	hairu	hai-tte	haira-nai
exhaust, use up	tr	tsukaikiri-masu	tsukaikiru	tsukaiki-tte	tsukaikira-nai
exhaust	intr	tsukare-masu	tsukareru	tsukare-te	tsukare-nai
expire/cut well	intr	kire-masu	kireru	kire-te	kire-nai
extend/spread out	tr	hiroge-masu	hirogeru	hiroge-te	hiroge-nai
fall out/miss/skip	tr	nuke-masu	nukeru	nuke-te	nuke-nai
feel	tr	kanji-masu	kanjiru	kanji-te	kanji-nai
frighten	intr	obie-masu	obieru	obie-te	obie-nai
get off/step down	intr	ori-masu	ori-ru	ori-te	ori-nai
go up	tr	age-masu	ageru	age-te	age-nai
grind	tr	kezuri-masu	kezuru	kezu-tte	kezura-nai
grow	tr	hae-masu	haeru	hae-te	hae-nai
hang up	tr	kake-masu	kakeru	kake-te	kake-nai
hang/carry in the arms	tr	kakae-masu	kakaeru	kakae-te	kakae-nai
harden	tr	katakunari-masu	katakunaru	katakuna-tte	katakunara-nai
have a heavy stomach	intr	motare-masu	motareru	motare-te	motare-nai
hurt	tr	itame-masu	itameru	itame-te	itame-nai
increase	intr	fue-masu	fueru	fue-te	fue-nai
inform/notify	tr	shirase-masu	shiraseru	shirase-te	shira-nai

English	Transitive Intransitive	**Masu** form Verb base	Stem verb Dictionary form	**Te**-form	Negative form
infect/transmit/ move	intr	**utsuri-masu**	utsuru	utsu-tte	utsura-nai
insert	tr	**ire-masu**	ireru	ire-te	ire-nai
investigate/ examine	tr	**shirabe-masu**	shiraberu	shirabe-te	shirabe-nai
kick	tr	**keri-masu**	keru	ke-tte	kera-nai
know/detect	tr	**shiri-masu**	shiru	shi-tte	shira-nai
leak	intr	**more-masu**	moreru	more-te	more-nai
lift up/raise	tr	**age-masu**	ageru	age-te	age-nai
lift up/rise	intr	**agari-masu**	agaru	agatte	agara-nai
make/allow/do	tr	**sase-masu**	saseru	sase-te	sase-nai
manifest/appear	intr	**araware-masu**	arawareru	araware-te	araware-nai
measure	tr	**hakari-masu**	hakaru	haka-tte	hakara-nai
mix	tr	**maze-masu**	mazeru	maze-te	maze-nai
open	tr	**ake-masu**	akeru	ake-te	ake-nai
paint/put/spread	tr	**nuri-masu**	nuru	nu-tte	nura-nai
rebound/turn back	intr	**modori-masu**	modoru	modo-tte	modora-nai
receive	tr	**uke-masu**	ukeru	uke-te	uke-nai
recommend	tr	**susume-masu**	susumeru	susume-te	susume--nai
recover/heal	tr	**naori-masu**	naoru	nao-tte	naora-nai
recover/heal	intr	**naoshi-masu**	naosu	naoshi-te	naose-nai
return/go back	intr	**kaeri-masu**	kaeru	kae-tte	kaera-nai
roll up	tr	**makuri-masu**	makuru	maku-tte	makura-nai
rub	tr	**kosuri-masu**	kosuru	kosu-ttte	kosura-nai
run	intr	**hashiri-masu**	hashiru	hashi-tte	hashira-nai
save/remain	intr	**nokori-masu**	nokoru	nook-tte	nokora-nai
see/look/check up/examine	tr	**mi-masu**	miru	mi-te	mi-nai
sew together, stitch	tr	**nui-masu**	nuu	nu-tte	nuwa-nai
shiver	intr	**furue-masu**	furueru	furue-te	furue-nai
show	tr	**mise-masu**	miseru	mise-te	mise-nai
sit down	intr	**suwari-masu**	suwaru	suwa-tte	suwara-nai
sleep	intr	**ne-masu**	neru	ne-te	ne-nai
slip	intr	**suberi-masu**	suberu	sube-tte	subera-nai

English	Transitive Intransitive	**Masu** form Verb base	Stem verb Dictionary form	**Te**-form	Negative form
slump	intr	**meiri-masu**	**meiru**	**mei-tte**	**meira-nai**
soften/relieve/ ease	tr	**yawarage-masu**	**yawarageru**	**yawarage-te**	**yawarage-nai**
stand up	intr	**tachiagari-masu**	**tachiagaru**	**tachiaga-tte**	**tachiagara-nai**
stiffen	intr	**kori-masu**	**koru**	**ko-tte**	**kora-nai**
stick in	tr	**hikkakari-masu**	**hikkakaru**	**hikkaka-te**	**hikkakara-nai**
suppress/keep down	tr	**osae-masu**	**osaeru**	**osae-te**	**osae-nai**
swell	intr	**hare-masu**	**hareru**	**hare-te**	**hare-nai**
take off	tr	**tori-masu**	**toru**	**to-tte**	**tora-nai**
tight	tr	**shime-masu**	**shimeru**	**shime-te**	**shime-nai**
tighten/enlarge/ strain	intr	**hari-masu**	**haru**	**ha-tte**	**hara-nai**
tire	intr	**tsukare-masu**	**tsukareru**	**tsukare-te**	**tsukare-nai**
touch	intr	**sawari-masu**	**sawaru**	**sawa-tte**	**sawara-nai**
transmit/move	intr	**utsuri-masu**	**utsuru**	**utsu-tte**	**utsura-nai**
turn on	tr	**tsuke-masu**	**tsukeru**	**tsuke-te**	**tsuke-nai**
understand	intr	**wakari-masu**	**wakaru**	**waka-tte**	**wakara-nai**
wake up	intr	**oki-masu**	**okiru**	**oki-te**	**oki-nai**
warm, warm up	tr	**atatame-masu**	**atatameru**	**atatame-te**	**atatame-nai**
wear (clothes)	tr	**ki-masu**	**kiru**	**ki-te**	**ki-nai**

* Irregular verbs

6. Onomatopoetic Expressions for Pains and Complaints

Expressions for the Head

hidoi zutsū	severe headache
karui zutsū	light/mild headache
zuki-zuki suru zutsū	throbbing headache
hen-zutsū	migraine
wareru yōna zutsū	splitting headache
gan-gan suru zutsū	intense/pounding headache
zujyū-kan	heaviness of the head
atama ga guru-guru mawaru	have a spinning head
atama ga furatsuku	dizziness

Expressions for the Ears

mimi-nari	ringing in ears
mimi ga zuki-zuki	have a throbbing pain in ears
mimi ga kiri-kiri	have a tingling in ears
mimi ga fusagatte iru kanji	feeling of plugged-up ears
mimi ga yoku kikoe-nai	have trouble hearing

Expressions for the Eyes

me no itami	sore eyes
me no kayumi	itchy eyes
mabuta ga piku-piku	eyelid is twitching
me ga goro-goro	feel gritty/sandy
me ga chika-chika	see a flickering
me ga hiri-hiri	sting
me ga chiku chiku	have/feel a prickling sensation
me ga atsui kanji	feel hot
me no jyūketsu	bloodshot
me no kasumi	bleary
bonyari mieru	see things dimly
kasunde mieru	distant things look blurry

Expressions for the Nose

hana-mizu ga zuru-zuru	runny nose
hana-zsumari	stuffed-up nose
hana no naka no haremono	swelling in the nose
kushami	sneezing
hana-ji	nosebleed
ibiki o gū-gū kaku	snore

Expressions for the Throat

hentōsen no hare	swollen tonsils
nodo no kawaita kanji	feeling of a dry throat
nodo ga igarapoi kanji	feeling of a dry, raw, and scratchy throat
nodo ga tsumatta kanji	feeling of a clogged-up throat
nodo ga kara-kara	thirsty
nodo ga gara-gara	raspy throat
nodo ga hiri-hiri	sore throat
nodo ga chiku-chiku	prickly pain
nodo no hare	swollen throat
koe ga denai	lost voice
koe gare	hoarse voice
seki	coughing
tsuba o nomikomu to itai	pain when swallowing
museru	choking

Expressions for the Teeth

ha ga zukin-zukin	sharp pain (in a tooth)
ha ga shimiru	The tooth is sensitive.

ha ga gura-gura	loose tooth
ha ga gaku-gaku	wobbly tooth
hagishiri	gnash teeth

EXPRESSIONS FOR THE CHEST/HEART

mune ga zei-zei	wheezing in chest
mune ga doki-doki	heart is beating fast
mune/shinzō ga zuki-zuki	throbbing chest/heart
mune ga chiku-chiku	prickly pain in the chest
mune ga muka-muka	feel like vomiting
mune/shinzō ga shimetsuke-rareru	squeezing pain in chest/heart
mune/shinzō ga appaku sareru	pressed pain in chest/heart

EXPRESSIONS FOR THE STOMACH

i no geki-tsū	sharp pain in stomach
i no don-tsū	dull pain in stomach
i ga kiri-kiri	piercing pain
i ni sashi-komu itami	gripping pain in stomach
i no motare	heavy-pressing feeling in stomach
i ga omoi	heavy feeling in stomach
i ga chiku-chiku	prickly pain in stomach
i ni ana ga akisō na itami	feel pain like having a hole in stomach
i no appaku-kan	pressing feeling in stomach
i ga zuki-zuki	throbbing pain in stomach
gero-gero to haku	throw up/vomit

EXPRESSIONS FOR THE ABDOMEN

geki-tsū	severe pain/excruciating pain
don-tsū	dull pain
atsu-tsū	pressing pain
surudoi itami	sharp pain
shitsukoi itami	persistent pain
jizoku suru itami	continuous pain
sakeru-yōna itami	tearing pain
sasu itami	piercing pain
shiku-shiku suru itami	mild piercing pain
zukin to suru itmi	biting/pounding pain
zuki-zuki suru itami	throbbing pain
chiku-chiku suru itami	pricking pain
onaka ga pan-pan	fully enlarged stomach
onaka ga peko-peko	hungry
onaka ga pī-pī	diarrhea

EXPRESSIONS FOR URINE/URINATION

shimiru yōna itami	penetrating pain
yakeru yōna itami	burning pain
karui itami	mild pain
tsuyoi itami	severe pain

geki-tsū	very severe pain
sasaru itami	piercing pain
shitsukoi itami	persistent pain
nibui itami	dull pain
hai-nyō kon-nan	urination trouble
hin-nyō	frequent urination
zan-nyō kan	feeling of incomplete urination

Expressions for the Skin

mizu-bukure	blister
kabure	skin irritant
hada-are	rough skin
hada ga zara-zara	rough skin
hada ga kasa-kasa	dry skin
hada ga hiri-hiri	sore skin
hada ga beta-beta	oily skin
hada ga sube-sube	smooth skin
hada ga shito-shito	moist skin

Expressions for the Legs

komura-gaeri	leg cramp
ashi ga piku-piku	leg cramp
ashi no tsuri	leg cramp
ashi ga pan-pan	fully stretched leg muscles

Expressions for Children

ogyā-ogyā to naku	mewl (for babies, baby's cry)
meso-meso to naku	whimper
wan-wan to naku	howl with pain
eēn-eēn to naku	cry
yochi-yochi to aruku	toddle
niko-niko to warau	smile and laugh with happiness
chū-chū to nomu/suu	suck (for infants)
goku-goku to nomu	gulp
hai-hai suru	crawl (for baby)
guzu-guzu suru	do something slowly and hesitantly
chan to suru	meet a certain standard
choro-choro suru.	move with quick movement
gero-gero suru	vomit/throw up
pero-pero suru	licking
taion ga poka-poka (to) suru	body temperature feels pleasant (for babies)
hada ga gasa-gasa	dry skin
hada ga fuwa-fuwa	soft skin
onaka ga peko-peko	hungry
onaka ga pī-pī	diarrhea
me no pachi-kuri	open and close eyes
karada o nobi-nobi	stretch body
te o gū-pā	open and close hands

7. List of Illustrations

8. Answers to Comprehension Quizzes

Lesson 1.   1) c, 2) b, 3) d, 4) d, 5) c, 6) a, 7) b.
Lesson 2.   1) c, 2) b, 3) c, 4) a, 5) b, 6) a, 7) b, 8) b, 9) b, 10) c, 11) b, 12) b, 13) c.
Lesson 3.   1) a, 2) b, 3) b, 4) b, 5) c, 6) b, 7) a, 8) b, 9) a, 10) c, 11) c, 12) a, 13) b, 14) c, 15) b.
Lesson 4.   1) c, 2) c, 3) d, 4) c, 5) a, 6) b, 7) c, 8) a, 9) c, 10) b, 11) a, 12) c, 13) b, 14) a.
Lesson 5.   1) a, 2) b, 3) b, 4) b, 5) a, 6) b, 7) a, 8) b, 9) c, 10) c, 11) a, 12) b, 13) c, 14) a, 15) c.
Lesson 6.   1) d, 2) b, 3) c, 4) b, 5) c, 6) c, 7) b, 8) a, 9) c, 10) b.
Lesson 7.   1) b, 2) d, 3) d, 4) b, 5) b, 6) b, 7) a, 8) c, 9) d, 10) d.
Lesson 8.   1) d, 2) a, 3) b, 4) d, 5) c, 6) c, 7) a, 8) b, 9) c, 10) a.
Lesson 9.   1) a, 2) c, 3) c, 4) c, 5) c, 6) c, 7) b, 8) c, 9) a, 10) c, 11) b, 12) e, 13) c, 14) d, 15) a.
Lesson 10. 1) b, 2) c, 3) b, 4) a, 5) a, 6) b, 7) a, 8) c, 9) b, 10) c, 11) d, 12) c, 13) a, 14) c, 15) b.
Lesson 11. 1) a, 2) b, 3) c, 4) d, 5) a, 6) c, 7) b, 8) c, 9) a, 10) c, 11) b, 12) e) 13) c, 14) a, 15) d.

Lesson 12. 1) c, 2) a, 3) b, 4) d, 5) c, 6) g, 7) a, 8) c, 9) e, 10) b, 11) f, 12) d.
Lesson 13. 1) b, 2) a, 3) b, 4) c, 5) e, 6) f, 7) b, 8) c, 9) a, 10) d.
Lesson 14. 1) c, 2) b, 3) b, 4) a, 5) b, 6) d, 7) e, 8) a, 9) c.
Lesson 15. 1) a, 2) c, 3) b, 4) d, 5) d, 6) e, 7) c, 8) b, 9) a.
Lesson 16. 1) d, 2) d, 3) d, 4) c, 5) d, 6) c, 7) a, 8) b, 9) e.
Lesson 17. 1) c, 2) b, 3) a, 4) a, 5) e, 6) c, 7) d, 8) b, 9) a.
Lesson 18. 1) c, 2) d, 3) b, 4) b, 5) c, 6) b, 7) e, 8) a, 9) d.
Lesson 19. 1) c, 2) c, 3) d, 4) d, 5) c, 6) b, 7) a, 8) e, 9) d.
Lesson 20. 1) d, 2) c, 3) b, 4) b, 5) d, 6) e, 7) a, 8) b, 9) c.
Lesson 21. 1) d, 2) b, 3) b, 4) a, 5) a, 6) d, 7) c, 8) e, 9) b.
Lesson 22. 1) c, 2) b, 3) d, 4) a, 5) b, 6) e, 7) c, 8) a, 9) d.
Lesson 23. 1) a, 2) b, 3) d, 4) b, 5) c, 6) b, 7) d, 8) a, 9) e.
Lesson 24. 1) b, 2) b, 3) b, 4) c, 5) d, 6) b, 7) e, 8) a, 9) c.
Lesson 25. 1) b, 2) c, 3) a, 4) a, 5) b, 6) d, 7) e, 8) c, 9) a.
Lesson 26. 1) d, 2) b, 3) a, 4) b, 5) d, 6) e, 7) b, 8) c, 9) a.
Lesson 27. 1) b, 2) c, 3) a, 4) b, 5) b, 6) e, 7) a, 8) c, 9) d.
Lesson 28. 1) a, 2) d, 3) d, 4) b, 5) b, 6) e, 7) a, 8) c, 9) d.
Lesson 29. 1) b, 2) b, 3) d, 4) a, 5) e, 6) b, 7) a, 8) c, 9) d.
Lesson 30. 1) b, 2) c, 3) b, 4) c, 5) a, 6) d, 7) b, 8) c, 9) e.

9. Answers to Practices

LESSON 1

1. 1) **Ohayō gozaimasu,** 2) **Kon-nichi wa,** 3) **Konban wa,** 4) **Oyasumi nasai,** 5) **Sayōnara.**
2. 1) **Kon-nichi wa. Hajime-mashite,** 2) **Your name desu,** 3) Affiliation **no** your name **desu.**
3. 1) Your name **desu,** 2) Affiliation **no** your name **desu.**
4. 1) **Onamae wa nan-desu ka,** 2) **Oshigoto wan an-desu ka,** 4) **Onamae wa nan-desu ka.**
5. 1) **Suzuki-san desu,** 2) **Sandra-san desu,** 3) **Hai, shoshin desu,** 4) **Iie, oisha dewa arimasen,** 5) **Iie, kango-shi dewa arimasen.**
6. Sample answers: 1) Affiliation **no** your name **desu,** 2) Your occupation **desu,** 3) **Hai, Nihon-jin desu,** or **Iie, Nihon-jin dewa arimasen,** 4) **Hai, uketsuke desu,** or **Iie, uketsuke dewa arimasen,** 5) **Hai, byōki desu,** or **Iie, byōki dewa arimasen.**

LESSON 2

1. 1) **Onamae wa nan desu ka,** 2) **Netsu wa nan-do desu ka,** 3) **Odenwa-bangō wa nan-desu ka,** 4) **Go-jūsho wa doko desu ka,** 5) **Hoken-gaisha wa doko desu ka,** 6) **Hoken no shurui wa nan-desu ka,** 7) **Seibetsu wa nan-desu ka,** 8) **Kokoseki wa nan-desu ka.**
2. 1) **Hachi-zero-ni no nana-roku-san no yon-kyū-san-zero,** 2) **Hachi-zero-hachi no gō-kyū-ni no zero-yon-go-ichi,** 3) **Ni-zero-ichi no yon-roku-kyū no san-nana-zero-zero.**
3. 1) **Kashi kyū-jyū-hachi-do desu,** 2) **Kashi kyū-jyū-kyū-do gurai desu,** 3) **Sesshi san-jyū-kyū ten san-do desu,** or **sesshi san-jyū-kyū do san-bu desu,** 4) **Roku-jyū-ni desu,** 5) **Hachi-jyū-go desu.**
4. 1) **Suzuki-san desu,** 2) **802-773-9801 (Hachi-zero-ni no nana-nana-san no kyū-hachi-zero-ichi) desu,** 3) **Netsu ga arimasu,** 4) **101 (Hyaku-ichi) do gurai desu,** 5) **Iie, hoken wa arimasen.**
5. Sample answers. 1) Your name **desu,** 2) Your telephone number **desu,** 3) Your address **desu,** 4) Your nationality **desu,** 5) **Odaiji-ni.**

LESSON 3

1. 1) **Nan-nichi ga aite imasu ka**, 2) **Iie, yoyaku de ippai desu**, 3) **Hai, nan-ji ga ii desu ka**, 4) **Gogo yo-ji dake aite imasu**, 5) **Hai, aite imasu.**
2. 1) **Hai, aite imasu**, 2) **Iie, ippai desu**, 3) **Hai, aite imasu**, 4) **Iie, ippai desu.**
3. 1) **Koko-no-ka wa dōdesu ka**, 2) **Assate wa dō desu ka**, 3) **Gozen jyū-ichi-ji wa dō-desu ka.**
4. 1) **Sen-Kyū-hyaku-Kyū-jyū-San nen desu.**, 2) **Jyū-gasu desu**, 3) **Jyū-ni ji desu**, 4) **San-jyū-go fun desu.**
5. **Suzuki-san desu**, 2) **Hoken-jo no Kim-sensei desu**, 3) **Ashita desu**, 4) **Gogo San-ji-Han desu**, 5) **Iie, yoyaku de ippai deshita.**
6. Sample Answers: 1) Today's month and date **desu**, 2) Your birthdate (Year, Month, and Day) **desu**, 3) Your age **desu**, 4) Tomorrow's date **desu**, 5) Present time **desu**.

LESSON 4

1. 1) **Yoyaku wa shite arimasu ka**, 2) **Yoyaku wa shite arimasu ka**, 3) **Kinyū shite arimasu ka**, 4) **Kinyū shite arimasu ka.**
2. 1) **Kenkō-hoken ga arimasu ka**, 2) **Hoken-gaisha wa doko desu ka**, 3) **Hoken-kanyū-sha wa dare desu ka**, 4) **Tanjyō-bi wa itsu desu ka (Sei-nen-gappi wa itsu desu ka)**, 5) **Sei-betsu wa nan desu ka.**
3. 1) **Nui-de kudasai**, 2) **Nui-de kudasai**, 3) **Hazushi-te kudasai**, 4) **Hazushi-te-kudasai**, 5) **Nui-de kudasai.**
4. 1) **Ki-te kudasai**, 2) **Hai-te kudasai**, 3) **Tsuke-te kudasai**, 4) **Kake-te kudasai.**
5. 1) **X hoken-gaisha desu**, 2) **Hai, shite arimasu**, 3) **Gogo San-ji Han no yoyaku desu.** 4) **Oku-san desu (Suzuki-san no kanai desu)**, 5) **Iie, arimasen.**
6. Sample Answers: 1) **Hai, shite arimasu**, or **Iie, shite arimasen**, 2) **Hai, arimasu**, or **Iie, arimasen**, 3) Name of your country of origin **desu**, 4) Your employer's name **desu**.

LESSON 5

1. 1) **Atama ga itai(n) desu ka**, 2) **Shita ga itai(n) desu ka**, 3) **Senaka ga kayui(n) desu ka**, 4) **Kubi ga darui(n) desu ka.**
2. 1) **Itsu kara karada ga itai(n) desu ka**, 2) **Itsu kara kubi ga darui(n) desu ka**, 3) **Itsu kara itai(n) desu ka**, 4) **Itsu kara sono shōjyō ga arimasu ka.**
3. 1) **Ikka-getsu gurai desu**, 2) **Ni-shū-kan gurai desu**, 3) **San-ka-getsu-kan gurai desu.**
4. 1) **Nichi-yōbi deshita**, 2) **Ka-yōbi desu**, 3) **Do-yōbi deshita**, 4) **Sui-yōbi desu.**
5. 1) **Iie, mune wa itaku nai(n) desu**, 2) **sakuya kara desu**, 3) **Hai, sukoshi arimasu**, 4) 100.5°F (**Hyaku-ten go do gurai deshita**). 5) **Kesa desu.**
6) Sample Answers: 1) Today's date with past tense **deshita**, 2) Today's month with present tense **desu**, 3) What will you do this week with present/future tense **desu**, 4) **Hai, Nihon ni ikimasu**, or **Iie, Nihon ni ikimasen**, 5) What did you do in the last week with past tense **shimashita**.

LESSON 6

1. 1) **Hiza wa dō-desu ka**, 2) **Koshi wa dō-desu ka**, 3) **Te wa dō-desu ka**, 4) **Ashi-kubi wa dō-desu ka.**
2. 1) **Hare-te imasu (ne)**, 2) **Kanō shi-te imasu (ne)**, 3) **Kire-te imasu (ne)**, 4) **Ore-te imasu (ne).**
3. 1) **Yoku tai(n) desu ka/ne**, 2) **Itsumo desu ka/ne**, 3) **Tamani shibirete imasu ka/ne.**
4. 1) **Geki-tsū desu**, 2) **Surudoi itami desu**, 3) **Sasu itami desu**, 4) **don-tsū ga aimasu.**
5. 1) **Kafukubu desu**, 2) **Kinō no asa kara desu**, 3) **Iie, wakarimasen**, or **iie, arimasen**, 4) **Sasu itami desu**, 5) **Iie, tokuni arimasen.**
6. Sample Answers 1) **Hai**, body part **ga itai(n) desu**, or **Iie, tokuni arimasen**, 2) **Hai, ashi wa harete imasu**, or **Iie, harete imasen**, 3) Body part **ga** adverb **ita(n) desu**, 4) **Hai**, adverb **itaku arimasen**, or **Iie**, adverb **itai(n) desu**, 5) Adverb **ii desu**, or adverb **yoku arimasen**.

LESSON 7

1. 1) **Geri o shite imasu ka,** 2) **Tai-on o hakari-mashō,** 3) **Nani-ka kusuri o nonde imasu ka,** 4) **Shinchō wa ikutsu desu ka.**
2. 1) **Shoku-yoku ga arimasu ka,** 2) **Seiri ga arimasu ka,** 3) **Hie-shō desu ka,** 4) **Horō desu ka.**
3. 1) **Myaku o totte imasu,** 2) **Ketsu-atsu o hakatte imasu,** 3) **Ninshin o kensa shite imasu.**
4. 1) 120 (**Hyaku ni-jyū**) 80 (**Hachi-jyū**), 2) 105 (**Hyaku go**) 70 (**Nana-jyū**), 3) 133 (**Hyaku san-jyū san**) 65 (**Roku-jyū go**), 4) 154 (**Hyaku go-jyū yon**) 58 (**Go-jyū hachi**).
5. 1) **Onaka ga itai(n) desu,** 2) **Kinō kara desu,** 3) **Taion to ketsu-atsu desu,** 4) **Iie, geri wa shite imasen,** 5) **Iie, nanimo nonde imasen.**
6. Sample Answers: 1) **Hai, arimasu,** or **Iie, arimasen,** 2) Number **kiro desu,** 3) Number **senchi desu,** 4) **Ue wa** number **de, shita wa** number **desu,** 5) **Hai,** name of medicine **o nonde imasu,** or **Iie, nanimo nonde imasen.**

LESSON 8

1. **Hanaji ga demasu ka,** 2) **Kettan ga demasu ka,** 3) **Ketsu-nyō ga demasu ka,** 4) **Ketsu-ben ga demasu ka.**
2. 1) **Itsu shoku-yoku-fushi ga hajimari mashie ka,** or **Itsu kara shoku-yoku-fushin desu ka,** 2) **Itsu benpi ga hajimari mashita ka,** or **Itsu kara benpi desu ka,** 3) **Itsu shukketsu ga hajimari mashita ka,** or **Itsu kara shukketsu desu ka.** 4) **Itsu hasshin ga hajimari mashie ka,** or **Itsu kara hasshin desu ka.**
3. 1) **Hukide-mono wa dō-desu ka,** 2) **Yakedo wa dō-desu ka,** 3) **Shisshin wa dō-desu ka.**
4. 1) **Futsu-ka mae kara desu,** 2) **Mikka mae kara desu,** 3) **Isshu-kan mae kara desu,** 4) **Ikka-getsu mae kara desu.**
5. 1) **Hai, shimasu,** 2) **Hai, sukoshi arimasu,** 3) **Kinō kara desu,** 4) **Iie, shite imasen,** 5) **Mikka-mae kara desu.**
6. Sample Answers: 1) **Hai, himan-gimi desu,** or **Iie, himan-gimi dewa arimasen,** 2) **Hai, hinketsu gimi desu,** or **Iie, hinketsu gimi dewa arimasen,** 3) **Hai, imasu,** or **Iie, imasen,** 4) **Hai, netsu ga arimasu,** or **Iie, netsu wa arimasen,** 5) **Iie, arimasen,** or **Hai, arimasu.**

LESSON 9

1. 1) **Koshi no shōjyō wa dō-desu ka,** 2) **Kansetsu-tsū wa dō-desu ka,** 3) **Nikibi wa wa dō-desu ka,** 4) **Okan wa dō-desu ka.**
2. 1) **En-shō mitai desu,** 2) **uchimi mitai desu,** 3) **Mushi-uchi-shō kamo shiremasen,** 4) **Hen-zutsū kamo shiremasen.**
3. 1) **Watakushi no hō o mite kudasai,** 2) **Ugokanai de kudasai,** 3) **Watakushi no yubi o mite kudasai.**
4. 1) **Tachi-kurami mitai desu,** 2) **Dōki mitai desu,** 3) **Seiri-tsū mitai desu,** 4) **Mune-yake mitai desu.**
5. 1) **Mune ga itai(n) desu,** 2) **Kinō kara desu,** 3) **Hai, tokidoki arimasu,** 4) **Ikigire to dōki to iki-gurushii(n) desu,** 5) **Shinzō mitai desu.**
6. Sample Answers: 1) **Hai, arimasu,** or **Iie, arimasen,** 2) **Hai, itai(n) desu,** 3) **Hai,** body part **ga itai(n) desu,** or **Iie, arimasen,** 4) **Hai, shimasu,** or **Iie, shimasen,** 5) **Hai, tottemo ii desu,** or **Iie, yoku nai desu.**

LESSON 10

1. 1) **Eiyō-busoku no yō desu,** 2) **Undō-busoku no yō desu,** 3) **Tabe-sugi mitai desu,** 4) **Nomi-sugi mitai desu,** 5) **Kusuri no nomi-sugi mitai desu.**
2. 1) **Iie, dame desu yo,** 2) **Hai, ii desu yo,** 3) **Denwa o shite kudasai,** 4) **Hai, shite kudasai,** 5) **Hai, ie de ryōyō shite kudasai.**

3. 1) **Kono kensa-gi ni kigaete kudasai,** 2) **Ao-muke ni natte kudasai,** 3) **Makuttte kudasai,** 4) **Muki o kaete kudasai,** 5) **Shinsatsu-dai kara orite kudasai.**
4. 1) **Kaikei de onegai shimasu,** or **Kaikei de haratte kudasai,** 2) **Shohōsen o moratte kudasai,** 3) **Raigetsu kite kudasai,** 4) **Odaiji ni.**
5. 1) **Seijyō deshita,** 2) **Hai, ii desu,** 3) **Hai, jyū-bun totte kudasai,** 4) **Sugi-ni naorimasu.**
6. 1) Sample Answers: 1) **Hai, jyū-bun totte kudasai,** or **Iie, tora-nai-de kudasai,** 2) **Hai, non-de kudasai,** or **Iie, noma-nai-de kudasai,** 3) **Hai, ii desu,** or **Iie, tai-in shitemo ii desu yo,** 4) **Hai, ii desu yo,** or **Iie, mada desu.**

Lesson 11

1. 1) **Hai wa dō-desu ka,** 2) **I wa dō-desu ka,** 3) **Shinzō wa dō-desu ka,** 4) **Kikanshi wa dō-desu ka.**
2. 1) **Kōmon o mite mimashō,** or **Kōmon o kensa shimashō,** 2) **Ketsu-eki kensa o shimashō,** 3) **Nyō-kensa o shimashō.** 4) **Rentogen o torimashō.**
3. Sample Answers: 1) **I-en dato omoimasu,** 2) **Mōchō-en no utagai ga airmasu,** 3) **Bōkō-en no yō desu.**
4. 1) **Shinzō o kensa shimashō,** or **Shinzō o mimashō,** 2) **Shikyū o kensa shimashō,** or **Shikyū mimashō,** 3) **Kanzō o kensa shimashō,** or **Kanzō o mimashō,** 4) **Suizō o kensa shimashō,** or **Suizō o mimashō,** 5) **Daichō o kensa shimashō,** or **Daichō o mimashō.**
5. 1) **I ga itai(n) desu,** 2) **kiri-kiri suru itami desu,** 3) **Onaka ga sukuto itai(n) desu,** 4) **Iie, shita koto ga arimasen,** 5) **I-kaiyō dato omowaremasu.**
6. Sample Answers: 1) **Hai, arimasu,** or **Iie, arimasen,** 2) **Hai, itai(n) desu,** or **Iie, itaku arimasen,** 3) **Hai,** body part **ga warui(n) desu,** or **Iie, waruku arimasen,** 4) **Hai, daijōbu desu,** or **Iie, dame desu,** or **Iie, yoku arimasen,** 5) **Hai,** name of medicine **o non-de imasu,** or **Iie, nanimo non-de imasen.**

Lesson 12

1. 1) **Ketsu-eki kensa ga hitsuyō desu,** 2) **Shinden-zu kensa ga hitsuyō desu,** 3) **Nō-ha kensa ga hitsuyō desu,** 4) **I-kamera kensa ga hitsuyō desu,** 5) **Rentogen kensa ga hitsuyō desu.**
2. 1) **Nyō o san-bun no ichi, totte kudasai/onegai shimasu,** 2) **Sode o makutte kudasai/agete kudasai,** 3) **Fuku o nuide kudasai.**
3. 1) **Hidari o mite kudasai,** 2) **Migi o mite kudasai,** 3) **Kuchi o akete kudasai,** 4) **Rirakkusu shite kudasai,** 5) **Shita o misete/dashite kudasai.**
4. 1) **Nyō/oshikko o kappu han-bun totte kudasai,** or **Kappu ni-bun-no ichi nyō/oshikko o onegai shimasu,** 2) **Nyō o kappu san-bun no ichi totte kudasai,** or **Kappu san-bun-no ichi nyō o onegai shimasu,** 3) **Nani-yorimo tabe-tari non-dari shite kudasai,** 4) **Nani-yorimo, yasun-dari, ne-tari shite kudasai.**
5. 1) **Hidoi ne-ase ga demasu,** 2) **Hai, tokidoki kettan ga demasu,** 3) **Saikin desu,** 4) **Rentogen kensa desu.**
6. Sample Answers: 1) **Hai, arimasu,** or **Iie, arimasen,** 2) Day **mae desu,** 3) **Hai, shite imasu,** or **Iie, shite imasen,** 4) **Mondai wa arimasen deshita,** or **Sukoshi takai desu,** or **Sukoshi yoku-nakkata desu.**

Lesson 13

1. 1) **Kūyō ga hitsuyō desu,** 2) **Eiyō o jyūbun totte kudasai,** 3) **Tsumetai-mono wa hikaete kudasai,** 4) **Nyūin ga hitsuyō desu,** 5) **Tsūin ga hitsuyō desu,** or **Tsūin suru hitsuyō ga arimasu,** 6) **Saihatsu ni kiotsukete kudasai,** 7) **Kekka wa yōsei desu,** 8) **Kekka wa insei desu,** 9) **Kekka wa giji-yōsei desu,** 10) **Kono kusuri wa fuku-sayō ga arimasu.**
2. 1) **Hai, kite kudasai,** 2) **Sono-mama chotto matte kudasai,** 3) **Suguni yoku narimasu yo,** 4) **Tsugi desu yo,** 5) **Kaikei de (o)shikarai kudasai.**
3. 1) **Ansei ni shite-ite kudasai,** 2) **Nyūin no hitsuyō ga arimasen,** 3) **Kensa no kekka ga detara denwa (o) shimasu.**

4. 1) Iie, ikimasen, 2) Shindan-sho ga hitsuyō desu, 3) Ni-shū-kan desu, 4) Tsūin suru hitsuyō ga ari-masu, 5) Sai-hatsu ga shinpai desu.
5. Sample Answers: 1) Hai, shite imasu, or Iie, shite imasen, 2) Hai, sukoshi/takusan arimasu, or Iie, arimasen, 3) Hai, shite imasu, or Iie, shite imasen, 4) Hai, arimasu, or Iie, arimasen, 5) Hai, ari-masu, or Iie, arimasen.

Lesson 14
1. 1) (Hifu ni) nutte kudasai, 2) Koshi ni hatte kudasai, 3) Mizu de nonde kudasai, or Mizu de fukuyō shite kudasai, 4) Jūsu to issho ni nonde kudasai, 5) Kōmon ni irete kudasai.
2. 1) Chintsū-zai desu, 2) Shōka-zai desu, 3) Genetsu-zai desu, 4) Kaze-gusuri desu.
3. 1) Shohōsen o omochi desu ka, or Shohōsen o kudasai, 2) Hai, yoku kikimasu yo, 3) Suguni de-masu, 4) Shinpai wa arimasen, 5) Nakunaru made nonde kudasai.
4. 1) Kore wa dō-desu ka, or Kore wa ikaga desu ka, 2) Kakasazu mai-nichi nonde kudasai, 3) Hai, gozai-masu.
5. 1) Hai, arimasu, 2) 808-509-8349 (Hachi-zero-hachi no gō-zero-kyū no hachi-san-yon-kyū) desu, 3) Iie, arimasen, 4) Sukoshi nemuku-naru kamo shiremasen, 5) Ni-jyuppun go desu.
6. Sample Answers: 1) Hai, arimasu, or Iie, arimasen, 2) Funmatsu-zai desu, or Kapuseru-zai desu, 3) Hai, arimasu, or Iie, arimasen, 4) Hai, nonde imasu, or Iie, nonde imasen, 5) Hai, sashite imasu, or Iie, sashite imasen.

Lesson 15
1. 1) Shoku-zen ni onomi kudasai/fukuyō shite kudasai, 2) Shokkan ni onomi kudasai/fukuyō shite kudasai, 3) Shoku-go ni onomi kudasai/fukuyō shite kudasai, 4) Kūfuku-ji ni fukuyō shite kudasai, 5) Kūfuku-ji ni fukuyō shinaide kudasai.
2. 1) Supūn ni-hai desu, 2) Tēburu-supūn ippai desu, 3) San-jyō desu, 4) Ni-jyō desu.
3. 1) Kono kusuri o fukuyō-go/nondara, ni-jikan wa unten shinaide kudasai, 2) Kono kusuri o non-dara, arukōru wa noma-naide kudasai, 3) Kodomo no te no todokanai tokoro ni hokan shite ku-dasai, 4) Kono kusuri wa suzushii tokoro ni hokan shite kusasai, 5) Kono kusuri o nonde, ijyō o kanjitara, sugu ni i-shi ni sōdan shite kudasai.
4. 1) Shoku-go sanjyuppun inai desu, 2) San-kai desu, 3) Ni-jyō desu, 4) Iie, nome-masen, 5) Jiko-futan kihon-ryōkin desu, 6) Hai, hoken ga kikimasu.
5. Sample Answers: 1) Hai, nomimasu, or Iie, nomimasen, 2) Hai, setsumei shimasu, or Iie, setsumei shimasen, 3) Iie, yasui desu, or Iie, takaku nai desu, 4) Hai, yasui desu, 5) Hai, nonde imasu, or Hai, fukuyō shite imasu, or Hai, nonde imasu, or Iie, fukuyō shite imasen, or Iie, nonde imasen.

Lesson 16
1. 1) Yōren-kin kansen-shō desu, 2) Uirusu desu, 3) Bakuteria desu, 4) Shin-gata uirusu desu, 5) Kisetsu-fūdesu.
2. 1) Mune ni hosshin ga dete imasu/araware-te imasu, 2) Kubi ni suihō ga dekite imasu, 3) Senaka ni shisshin ga dekite imasu, 4) Kuchi ni kizu ga airmasu, 5) Kō-netsu desu.
3. 1) Kensa ga hitsuyō desu, 2) Kyūyō ga hitsuyō desu, 3) Sui-bun ga hitsuyō desu, 4) Kōsei-bushitsu o nonde kudasai, 5) Hiyashite kudasai.
4. 1) Kato-san no musuko-san desu, 2) Saku-ya kara desu, 3) Suihō ga kayui desu, 4) 38.8 (san-jyū hachi-ten hachi-do) desu, 5) Mizu-bōsō desu.
5. Sample Answers:1) Hai, uke-mashita, or Iie, ukete imasen, 2) Hai, imasu, or Iie, imasen, 3) Hai, kakari-mashita, or Iie, kakarimasen deshita, 4) Hai, ukemashita, or Iie, ukete imasen, 5) Hai, shi-mashita, or Iie, shite imasen.

LESSON 17

1. 1) Taion-kei o shita no shita ni irete kudasai, 2) Kuchi o akete aā to itte kudasai, 3) Nyūin ga hitsuyō desu, 4) Hentō-sen ga harete imasu.
2. Sample Answers: 1) Hai-kekkaku kamo shiremasen/mitai desu, 2) Hai-en no yō desu, 3) Kikanshi-en mitai desu, 4) Zensoku kamo shiremasen.
3. 1) Shoki no yō desu, 2) Chūki no yō desu, 3) Makki no yō desu.
4. 1) Chiku-chiku shimasu, 2) zei-zei shimasu, 3) zukin-zukin shimasu, 4) doki-doki shimasu.
5. 1) Futsu-ka mae kara desu, 2) Zei-zei to seki ga dete, tan ga tsuzuite, netsu-poi(n) desu, 3) Mune desu, 4) sasu-yō na itami desu, 5) Ketsu-eki kensa to CRP kensa desu.
6. Sample Answers: 1) Hai, fumin-shō mitai desu, or Iie, fumin-shō dewa arimasen, 2) Hai, arimasu, or Iie, arimasen, 3) Hai, imasu, or Iie, imasen, 4) Hai, harete imasu, or Iie, harete imasen, 5) Hai, kakatta koto ga arimasu, or Iie, kakatta koto ga arimasen.

LESSON 18

1. 1) Fukai-kan desu, 2) Sōkai-kan desu, 3) Datsu-ryoku-kan desu, 4) Fuan-kan desu, 5) Anshin-kan desu.
2. Sample Answers: 1) Doko ga itai(n) desu ka, 2) Shōjyō wa dō-desu ka, 3) Kokyū wa dō-desu ka, 4) Shōjyō wa dō-desu ka/nan-desu ka, 5) Shinzō wa dō-desu ka, 6) Don-na itami desu ka, 7) Itami wa dō-desu ka.
3. 1) Enbun ni ki o tsukete kudasai, 2) Amai-mono ni ki o tsukete kudasai, 3) Osake ni ki o tsukete kudasai, 4) Und dō ni ki o tsukete kudasai, 5) Karada ni ki o tsukete kudasai.
4. 1) Dōki ga shimasu, 2) Kibun ga warukute, kokyū ga shinikui desu, 3) Shinden-zu kensa to Toro-ponin tesuto desu, 4) Kyū-sei shinkin kōsoku desu, 5) Nyūin ga hitsuyō desu.
5. Sample Answers: 1) Hai, shimasu, or Iie, shimasen, 2) Hai, hinketsu-gimi desu, or Iie, hinketsu-gimi dewa arimasen, 3) Ketsu-atsu wa takai desu, or Ketsu-atsu wa hikui desu, 4) Hai, tokidoki/sukoshi itaku narimasu, or Iie, itaku wa narimasen, 5) Hai, saserare-mashita, or Iie, saserare-masen.

LESSON 19

1. 1) I-keiren wa dō-nasare mashita ka, 2) I-kaiyō wa dō-nasare-mashita ka, 3) Tanseki wa ikaga desu ka, 4) Mōchō-en wa dō nasare mashita ka, 5) Ji wa dō-nasare mashita ka.
2. Sample Answers: 1) I ga motarete imasu ka, 2) I ni appaku-kan ga arimasu ka, 3) I ni zuki-zuki suru itami ga arimasu ka, 4) I ni chiku-chiku suru itami ga airmasu ka, 5) I ni don-na itami ga arimasu ka.
3. 1) Geki-tsū ga shimasu, 2) Motare-te imasu, 3) Kiri-kiri suru itami desu, 4) Omoi-kanji desu, 5) Don-tsū ga arimasu.
4. 1) Onaka ga itai(n) desu, 2) Kinō kara desu, 3) Hanasu to itai(n) desu, 4) Kūsei-chūsui-en desu.
5. Sample Answers:1) Hai, tottemo/sukoshi ii desu, or Chotto/sukoshi warui(n) desu, 2) Hai, arimasu, or Iie, arimasen, 3) Hai, sukoshi itai(n) desu, or Iie, itakuwa arimasen, 4) Benpi-gimi desu, or Chōshi ga ii desu, 5) Iie, narimasen, or Hai, narimashita.

LESSON 20

1. 1) Oshikko ga demasu ka, 2) Oshikko wa gaman shinaide kudasai, 3) Isshu-kan gurai de yoku na-rimasu, 4) Osake wa hikaete kudasai, 5) Seikō o suru toki ni itai(n) desu ka, or Seikō no toki itami o tomonai masu ka.
2. 1) Kanzō no en-shō no koto desu, 2) Tochū no nyō no koto desu, 3) Nyō no koto desu, 4) Bokki-fuzen no koto desu, 5) Sei-byō no koto desu.
3. 1) Yakeru yō na itami desu, 2) Karui itami desu, 3) Nibui itami ga arimasu, 4) Hin-nyō desu, 5) Hai-nyō-shōgai desu.

4. 1) **Nyō ni chi ga majirimasu,** 2) **Fukubu-ekō kensa o shimashita,** 3) **Hai-nyō ga owaru toki ni itami o tomonaimasu,** 4) **Kyū-sei bōkō-en desu,** 5) **Mikka teido desu.**
5. Sample Answers: 1) **Hai, sukoshi/chotto arimasu,** or **Iie, arimasen,** 2) **Hai, arimasu,** or **Iie, arimasen,** 3) **Hai, shimashita,** or **Iie, shite imasen,** 4) **Iie, arimasen,** or **Sukoshi mondai ga aruyō desu,** 5) **Iie, arimasen,** or **Hai, natta koto ga arimasu.**

LESSON 21
1. 1) **Doko mo waruku arimasen,** 2) **Sukoshi mo waruku arimasen,** 3) **Nani mo shinpai shinai de kudasai,** 4) **Mettani arimasen,** 5) **Kesshite arimasen.**
2. 1) **Bitamin ketsubō-shō no yō desu,** 2) **Kakke mitai desu,** 3) **Ryūmachi no yō desu,** 4) **Arukōru chū-doku kamo shiremasen,** 5) **Himan no yō desu.**
3. 1) **Hidoi zutsū desu ne,** 2) **karui zutsū desu ne,** 3) **Hen-zutsū desu ka,** 4) **Zujyū-kan desu ne,** 5) **Zuki-zuki suru zutsū desu ne,** 6) **Gan-gan suru zutsū desu ne,** 7) **Wareru yō na zutsū desu ne.**
4. 1) **Memai to mimi-nari ga airmasu,** 2) **Takai desu,** 3) **Ue wa 175 (Hyaku nana-jyū go) de, shita wa 105 (Hyaku go) desu.** 4) **Zatsu-on ga shimasu,** 5) **Dōmyaku-kōka no chōkō desu.**
5. Sample Answers: 1) **Hai, arimasu,** or **Iie, arimasen,** 2) **Hai, sukoshi himan-shō gimi desu,** or **Iie, himan-shō dewa arimasen,** 3) **Hai, jikaku-shōjyō ga gozaimasu,** or **Iie, gozaimasen,** 4) **Hai, toki-doki mimi-nari ga shimasu,** or **Iie, shimasen,** 5) **Hai, shimashita,** or **Iie, shimasen deshita.**

LESSON 22
1. 1) **Aza ga airmasu,** 2) **Hidari hiza ga oregte imasu,** 3) **Tabun dakkyū desu ne,** 4) **Migi-ashi-kubi ga nenza shite imasu,** 5) **Hito-sashi-yubi ga tsuki-yubi desu ne.**
2. 1) **Ashi o magete kudasai,** 2) **Koshi o nobashite kudasai,** 3) **Kubi o mawashite kudasai,** 4) **Kata o ue to shita ni ugokashite kudasai,** 5) **Yukkuri koshi o ugokashite kudasai.**
3. 1) **Kenin ryōhō ga hitsuyō desu ne,** 2) **Rei-shippu o nutte kudasai,** 3) **Gibusu o shite kudasai,** 4) **Korusetto o tsukete kudasai,** 5) **Undō no shi-sugi ni ki o tsukete kudasai.**
4. 1) **Koshi o itame mashita,** 2) **Iie, shibirete imasen,** 3) **Ashi o ageru toki ni itami masu,** 4) **Hai, ari-masu,** 5) **Migi-ashi desu,** 6) **Tsuikanban herunia dewa naikato omoimasu.**
5. Sample Answers: 1) **Hai, shimasu,** or **Iie, shimasen,** 2) **Hai, seijyō dato omoimasu,** 3) **Hai, itakkata desu,** or **Iie, itakuwa arimasen deshita,** 4) **Hai, arimasu,** or **Iie, arimasen,** 5) **Hai, arimasu,** or **Iie, arimasen.**

LESSON 23
1. 1) **Mabataki no toki itami masu ka/itai(n) desu ka,** 2) **Ōkiku ryō-me o akete kudasai,** 3) **Me-gusuri o sashi masu ka,** 4) **Me ni sawattari kosuttari shimashita ka,** 5) **Nijyū ni miemasu ka.**
2. 1) **Ue o mite kusasai,** 2) **Shita o mite kudasai,** 3) **Hidari-gawa o mite kudasai,** 4) **Migi-gawa o mite kudasai,** 5) **Sensei no yubi o mite kudasai.**
3. 1) **Me ga chiku-chiku shite imasu ka,** 2) **Me ga chika-chika shite imasu ka,** 3) **Me ga hiri-hiri shite imasu ka,** 4) **Me ga piku-piku shite imasu ka.**
4. 1) **Sujitu-mae kara desu,** 2) **Enshō o okoshite imasu,** 3) **Ni-san-shū-kan desu,** 4) **Ni-san-shū-kan teido desu,** 5) **Taoru nado o hoka no hito to kyoyū shinai de kudasai,** 6) **Isshū-kan-go desu.**
5. Sample Answers: 1) **Hai, shiryoku kensa o uke-mashita,** or **Iie, mada desu,** 2) **Hai, arimasu,** or **Iie, arimasen,** 3) **Hai, shimasu,** or **Iie, shimasen,** 4) **Kinshi desu,** or **Enshi desu,** 5) **Hai, kakemasu,** or **Iie, kakemasen.**

LESSON 24
1. 1) **Nodo ga hiri-hiri desu,** 2) **Nodo ga gara-gara desu,** 3) **Mimi ga zukin-zukin itami masu,** 4) **Mimi ga fusagatte iru kanji desu,** 5) **Nodo ga tsumatta kanji desu.**

2. 1) **Kuchi o akete (kudasai),** 2) **Hana-no-ana o misete (kudasai),** 3) **Hidari o mite (kudasai),** or **Hi-dari ni atama o mukete (kudasai),** 4) **Mimi o misete (kudasai),** 5) **Kafun-shō wa naori-nikui desu.**

3. 1) **Hidari-mimi kara mimi-dare ga dete imasu (yo),** 2) **Mimi-aka wa katai desu (yo),** 3) **Hidari-mi-mi ni porīpu ga dekite imasu (yo),** 4) **Nodo ga harete imasu kara nomikomu toki itai to omoi-masu,** 5) **Hana-no-ana ni en-shō ga arimasu (ne).**

4. 1) **Miminari to memai ga shite tatte iraremasen,** 2) **Karada ni shibire wa arimasen,** 3) **Kō-on no miminari ga shite, oto ga kikoe nikui desu,** 4) **Mā-mā desu,** 5) **Naiji no kinō-shōgai desu,** 6) **Ondo-ganshin kensa desu.**

5. Sample Answers: 1) **Hai, shimasu,** or **Iie, shimasen,** 2) **Hai, uke-mashita,** or **Iie, ukete imasen,** 3) **Hai, kafun-shō desu,** or **Iie, kafun-shō dewa arimasen,** 4) **Hai, kakuto omoimasu,** or **Iie, kaka-nai to omoimasu,** 5) **Hai, narimasu,** or **Iie, narimasen.**

LESSON 25

1. 1) **Suihō ga arimasu,** or **Mizu-bukure desu (ne),** 2) **Tōshō desu (ne),** 3) **Hasshin desu (ne),** 4) **Kansō-hada desu (ne),** 5) **Shisei-hada desu (ne),** or **Abura-ppoi desu (ne).**

2. 1) **Tsume o mijikaku kitte kudasai,** 2) **Ashi o misete kudasai,** 3) **Ashi o kirei ni shite-ite kudasai,** 4) **Nuri-gusuri o agemasu,** or **Nankō o dashimasu,** 5) **Kao o aratte kudasai.**

3. 1) **Oshiri ni odeki ga arimasu,** or **Denbu ni fukude-mono ga arimasu (ne),** 2) **Hidoi fuke desu (ne),** 3) **Keshō-hin ga gen-in no hasshin ga airmasu,** 4) **Kadada zentai ni hasshin ga dete imasu,** 5) **Kubi ni shisshin ga dekite imasu,** or **Kubi ni shisshin ga airmasu (ne).**

4. 1) **Wakino-shita ni hasshin ga dekite/dete imasu,** 2) **Sakana o tabemashita,** 3) **densen-sei nōkashin desu,** or **Tobihi desu,** 4) **Kōsei-bushitsu no nankō to kō-hisutamin no nomi-gusuri desu,** 5) **Te-arai ya, tsume ya, karada no seiketsu ni ki o tsukemasu.**

5. Sample Answers: 1) **Hai, tokidoki demasu,** or **Iie, demasen,** 2) **Hai, hiyake o shite imasu,** or **Iie, hiyake wa shite imasen,** 3) **Hai, ki ni narimasu,** or **Iie, ki ni narimasen,** 4) **Hai, arimasu,** or **Iie, ari-masen,** 5) **Hai, arimasu,** or **Iie, arimasen.**

LESSON 26

1. 1) **Suimin-dōnyū-zai o nonde kudasai,** 2) **Nyūin o osusume shimasu,** 3) **Kyūyō o shite kudasai,** or **Kyūyō o osusume shimasu,** 4) **Yase dashimashita (ne),** 5) **Rirakkusu shite kudasai.**

2. 1) **Futori-gimi desu (ne),** 2) **Tsukare-gimi desu ne,** 3) **Utsu-(jyōtai)-gimi desu,** 4) **Fumin-shō-gimi desu,** 5) **Yaku-butsu ranyō-gachi desu (ne).**

3. 1) **Sutoresu ga arimasu ka,** 2) **Genchō ga arimasu ka,** or **Genchō ga shimasu ka,** 3) **Fuan-hossa ga arimasu ka,** 4) **Fumin-shō desu ka,** 5) **Zetsubō-kan ga shimasu ka.**

4. 1) **Koko san-ka-getsu-kan desu,** 2) **Yoru mo yoku nemure-nai shi, karada mo tsukare-gimi desu,** or **Shoku-yoku ga arimasen,** or **Kadara ga tsukare-yasuku, kuchi ga kawaite, benpi-gachi desu,** 3) **Ki ga meiri-masu,** 4) **Utsu-jyōtai desu,** 5) **Kyūyō to yaku-butsu ryōhō ga hitsuyō desu.**

5. Sample Answers: 1) **Hai, tokidoki arimasu,** or **Iie, zenzen arimasen,** 2) **Hai, kanji masu,** or **Iie, kanji masen,** 3) **Hai, narimasu,** or **Iie, narimasen,** 4) **Hai, sō desu,** or **Iie, chigai-masu,** 5) **Hai, omoi-masu,** or **Iie, omoi-masen.**

LESSON 27

1. 1) **Byōki no gen-in wa fumei desu,** or **Byōki no gen-in wa wakarimasen,** 2) **Byōki no gen-in ga wakari-mashita,** 3) **Kafukubu-tsū no gen-in wa uirusu desu,** 4) **Gan no gen-in wa fumei desu,** or **Gan no gen-in wa wakarimasen,** 5) **Surotesu ga funin-shō no gen-in ni natte iru gaai ga ōi desu,**

2. 1) **Yon bun-no ichi inchi desu,** 2) **San bun-no yon inchi desu,** 3) **Ni miri (mētoru) desu,** 4) **Kōsei-bushitsu o shohō shimasu,** 5) **Sukoshi kyūyō o osusume shimasu,** or **Sukoshi yasunde kudasai.**

3. 1) **Kutsu wa nuide kudasai,** 2) **Hai, shinsatsu-dai ni agatte kudasai,** 3) **Te wa mune no ue de kunde kudasai,** 4) **Karada no chikara o nuite kudasai,** 5) **Mō-shukoshi, sagatte kudasai.**

4. 1) **Yoku tsukarete, ikigire o kanshi masu, soreni, hinketsu-gimi desu,** 2) **Hai, ichiō jyunchō desu,** 3) **Koko sū-ka-getsu desu,** 4) **Naishin to chō-onpa de kensa o shimasu,** 5) **Chō-onpa kensa de chokkei ni-senchi hodo no kinshu ga mitsukari-mashita.**
5. Sample Answers: 1) **Hai, shimasu,** or **Iie, shimasen,** 2) **Hai, kekkō desu,** or **Iie, dame desu,** 3) **Hai, ita-gattari shite imasu,** 4) **Hai, daijyōbu desu,** or **Iie, daijyōbu dewa arimasen,** 5) **Hai, shinpai desu,** or **Iie, shinpai dewa arimasen.** 6) **Hai, hinin o suru yō ni shite imasu,** or **Iie, shite imasen.**

LESSON 28

1. 1) **Iki o yukkuri suttee kudasai,** 2) **Iki o yukkuri haite kudasai,** 3) **Iki o ōkiku suttee kudasai,** 4) **Iki o ōkiku/fukaku haite kudasai,** 5) **Iki o suttari, haitai shite kudasai.**
2. 1) **Ikinde kudasai,** 2) **Motto ikinde kudasai,** 3) **Tsuyoku ikinde kudasai,** 4) **Ikima-naide kudasai,** 5) **Ikimu no o yamete kudasai.**
3. 1) **Mune ga muka-muka shimasu ka,** or **Haki-ke ga shimasu ka,** 2) **Zukin-sukin shimasu ka,** 3) **Onaka ga pan-pan ni hatte imasu,** or **Onaka ga hatte imasu (ne),** 4) **Ashi ga tsutte imasu (ne),** 5) **Ashi ga pan-pan ni hatte imasu.**
4. 1) **Ninshin kensa desu,** 2) **Yon-ka-getsu-gurai mae deshita,** 3) **Mune ga muka-muka shimashita,** 4) **Suppai-mono ga tabe-tai desu,** 5) **Ryūzan o shimashita,** 6) **Shi-gatsu jyōjun gurai desu.**
5. Sample Answers: 1) **Hai, sō desu,** or **Iie, futago dewa arimasen,** 2) **Hai, arimasu,** or **Iie, arimasen,** 3) **Hai, hitokatta desu,** or **Iie, hidoku nakatta desu,** or **Iie, hidokuwa arimasen deshita,** 4) **Hai, komura-gaeri ga arimashita,** or **Iie, arimasen deshita,** 5) **Hai, totte arimasu,** or **Iie, totte arimasen.**

LESSON 29

1. 1) **Aān shite (kudasai),** 2) **Bē shite (kudasai),** 3) **Nobi-nobi shite (kudasai),** 4) **Me o pachi-kuri shite (kudasai),** 5) **Te o gū-pā shite (kudasai).**
2. 1) **Aka-chan wa nemure-nai yō desu ne,** 2) **Kigen ga warui yō desu ne,** 3) **Omutsu-kabure mitai desu ne,** 4) **Porio wakuchin o shite-inai yō desu ne,** 5) **Tamago arerugī no utagai ga arimasu.**
3. 1) **Mune wa kirei desu,** 2) **Zei-zei shite imasu,** 3) **Yōsei desu,** 4) **Giji- yōsei desu,** 5) **Insei desu.**
4. 1) **Ni-san-nichi mae kara desu,** 2) **zei-zei shite imasu,** 3) **Nodo ga harete akaku-natte imasu,** 4) **Uirusu-sei no kikanshi-en desu,** 5) **Kyōbu rentogen desu,** 6) **Seigo ni-nen-me goro kara desu.**
5. Sample Answers: 1) **Hai, suibun-hokyjū wa yūbun desu,** or **Iie, jyūbun dewa arimasen,** 2) **Kyō wa kigen ga ii desu,** or **Kyō wa kigen ga warui desu,** 3) **Hai, arimasu,** or **Iie, arimasen,** 4) **Hai, kyojyaku-taishitsu desu,** or **Iie, kyojyaku-taishitsu dewa arimasen,** 5) **Hai, arimasu,** or **Iie, gengo-shōgao wa arimasen.**

LESSON 30

1. 1) **Mushi-ba wa airmasen,** 2) **Oku-ba ni mushi-ba ga arimasu,** 3) **Tsumetai-mono ni shimi-masu,** 4) **Ha-guki kara no shukketsu ga arimasu,** or **Ha-guki kara chi ga dete imasu,** 5) **Fusso o nuru hitsuyō ga airmasu.**
2. 1) **Rinsu o shite (kudasai),** or **Kuchi o susuide (kudasai),** 2) **Itai-toki wa oshiete (kudasai),** 3) **Kuchi o akete (kudasai),** 4) **Shita o agete (kudasai),** 5) **Chotto matte (kudasai).**
3. 1) **Ha ga shimi-masu ka,** 2) **Ha ga itai(n) desu ka,** 3) **Ha ga tottemo itai(n) desu ka,** or **Ha ni geki-tsū ga arimasu ka,** 4) **Ha ga gura-gura shite imasu ka,** 5) **Ha ga nuke-sō desu ka.**
4. 1) **Hidari-gawa no oku-ba desu,** 2) **Ōkina mushi-ba o mitsuke-mashita,** 3) **Hai, basshi suru hitsuyō ga arimasu,** 4) **Hai, nokoshi-tai desu,** 5) **Kōsei-zai to chintsū-zai desu,** 6) **Mikka-kan wa ugai o tsu-zuke nakereba narimasen.**
5. Sample Answers: 1) **Hai, ha no teiki-kenshin o shite imasu,** or **Iie, shite imasen,** 2) **I-kkai desu,** or **Ni-kai desu,** or **San-kai desu,** 3) **Hai, I-ppon arimasu,** or **Hai, arimasu,** or **Iie, zenzen arimasen,** 4) **Hai, ire-ba o shite imasu,** or **Hai, Ire-ba to sashi-ba o shite imasu,** or **Iie, shite imasen,** or **Iie, dochira-tomo shite imasen.**

10. Answers to Exercises

LESSON 1

1. A) **Ohayō gozaimasu**, B) **Kon-nichi wa**, C) **Kon-ban wa**, E) **Sayōnara**, F) **Dō shimashita ka**, G) **Odai-ji ni**, H) **Onamae wa nan desu ka**.
2. Your name **desu**.
3. Your postion **no** your name **desu**.
4. **Hai** or **Iie** (Free response).
5. A) Name, B) Doctor, C) Emergency, D) Mother, E) Translator.
6. A) **(Watakushi wa) ishi desu**, B) **(Anata wa) kango-shi dewa arimasen**, C) **Uketsuke desu ka**, D) **Shoshin desu ka**.

LESSON 2

1. A) Health insurance. B) Health center, C) Telephone number, D) General hospital, E) Ambulance.
2. A) **Yoyaku ga arimasu ka**, B) **Netsu ga arimasu ka**, C) **Hoken ga arimasu ka**, D) **(O)namae wa nan desu ka**, E) **(O)denwa-bangō wa nan desu ka**, F) **(Go)jyūsho wa doko desu ka**, G) **Taion wa nan-do desu ka**, H) **Dōitashi-mashite**.
3. A) Do you have insurance? B) What is your name? C) What's your telephone number? D) What is your address? E) What is your approximate temperature?
4. A) **Hachi-Zero-Nana-no, Go-Kyū-Yon-no, San-Roku-Go-Zero desu**, B) **Ni-Zero-Ichi-no, Hachi-Go-Nana-no, Ni-Zero-Hachi-Kyū desu**, C) **Ichi-Happyaku** (or **Hachi-Zero-Zero-no**), **Ni-Zero-Ichi-no, Kyū-Hachi-Roku-no, Kyū-Nana-Ichi-San desu**.
5. A) **Kyū-jyū-nana**, B) **San-jyū-Nana ten Ni**, C) **Hyaku**, D) **San-jyū-Hachi ten Nana**, E) **Hyaku-Ni**.

LESSON 3

1. A) **Shoshin desu ka**, B) **Nan-sai desu ka**, C) **Tanjyō-bi wa itsu desu ka**, D) **San-ji ni omachi shite imasu**, E) **Nan-ji ga ii desu ka**.
2. A) **Sen-Kyū-Hyaku-Nana-jyū-Nen, Hachi-gatsu-futsu-ka desu**, B) **Sen-Kyū-hyakyu, Roku-jyū-Hachi-nen, Shi-gatsu, Tō-ka desu**, C) **Ni-sen-Ichi-nen, Ichi-gatsu, Jyū-go-nichi desu**, D) **Gogo Ku-ji Yon-jyū-go fun desu**, E) **Yo-ji San-jyu-ppun** (or **han**) **desu**.
3. A) **Kyō**, B) **Kinō**, C) **Ashita**, D) **Asatte**, E) **Mai-nichi**.
4. A) **I-ssai (Hitotsu)**, B) **San-sai (Mittsu)**, C) **Yon-sai (Yottsu)**, D) **Kyū-sai (Kokonotsu)**, E) **Jyu-ssai (Tō)**.
5. A) **Seibetsu wa nan desu ka**. B) **Go)jyūsho wa doko desu ka**, C) **(O)denwa-bangō wa nan desu ka**, D) **Shi-gatsu Itsu-ka, Gogo San-ji ni kite kudasai**, E) **Ashita, Gozen Ku-ji ni kite kudasai**.

LESSON 4

1. A) **Shussei-chi**, B) **Hoken-gaisha**, C) **Shokugyō** (or **shigoto**), E) **Kaikei**, E) **Fuku**.
2. A) Take off, B) Wear, C) Wait, D) Insured person, E) Fill in.
3. A) **Shussei-chi wa doko desu ka**, B) **Hoken-gaisha wa nan-desu ka**, C) **Haigū-sha wa dare desu ka**, D) **Shatsu o nuide kudasai**, E) **Matte kudasai**.
4. A) **Hai, shimashita**. B) Your address (Free responses), C) **Hai, Hoken ga arimasu**, D) **Hai**, or **Iie** (Free responses).

LESSON 5

1. A) **Ka-han-shin**, B) **Komekami**, C) **Kao**, D) **Matsu-ge**, E) **Kuchi-biru**, F) **Kubi**, G) **Senaka**, H) **Ago**, I) **Haguki**, J) **Kata**.
2. A) **Me ga kayui(n) desu**, B) **Kesa kara mimi-tabu mo itai(n) desu**, C) **Saku-ban kara hitai ga itai(n) desu**, D) **Kuchi wa tsukarete -imasen**, E) **Mimi ga itai(n) desu**.

3. A) **Onaka ga itai(n) desu ka,** B) **Asa kara ha mo itai(n) desu ka,** C) **Nichiyō-bi kara kata ga itai(n) desu ka,** D) **Itsu kara kubi ga itai(n) desu ka,** E) **Sakuya kara, mune ga itai(n) desu ka,** F) **Raishū yoyaku o shimasu ka.**

Lesson 6
1. A) **Hiji,** B) **Hiza,** C) **Fukurahagi,** D) **Ude,** E) **Te-kubi,** F) **Kakato.**
2. A) **Hiza o tsuyoku uchi-mashita ka,** B) **Don-na itami desu ka,** C) **Sasu itami desu ka,** D) **Hokani dokoka itai tokoro ga arimasu ka,** E) **Yubi ga harete imasu,** F) **Doko ga shibirete imasu ka.**
3. Sample answers: A) **Dōshimashita ka,** B) **Dōka shimashita ka,** C) **Doko ga warui(n) desu ka,** D) **Doko o uchimashita ka,** E) **Doko o surimuki-mashita ka.**
4. A) **Surudoi itami,** B) **Shitsukoi itami,** C) **Dontsū,** D) **Zukin-zukin suru itami,** E) **Chiku-chiku suru itami.**
5. A) **Zenzen kafukubu wa itaku arimasen,** B) **Hotondo kansetsu wa itaku arimasen,** C) **Amari ashi-kubi wa itaku-naidesu,** D) **Hontōni kayuku nai(n) desu.**

Lesson 7
1. A) **Taijyū,** B) **Shinchō (Se no takasa),** C) **Taion,** D) **Ketsu-atsu,** E) **Myaku(haku)**
2. A) **Nanika kusuri o nonde imasu ka,** B) **Taion o hakari-mashō,** C) **Myaku(haku) o tori-mashō ka,** D) **Tabako o sui-masu ka,** E) **Arerugī ga arimasu ka.**
3. A) **Itsu kara desu ka,** B) **Kuchi o akete kudasai.**
4. A) **Taijyū wa Hyaku-jyū-ni-pondo de, Go-jyū-kiro desu,** B) **Shinchō wa Go-fīto go-inchi de, Hyaku nana-jyū-ssenchi desu.** C) **Taion wa Kyū-jyū Hachi-ten, roku-do de, Sanjyū-nana-do desu,** D) **Ketsu-atsu wa ue wa Hyaku-jyū de, shita wa nana-jyū hachi desu.**

Lesson 8
1. A) **Hakike,** B) **Mimi-nari,** C) **Zutsū,** D) **Seki,** E) **Tan.**
2. A) **Nani-ka shōjyō ga arimasu ka,** B) **Atama ga itai(n) desu ka, or Zutsuu ga shimasu ka,** C) **Benpi desu ka,** D) **Ketsu-nyō ga demasu ka,** E) **Hokani nani-ka shōjyō ga arimasu ka.**
3. A) **Mimi-nari ga shite, fukai desu, or Mini-nari ga shite fukai-kan ga arimasu,** B) **Geri de, onakaga itai(n) desu,** C) **Benpi-gimi desu,** D) **Hinketsu-gimi desu,** E) **Geri wa itsu hajimari-mashita ka.**
4. A) **I-sshū-kan mae kara desu,** B) **Kinō kara desu.**
5. QA) **Itsu kara shukketsu ga hajimari-mashita ka,** QB) **Itsu kara ketsu-nyō ga hajimari-mashita ka.**

Lesson 9
1. A) **Hare-mono, or hareru,** B) **Samuke,** C) **Mukuni,** D) **Uchimi, or Daboku,** E) **Shikori**
2. A) **Don-na shōjyō desu ka,** B) **Kono shōjyō wa itsu kara desu ka,** C) **Kono shōjyō wa hajimete desu ka,** D) **Onaji shōjyō ga yoku arimasu ka,** E) **(Nani-ka) omoi-atari masu ka, Omoi-atari ga arimasu ka, or Genin ga wakari-masu ka.**
3. A) **Shinpai (wa) nai desu yo,** B) **Jyōtai wa warukuwa nai desu,** C) **Nani mo warukuwa nai desu,** D) **Warui-kamo shiremasen,** E) **Kensa ga hitsuyō kamo shiremasen.**
4. A) **Dōki ga shimasu,** B) **Mikka mae kara desu,** C) **Hai, tokidoki arimasu.** D) **Hai, onegai shimasu.**

Lesson 10
1. A) **Ansei,** B) **Seiyō,** C) **Tantō-i,** D) **Suibun,** E) **Ryōyō.**
2. A) **Suguni yoku nari-masu yo,** B) **Ansei ni shiteite kudasai,** C) **Gakkō wa yasunde kudasai,** D) **Kensa kekka wa seijyō desu,** E) **Nani-ka shitsumon ga arimasu ka.**
3. A) You should drink a lot of liquid, B) I will refer you to a specialist, C) I'm telling you not to worry, D) You should not go to school, E) If you have any problems, please inform us immediately.

4. A) **Iie, shigoto wa yasunde kudasai,** B) **Hai, suimin o jyūbun totte kudasai,** C) **Hai, suibun o jyūbun totte kudasai,** D) **Seikyū-sho o age-masu (sashiage-masu).**

Lesson 11

1 A) **Chūsui-en,** or **Mōchō(en),** B) **Shinzō,** C) **Kanzō,** D) **Daichō,** E) **Hai.**
2. A) **I no atari ga itai(n) desu ka,** B) **Kōmon kara jiketsu ga arimasu/demasu ka,** C) **Tannō o kensa shimashita ka,** D) **Shoku-zen ni I ga itai(n) desu ka,** E) **Kikan no kensa o shimashō ka.**
3. A) It may be the appendix, B) It looks like pneumonia, C) I suspect it may be rectum cancer, D) Your duodenum looks like something is wrong, E) I think that you have bronchitis.
4. A) Chronic pain, B) Acute pain, C) Continuous pain, D) Persistent pain, E) Stinging pain, F) Throbbing pain, G) Prickling pain, H) Burning pain, I) Gripping pain, J) Squeezing pain.
5. A) **Hai-en no utagai ga arimasu,** B) **Dono atari ga itan(n) desu ka,** C) **Kikanshi ga enshō o okoshite iru mitai desu.**

Lesson 12

1. A) **Byōreki,** B) **Nyō-kensa,** C) **Shujyutsu,** D) **Chōryoku-kensa,** E) **Shoku-shin.**
2. A) **Byōreki o oshiete kudasai.** B) **Nyō-kensa o shitari, shinden-zu o tottrai shimasu,** C) **Mune ga itai(n) desu ka (Mune no atari ni itami ga arimasu ka),** D) **Kyō wa kensa ga aru-node, (nani-mo) tabenai-de kudasai,** E) **Rentogen kensa no kekka wa mada wakarimasen.**
3. A) **Kenkō-shinadan o shimasu ka,** B) **Kagaku-ryōhō o shimashō (shite mimashō),** C) **Rentogen o torimasu kara, rentogen-shitsu ni itte kudasai,** D) **Tenteki o shimasu kara sode o makutte kudasai.** E) **Chiryō o shimasu kara, utsubuse ni natte kudasai.**
4. A) **Iie, mada kensa-kekka wa wakarimasen,** B) **Kensa no kekka wa ii desu yo (to omoimasu).**

Lesson 13

1. A) **Yobō,** B) **Kansen-shō,** C) **Saihatsu,** D) **Fukusayō,** E) **Yōsei.**
2. A) **Zettai-ansei ga hitsuyō desu,** B) **Shi-go nichi mo sureba yoku-nari masu,** C) **Teiki-kenshin ga hitsuyō desu,** D) **Shōjyō wa karui desu ga, naoru no ni shibaraku (jikan ga) kakarimasu yo,** E) **Shi-zen ni naorimasu.**
3. A) **Kyō kensa suru tsumori desu ka,** B) **(Jyūbun) eiyō o totte kudasai,** C) **Senmon-i o shōkai shimasu (Senmon-i no namae o agemashu),** D) **(Sugu ni) nyūin ga hitsuyō desu,** E) **Shibaraku tsuuin shite kusasai.**
4. A) **Ashita niwa genki ni narimasu yo,** B) **Karui kaze no yō desu ga, gakkō wa yasunde kudasai,** C) **Sugu ni kensa o suru hitsuyō ga airmasu.**

Lesson 14

1. A) **Kaze-gusuri,** B) **Genetsu-zai,** C) **Wakuchin,** D) **Shohōsen,** E) **I-gusuri.**
2. A) **Don-na kusuri ga hoshii desu ka (hitsuyō desu ka/irimasu ka),** B) **Shohōsen o omochi desu ka,** C) **Nemuku-naru kamo shiremasen,** D) **Jyuu-go fun go ni, torini kite kudasai,** E) **Sugu-ni demasu. Chotto matte kudasai (Shōshō omachi kudasai).**
3. A) **Nomi-owaru made (Nomi-kiru made), nonde kudasai,** B) **Otona wa San-jyō, Kodomo wa ichi-jyō nonde kudasai,** C) **Mainichi tsuzukete nonde kudasai,** D) **Kono kusuri o nomu to, onaka ga itaku naru kamo shiremasen,** E) **Kono kusuri wa kaze ni yoku kikimasu.**

Lesson 15

1. A) **Kō-gan-zai,** B) **Ichō-yaku,** C) **Kayumi-dome,** D) **Kōsei-bushitsu,** E) **Hinin-yaku.**
2. A) **Sakkin-zai no shiyō hōhō o setsumei shimasu,** B) **Kono kōatsu-zai wa mai-shoku-go sanjyuppun inai ni onomi kudasai,** C) **Kono geri-dome wa geri ni yoku-kikimasu,** D) **Kono suimin dōnyū-zai**

wa hitsuyo no toki-ni onomi kudasai, E) Kono chintsuu-zai wa hitsuyō no toki-dake onomi kudasai.

3. A) Kono kusuri o nondara, Ni-ji-kan wa unten o shinaide kudasai, B) Kono kusuri o fukuyō-chū wa, osake o nomanai de kudasai, C) Kodomo no te no todokanai tokoro-ni hokan shite kudasai, D) Kono kusuri o nonde ijyō o kanjitara suguni oshirase kudasai, E) Kono kusuri wa suzushii tokoto-de hokan shite kudasai.

4. A) Kono jyō-zai wa otona wa san-jyō, kodomo wa ni-jyō, go-zai ika wa nomanai-de kudasai, B) (Kono kusuri wa) neru-mae ni nonde kudasai.

Lesson 16

1. A) Saikin (Bakureria), B) Hashika, C) Hashōfū, D) Yobō-sesshu, E) Yōren-kin.

2. A) Kafuku-bu ni shuyō ga arawarete kimashita, B) Kanjya wa senaka o kayu-gatte imasu, C) Hyaku-nichi-zeki ga gakkō no mawari de ryūkō shite imasu. D) Kono shōjyō wa Ryūkōsei kan-en ni chigai arimasen, E) Infuruenza ni kono kōsei-bushitsu o fukuyō shite kudasai.

3. A) Chi o haitari ketsuben ga detari shimasu ka, B) Karui netsu ga detemo shinpai wa irimasen, C) (Zenzen) itaku arimasen node, rirakkusu shite kudasai, D) Sugu-ni byōin ni tsurete-kita hō ga ii desu, E) Infuruenza no kensa o suru node, hana ni menbō o irete kentai o torimasu.

4. A) (Kono shōjyō wa) Hashika-ni chigai arimasen, B) (Oko-san wa) karui netsu ga aruyō desu, C) Hai, suibun o takusan totte kudasai.

Lesson 17

1. A) Hai-gan, B) Kyōmaku-en, C) Kekkaku, D) Hai-en, E) Kikanshi-en.

2. A) Toriaezu, ketsueki-kensa o shite mimasu, B) Kinō-kara koshi ga itakute, chōshi ga yoku-nai desu, C) Tashikani, kyōmaku-en no shōjyō no yōni seki ga dete imasu ne, D) Kesa kara tashikani okan mitai desu, E) Toriaezu, hai-gan ni natte inai ka kensa shite mimasu.

3. A) Kuchi o akete "Aā" to itte kudasai, B) Taion-kei o shita no shita ni irete kudasai, C) Sūjitsu kan keika-kansatsu o shimasu, D) Shatsu o agete (makutte), iki o suttee, tomete, haite kudasai, E) Ima wa ii kusuri ga arimasu kara, nyūin shinaide ii desu yo.

Lesson 18

1. A) Kankōhen, B) Fusei-myaku, C) Nō-socchū, D) Shin-fuzen, E) Kyōshin-shō.

2. A) Hakketsu-byō wa naori nikui desu, B) Kanjya wa sensei ni nai-shukketsu o mite moraimashita, C) Kensa o suru to hai-kekkaku deshita, D) Kessen-shō no toki wa dō sureba ii(n) desu ka, E) Hinketsu-sase-rareru yōna kibun desu.

3. A) Yoku memai ga shimasu ka, B) Shinzō-hossa o okoshita koto ga arimasu ka, C) Mune ni shime-tsuke raresu yōna itami ga arimasu ka, D) Dōki ga hayaku-naru koto ga arimasu ka. E) Donokurai osake o nomimasu ka.

4. A) Tetsubun no takai tabemono o totte kudasai, B) Iie, yomi yasui desu yo, C) Nō-socchu no yobō niwa seikatsu yōshiki no kaizen ga hitsuyō desu yo.

Lesson 19

1. A) Kiseichuu, B) I-en, C) I-kaiyō, D) Chūsui-en, E) Jyūnishichō-kaiyō.

2. A) Onaka ga itai(n) desu ka, B) Onaka no chōshi wa dōdesu ka, C) Kafukubu ga itakute kurushii desu ka, D) Mae no kensa kekka yori, yokunatte imasu, E) Kono kusuri wa yoku kikimasu ka.

3. A) I ga itakuwa arimasen ka, B) I ni appaku-kan ga arimasu ka, C) Onaka ni gasu ga tamatte imasen ka, D) Shoku-go i ga itami masu ka, E) Aruku to masu-masu itaku-nari masu ka.

4. A) Itsu itai(n) desu ka, B) Osake ya tabako o shimasu ka, C) Sukoshi no aida, osake ya tabako o herashita hō ga ii desu yo.

LESSON 20

1. A) **Nyōdoku-shō**, B) **Jin-en**, C) **Jinu-en**, D) **Nyōro-kesseki**, E) **Nyōdō-en**.
2. A) **Ichi-nichi ni nankai oteari ni ikitaku-narimasu ka** (Ichi-nichi ni nan-kai oshikko o shimasu ka), B) **Narubeki, omizu o takusan nonde kudasai**, C) **Oshikko wa nyō no koto desu**, D) **Sensei wa kanjya o beddo ni suwarase-mashita**, E) **Nyōdō-en wa san-shū-kan teido de yokunari-masu**.
3. A) **Saiketsu sezuni , ketsueki kensa wa dekimasen ne**, B) **Kesa okita toki [ni] bōkō ga totemo ita-katta deshita ka**, C) **Bōkō-kyō kensa wa itai(n) desu ka**. (Bōkō-kyō kensa o suru noni itami ga ari-masu ka), D) **Eizu tesuto no kekka ga wakaru noni, donokurai kakarimasu ka**, E) **Gohan o tabetaku nari-mashita ka**.

LESSON 21

1. A) **Kōjyōsen**, B) **Chuudoku**, C) **Taishitsu**, D) **Iden**, E) **Zōki-ishoku**
2. A) **Genki de ite kudasai**, B) **Hidari-hai ni itami ga arimasu ka**, C) **Kensa no kekka wa (doko-mo) waruku wa arimasen**, D) **Kensa no kekka ni yoruto tsūfū mitai desu**, E) **Kuhci o akete kudasi**
3. A) **Nyō ni chi ga majitte iru noni ki ga tsuki mashita ka**, B) **Mune ga doki-doki shite, ikigire mo shimasu ka**, C) **Beddo ni yokoni natte itadake masen ka**, D) **Netsu mo aruyō desu ne**, E) **Ichi-nichi ni ichi-ji-kan undō o shite imasu ka**.
4. A) **Zujyū-kan no jikaku-shōjyō ga arimasu ka**, B) **Monshin-hyō ni yoruto, ichido hossa o okoshi-mashita ne**, C) **Seikatsu-yōshiki ni chūi-shite kudasai** (or ki o tsukete kudasai).

LESSON 22

1. A) **Nenza**, B) **Dakkyū**, C) **Daboku** or **Uchimi**, D) **Kosettsu**, E) **Hibi**.
2. A) **Zakotsu-shinkei-tsuu dewa naika to omoimasu**, B) **Kanjya-san wa sensei kara Gibusu o mo-raimashita**, C) **Doā** (or to) **o akeyō to shita totan** (ni), **oya-yubi o doā** (or to) **ni hasami-mashita**, D) **Koko o utta dake de, hibiware o shimashita**, or **hibi ga hairi-mashita**, E) **Mita tokoro, migi-ashi no jintai ga kirete-iru yō desu**.

LESSON 23

1. A) **Shashi**, B) **Torime**, C) **Shikimō**, D) **Ranshi**, E) **Shitsumei**.
2. A) **Kensa no tame(ni) mazu hidari-me o ōkiku akete kudasai**, B) **Me ni Jyūketsu mo arushi, sarani me-yani mo arushi, yoku nai yō desu**, C) **Kono enshō wa utsuru koto ni narimasu** (or kanō-sei ga arimasu), D) **Ketsumaku-entoiu byōki ni natta** (or kakatta) **koto ga arimasu ka**, E) **Me o sawattari, kosuttari shinai-de kudasai**.
3. A) **Chiisai moji ga kasunde miemasu ka**, B) **Itsu mōmaku-hakuri ni narimashita ka**, C) **Migi-me no hakunaishō no naosu-noni shujyutsu o shimasu ka**, D) **Mabataki o shuruto itai(n) desu ka**, E) **(Mono ga) ni-jyuu ni miemasu ka**.
4. A) **Osoraku, enshō o okoshite-imasu**, B) **Kensa no tame(ni) migi-me o ōkiku akete kudasai**, C) **Me o kosuttari shinai-de kudasai**.

LESSON 24

1. A) **Ibiki**, B) **Bi-en**, C) **Kafun-shō**, D) **Chikunō-shō**, E) **Nan-chō**.
2. A) **Ōku no kanjya ga chū-ji-en ni kakatte imasu**, B) **Shita o dashite iraremasu ka**, C) **Zan-chō shōgai desu ka**, D) **Sukoshi** (or chotto) **tatte itadake masen ka**, E) **Dewa, kensa o hajime-mashō ka**.
3. A) **Mimi-nari ga shimasu ka**, B) **Yoku kushami ga demasu ka**, C) **Migi-mimi ni nanika haitte imasu ka**, D) **Me no kansen-shō ni yoku kakarimasu ka**, E) **Hana-mizu ga demasu ka**.
4. A) **Kensa o shimasu kara, kuchi o akete-ite kudasai** (or akete itadake masen ka), B) **Dewa, kensa o hajimemashō**, C) **Kokyū suru noga tamarania desu ka** (or kurushii desu ka).

LESSON 25

1. A) **Fuke,** B) **Ibo,** C) **Shimi,** D) **Hokuro,** E) **Mizu-mushi.**
2. A) **Kusuri o nondara, kaette yakushin ni narimashita,** B) **Sawatta baikin de, tobihj ni narimashita ka,** C) **Kono jinmashin ni tsuite omoiatari ga arimasu ka,** D) **Nantoka, hiyake o naoshite agetai desu,** E) **Kore wa mizu-mushi dato omowaremasu.**
3. A) **Shimi de komatte imasu ka,** B) **Mune ni hasshin ga demashita ka,** C) **Hidoi fuke ga arimasu ka,** D) **Nettō de yakedo o shimashita ka,** E) **Hiyake no ato wa kayui(n) desu ka.**
4. A) **Nantoka, shimi o naoshite agetai desu,** B) **Kono hasshin ni tsuite omoiatari ga arimasu ka,** C) **Kore wa nikibi dato omowaremasu.**

LESSON 26

1. A) **Tenkan,** B) **Sōgō-shichō-shō,** C) **Kyōhaku-shinkei-shō,** D) **Jisatsu,** E) **Jinkaku-shōgai.**
2. A) **Shinkei-en no kusuri o nomazuniwa iraremasen.** B) **Utsu-byō no chōkō ga arimasu,** C) **Sen-getsu kyū-ni futori-mashita,** D) **(Sukoshi) kyūyō o osusume shimasu,** E) **Sōgō-shichō-shō niwa yakuji ryōhō ga kakasemasen.**
3. A) **Tachi-agaru to, memai ga shimasu ka,** B) **Saikin, hidoi henzutsuu ga arimasu ka,** C) **Karada ga omoku(te), datsuryoku-kan ga shimasu ka,** D) **Neyō to suruto, (masu-masu) neraremasen ka,** E) **Sō-utsu-byō ni nayande imasu ka.**

LESSON 27

1. A) **Shikyū-tai-gan,** B) **Shikyū-kei-gai,** C) **Nyū-gan,** D) **Shikyū-gan,** E) **Ransō-gan.**
2. A) **Kensa no kekka wa ichiyō (or ima-no-tokoro) mondai nai desu yo,** B) **Jinkō-jyusei (o) shita hazu nano ni, mada ninshin shite imasen,** C) **Kanjya wa ima-no-tokoro daijyōbu desu yo,** D) **Ransō-shuyō ga mitsukari-mashita** E) **Kanōna kagiri, kayumi no chiryō o shimashō.**
3. A) **Chitsu kara orimono ga demasu ka,** B) **Saigo no seiri wa itsu deshita ka,** C) **Hidoi seiri-tsū ga arimasu ka (or Seiri no toki (ni) hidoi itami ga arimasu ka),** D) **Izen ni jinkō-jyusei o shimashita ka,** E) **Chibusa ni shikori ga arimasu ka.**
4. A) **Jiko-nyū-gan kensa wa ima-no-tokoro daijyōbu desu yo (or mondai arimasen),** B) **Kanō-na kagiri, fusei-shukketsu no chiryō o shimashō,** C) **Tokidoki dōki ga shimasu ka.**

LESSON 28

1. A) **Tsuwari,** B) **Taidō,** C) **Jintsū,** D) **Ikimi,** E) **Teiō-sekkai.**
2. A) **Masaka ryū-zan dato wa omowana katta desu,** B) **Sōki-hasui ga okitara, suguni renraku shite kudasai,** C) **Jitsuwa, [anata wa] teiō-sekkai ga hitsuyō desu,** D) **Itami mo, tsuwari mo mada airmasen,** E) **Tsuwari ya, shokuyoku-fushin ga arimasu ka.**
3. A) **Jintsū wa mada desu ka,** B) **Jintsū ga hajimari-mashita ka,** C) **Jintsū wa yaku 5 fun tsuzuki mashita ka,** D) **Jintsū wa dono-kurai (or nan-pun oki-ni) airmasu ka,** E) **Jintsū ga hayaku natte imasu ka.**
4. A) **Ninshin jyū-go ka getsu desu,** B) **Hā-hā-hā to itte kudasai, itami ga yawaragimasu,** C) **Moshi jintsū ga areba oshiete kudasai.**

LESSON 29

1. A) **Hattatsu-shōgai,** B) **Shōni-zensoku,** C) **Kin-jisutorohī,** D) **Nō-sei-mahi,** E) **Shirome.**
2. A) **Atopī-sei hifu-en ka dōka, sai-kensa shimasu,** B) **Hana-mizu ga dehajime mashita ka,** C) **Aka-chan ga nomete inai yō desu,** D) **Benpi desu kara, kanchō ga hitsuyō desu,** E) **Arerugī no kusuri o shohō shite okimasu.**
3. A) **Kanshaku desu ne,** B) **MMR no wakuchin o uke-mashita ka,** C) **Tamago o tabeta toki, fukide-mono ga dekimashita ka,** D) **Omutsu-kabure ga hidoi(n) desu ka,** E) **Karada zentai ni asemo ga arimasu ka.**

LESSON 30

1. A) **Haguki**, B) **Shiseki**, C) **Shikō**, D) **Ireba**, E) **Eikyūshi.**

2. A) **Oya-shirazu ga itakute itakute tamarimasen**, B) **Shika-gikō-shi wa kanjya ni sashi-ba o tsukura-sare-mashita** (or **Shika-gikō-shi wa kanjya ni sashi-ba o tsukuri mashita**), C) **Koshū ga niowanai yō(ni) ha o migaite kudasai**, D) **Dōshite mo nyuu-shi wa (or o) nokoshitai(n) desu ka**, E) **Basshi-go wa sukunaku-tomo i-sshuu-kan wa ugai o tsuzukete kudasai.**

3. A) **Mushi-ba ga yoku itami-masu ka**, B) **Kodomo no ha ni fusso o nurimasu ka**, C) **Hirari-shita no oya-shirazu ga itami-masu ka**, D) **Tsumetai tabe-mono ni shimi-masu ka**, E) **Dochira no ha ga itai(n) desu ka** (or **itami masu ka**).

4. A) **Hai, shikashi yoku hamigaki o sureba, mushi-ba o fusegu koto ga dekimasu,** (or **fusege-masu**), B) **Hai, takusan mushi-ba ga arimasu yo**, C) **Oku-ba ga mushi-ba desu yo.**

INDEX